Dancing

Dancing

A Guide for the Dancer You Can Be

Ellen Jacob

A DANCEWAYS BOOK

ADDISON-WESLEY PUBLISHING COMPANY

Reading, Massachusetts • Menlo Park, California

London • Amsterdam • Don Mills, Ontario • Sydney

Library of Congress Cataloging in Publication Data

Jacob, Ellen.
  Dancing, a guide for the dancer you can be

  Bibliography: p.
  Includes index.
  1. Dancing—Addresses, essays, lectures.
2. Dancing—United States—Addresses, essays,
lectures. I. Title.
GV1594.J33   793.3′2   80-66832
ISBN 0-201-04956-2
ISBN 0-201-04957-0 (pbk.)

Copyright © Ellen Jacob 1978, 1981

ISBN 0-201-04956-2 Hardback
ISBN 0-201-04957-0 Paperback

ABCDEFGHIJ-HA-8987654321

Book design by Barbara Hoffman.

Cover design by Iris Weinstein

Danceways is a nonprofit foundation dedicated to the promotion of dance and the education of dance consumers: 393 West End Avenue, New York, New York 10024, 212-799-2860.

Acknowledgments

Dancing is the result of over three years' research, numerous interviews, and a national survey of dance schools and organizations which would not have been possible without the aid and cooperation of many. I am deeply indebted to Chris Jonas, whose levelheaded advice and unflagging sense of humor kept me going through what seemed to be endless adversities; Joan Jacob, for giving up a summer vacation to critique and type an unwieldy manuscript; Frank Gimpaya for his eloquent photos; Barbara Hoffman for her sensitive design; editor David Trainer and research assistant Holly Williams; and for their wisdom and help at critical times: Margaret Pierpont, Bonnie Pastor, Roni and Richard Schotter, Ellen Kogan, Janet Reibstein, Ben Pomerantz, Joan Finkelstein, Sally Banes, Connie Allentuck, Ernie Smith, Dr. L. M. Vincent, Julius Nirenstein, Andy Chernuchin and Bob Kramer.

I would like to thank all the dancers, teachers, photographers, school administrators and company managers who contributed material and enriched this book immeasurably with their experiences, including Stuart Hodes, Gena Belkin, Bob Audy, Nat Horne, John Dayger, Barbara Roan, Susan Whelan, Don Redlich, Ernie Pagnano, Irene Feigenheimer and Karla Woolfangle; also Doris Hering and Paula Babalis of the National Association for Regional Ballet, Heidi von Obenauer at *Dancemagazine*, Barbara Earnest at Capezio Ballet Makers, orthopedists William Hamilton and Mark Schottenfeld, and Ted Striggles, Dave Jacobson, Steve Hamilton and Jerry Menikoff of the Volunteer Lawyers for the Arts for assistance above and beyond the call of duty.

for Harry Jacob

Contents

Part IV A Leg Up: Making the Most of Dance Classes

Part V The Finishing Touches

You don't wake up one morning and say,
I will become a dancer.
You wake up one morning and realize
you've been a dancer all your life . . .
and you say to yourself, I am a dancer.
I am dance.

—*SUSAN BOTNEY*

Introduction

This is a book for everyone who dances or wants to dance: for those who don't yet know they are dancers and those who have always known, for amateurs of all ages as well as aspiring professionals, for beginning through advanced dancers and for parents of children who dance.

What is a dancer? Most people would guess that a dancer is something they aren't, when in fact we are all dancers. I'm sure that even those who shrink at the thought of ever putting on leotards and tights can remember occasions in their lives when they have leaped into the air with a cry at hearing some especially good news, or swung a loved one in their arms, or improvised a little jig to keep warm on a wintry day.

Some of the best dancers I've seen have never been onstage; I doubt very much whether they would think of themselves as dancers at all. After a couple of drinks and a little coaxing, a favorite aunt of mine, who is good-natured and rotund, performs an expert belly dance. Once the music starts, this silver-haired matron becomes a marvel of sensuous curves and serpentine hand movements. Many times as I've stood waiting for a subway in Manhattan, I've watched black and Hispanic teenagers outdo each other with incredibly tricky inventions to the blare of their transistor radios. And I've seen superb partnering at a discotheque in Knoxville where office workers come to unwind at the end of the day. Once while visiting a teacher friend of mine in Charleston, I had the good fortune to walk in on a group of eight-year-olds at play during recess. Arranged in a circle on the grass (it was more mud than grass), they were practicing a synchronized routine they had made up, snapping their fingers, kicking and turning, and singing in rural accents I didn't understand. But I remembered those little girls from South Carolina long after many a glittering New York season had faded into oblivion.

In the early days of researching this book I tossed around a few ideas with Ellen Kogan, a close friend whom I'd met while working with the Cliff Keuter company. "What is a dancer, anyway?" I asked, half expecting her to chuckle at such an elemental question. But she surprised me with this poignant reply: "I'm a performer, I get up on a stage, but dance is bigger than that, much bigger than that," she said. "I have seen people break into tears from dancing, or laugh hysterically, reaching different places in themselves — not because they have technique but because they are somehow able to find expression in movement. I've taught recreational dancers and senior citizens and I've seen them have experiences with movement that are every bit as profound as I can imagine. That to me is dancing, because if you are expressing yourself that deeply, you're dancing; and whether or not it's on a stage, to me, is not the point."

Dance has always been as much a part of our human heritage as the ability to speak or walk or run. I don't know just how or when dancing became something other people did, a thing to be admired from a distance — perhaps the invention of the proscenium stage was partly to blame, for it literally put a wall between professional and amateur dancers, separating dance enthusiasts into performers and viewers. I do know there is no better way to see or enjoy dance than through the sinews of our own bodies, and that the time is ripe at last to reclaim our birthright.

It is no accident that the extraordinary burst of dance activity over the past decade got started during the 1960s, a period of vast social change in this land. "Do it" was the message of the sixties — do what you've always wanted to do, do your own thing. It was an age of liberation — for the races, the sexes, children and adults. Along with expanding consciousness there came a new respect for the body. Americans wanted more out of life, and a nation of spectators got out of their easy chairs and onto their feet.

As the sixties became the seventies more people were discovering dance for the first time and finding the courage to act on their secret desires. They danced in discotheques and at parties. They wandered into dancing from their exercise classes. They came to pick up their children from ballet lessons and stayed to dance themselves. Some, who had never before dreamed it possible, found themselves pursuing careers in dance.

More people began to attend dance events, and in response to the mounting public interest, dance became more available. An unprecedented number of private dance schools sprung up, while the established ones created special classes to accommodate the variety of new students they were attracting. Organizations emerged to foster the arts and bring quality dance to communities all over the nation. The media picked up the new craze and splashed dance and dancers on television, film and the covers of popular magazines, sparking an even greater demand for it.

Thus a chain reaction has erupted into a dance explosion. The National Endowment for the Arts reports that in the 1970s nationwide attendance at dance concerts shot up from one million to fifteen million. In 1977 the first National Dance Week was proclaimed and at present over 350 American colleges are offering degree programs in dance. What is most interesting to me — and the reason for this book — is that as we enter the 1980s, more people are dancing in America than ever before.

The rise in dance activity has been so rapid and widespread that in some respects we are footloose in a wilderness of new growth. There is no longer one kind of dancer. For the first time there are numerous recreational dancers and serious amateurs as well as professionals and aspiring professionals. We each have our own needs and concerns. So now, more than ever, we have to take our individual circumstances into account. With new dance schools cropping up every year, we need reliable guidelines to judge their competence. More than ever before, there are opportunities and resources for dancers, but in order to benefit we need to know how best to make use of them.

Whether dance is a big part of your life or only a yearning, this book will provide information and guidance to bring to full flower the dancer within you. It is not about bright lights and glitter — which are, after all, only a small, evanescent part of dance — but the day-to-day process of learning to dance and the growth of self-expression that is dancing. Since much of the book was prompted by questions I've heard and asked, myself, over the years, *Dancing* centers on practical issues that touch us all, from how to find a good teacher to how to cure the cramp in your big toe; from what to look for in a children's dance class to how much money professional dancers make. It is also about dancers: what they think, how they feel, how they live, and how they get good at dancing.

Frank Gimpaya

Part 1

Finding
the
dancer
within

The Man Who Walked on Water

A conventionally minded dervish, from an austerely pious school, was walking one day along a riverbank. He was absorbed in concentration on moralistic and scholastic problems. Suddenly his thoughts were interrupted by a loud shout: someone was repeating the dervish call. "There is no point in that," he said to himself, "because the man is mispronouncing the syllables. Instead of intoning YA HU, he is saying U YA HU."

Then he realized that he had a duty, as a more careful student, to correct this unfortunate person, who might have no opportunity to be rightly guided, and was therefore probably only doing his best to attune himself to the idea behind the sounds.

So he hired a boat, and made his way to the island in midstream from which the sound appeared to come. There he found a man sitting in a reed hut, dressed in a dervish robe, moving in time to his own repetition of the initiatory phrase. "My friend," said the first dervish, "you are mispronouncing the phrase. It is incumbent on me to tell you this, because there is merit for him who gives and for him who takes advice. This is the way in which you speak it," and he told him.

"Thank you," said the other dervish humbly.

The first dervish entered his boat again, full of satisfaction at having done a good deed. After all, it was said that a man who could repeat the sacred formula correctly could even walk on the waves: something that he had never seen, but had always hoped — for some reason — to be able to achieve.

Now he could hear nothing from the reed hut, but he was sure that his lesson had been well taken. Then he heard a faltering U YA as the second dervish started to repeat the phrase in his old way.

While the first dervish was thinking about this, reflecting on the perversity of humanity and its persistence in error, he suddenly saw a strange sight. From the island, the other dervish was coming toward him, walking on the surface of the water.

Amazed, he stopped rowing. The second dervish walked up to him, and said, "Brother, I am sorry to trouble you, but I have come out to ask you again the standard method of making the repetition you were telling me, because I find it difficult to remember it." *

---

* Adapted from Indries Shah, *The Exploits of the Incomparable Mulla Nasrudin.*

Your Individual Style

*what makes every dancer
unique and interesting*

If you stop to think about it, all great dancers have a one-of-a-kind quality that makes whatever they do unforgettable: Galina Ulanova's luminescence, Fred Astaire's style, Ethel Winter's warmth, Margot Fonteyn's purity of line, Clive Thompson's intelligence, Mikhail Baryshnikov's physical largesse and Merce Cunningham's animal alertness.

What makes you a good dancer is *not* trying to be someone you're not. You don't become good by wishing that you had longer legs or a wider turn-out, or that you were ten years younger or ten pounds lighter. Forcing your leg four inches higher than it will go won't make you special either. What makes you a good dancer is being yourself, but more so.

As Ted Shawn has said, "Dance is the only art in which we ourselves are the stuff of which it is made." Just as no two people have the same handwriting or gait, no two dancers look or move alike. Underneath all that you do ticks an individual style that makes you the inimitable person — and dancer — you are. The singular form and structure of your body, how they make you move, your sense of timing, your feelings and your experiences are the raw materials you have to work with as a dancer. However limiting they may seem sometimes, they are your lump of clay, ready to be kneaded and shaped into movement. Success — whether for yourself or before an audience — depends to a great extent on how effectively you can make your unique qualities of body and spirit work for you.

Many dancers stop far short of realizing their potential because they feel they don't fit some stereotyped notion of what a dancer should be. Or they make the mistake of trying to cram themselves into an ill-fitting mold. In doing

15

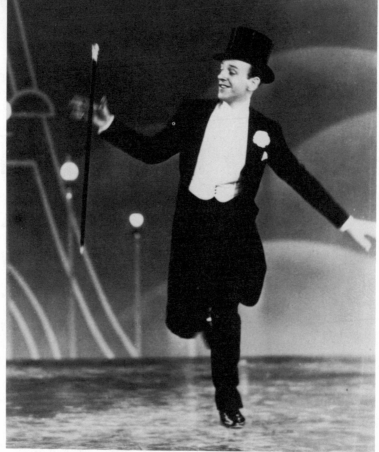
The one and only Fred Astaire. *Museum of Modern Art*

so they lose their greatest ally, the natural dancer within. For dancing is best and most enjoyable when you use it to express — not suppress — yourself. There is a mushrooming effect: The more of yourself you can put into dancing, the more satisfying it will be both for you and for others watching you.

Paul Taylor has remarked that it is not the size of the jump but the valor of the effort that makes a dancer exciting to watch. Without the dimension of personal expression dancing becomes mere movement and dances wither into empty husks of technique. Lamenting the present overemphasis on technical virtuosity, Antony Tudor recently said of the dancers on whom he staged his early works for American Ballet Theatre, "Then I had people who happened to be dancers. Now they are dancers who happen to be people."* In dance classes, your teachers are there not only to provide models you can imitate, but to help you discover those sides of yourself you want to express. In a similar way, the great performers who capture our imaginations should inspire us to search out in ourselves those individual attributes that make dancing a satisfying and full experience.

*From Anna Kisselgoff, "At 40, Ballet Theater Stands for 'Sheer Dance Power,' " in *The New York Times*, May 4, 1980.

I see people jumping to the sky and twisting their legs around their heads, but they don't dance. Ask them to walk! Ask them to waltz! Just to touch. We've got a whole society in which the average person doesn't know how to touch another, let alone dance together. [*]

—*ARTHUR MITCHELL*
director, Dance Theatre of Harlem

In today's burgeoning dance world there are so many ways to dance that there are no hard and fast rules about the correct age, build or physical condition you need to begin or continue dancing. You can find retired couples in their sixties learning how to tap dance, as well as children in preschool movement classes who have barely begun to walk and run. If you feel that one way of dancing is wrong for your personality or physique, you can always study another. When you come upon the right style you will know it because the true dancer in you will start to emerge and flourish.

I saw this happen onstage once, during the second act of a Broadway musical. Most of the cast was superb, but for some perverse reason I was fascinated that night by a dancer who seemed to fade into the woodwork, even when she was standing dead center. She did her steps competently, yet something was lacking. Toward the end of the evening she appeared in a lyrical jazz number. The choreography for it was unlike any other in the show. Suddenly she clicked with the movement, and out came a smoldering character in her dancing that held the audience spellbound.

The pages of dance history are filled with accounts of dancers who learned to capitalize on what they could do rather than be limited by what they couldn't change. Imagine if Fred Astaire had spent all his time working out with weights, desperately trying to make himself into the athletic sort of tap dancer that Gene Kelly was. What if he had vainly set his sights on joining a classical ballet company — for which he was equally unsuited? He probably would have quit long before his prime. Instead Astaire threw out all the rules. He became great by cultivating his cool, quicksilver way of moving and his flair for choreographic invention. He perfected an apt blend of ballroom and tap dancing, and he used his physical peculiarities — a light, unmuscular build — to put together the breezy, elegant personal style for which he is famous. Ballerina Anna Pavlova, whose admirers were legion, had turned-in hips. But her exquisite legs and feet, supple upper body, and magnetic stage personality more than made up for that flaw. Even the celebrated Danish ballet master August Bournonville, who devised a technique for brilliant jumping based on quick rebounds and fluent transitions, did so chiefly to conceal his own brittle landings from jumps and lack of elevation.

[*]From Brett Raphael and Tullia Bohen, "The Choreographer and the Public" in *The Wisdom's Child New York Guide*, January 22-28, 1979.

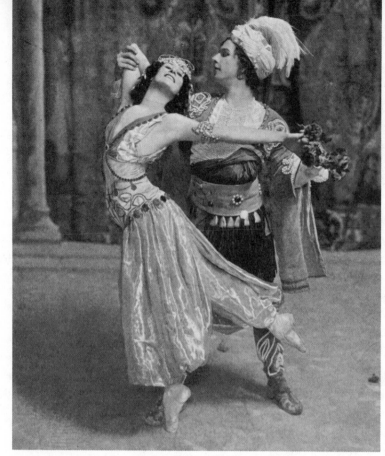

Anna Pavlova with partner Mikhail Mordkin. *New York Public Library*

I have seen more Swan Lakes *than I can count . . . Frequently, I am called upon to see a good many of them during a given ballet season, even as many as five four-acters in a row . . . That, I might point out, is an awful lot of Tchaikovsky and feathers (about sixteen hours) to take in such a short span of time. . . . And what makes it bearable, and very often exciting, is that no two ballerinas are the same. The steps are the same but the ways in which they do them are totally different.*

—*WALTER TERRY,*
The Ballet Companion

Right: Choreographer Gus Solomons, Jr. exploits his unusual body proportions to achieve extraordinary plastic shapes. *Guy Cross, courtesy of the Solomons Company/Dance*

Sometimes what starts out as a weakness can become a strength because you give it special attention. And sometimes a particular attribute, like a flexible back, is a limitation only until you understand how to work with it. Frequently, as in my own experience, physical idiosyncrasies can be turned to good advantage and help make your dancing distinctive. When I first started dancing my long, floppy feet and gangly arms were so conspicuous that I had to learn to use them well out of sheer embarrassment. Now I wouldn't change those outsized features for the world, since I'm often told they are part of what people like most about the way I move.

Ironically, many of the concert pieces we see today are the product of a certain dancer's inability to conform to the prevailing standards of his or her day. Steps, whole dances and entire movement styles have been invented out of a choreographer's personal oddities — which have, in fact, turned out not to be limitations but openings into new ways of moving. Pilobolus, the popular modern dance company, was formed by four male students from Dartmouth College who were interested in making dances but had no formal dance training when they started. Feeling that they didn't look like dancers (at least in the conventional sense), these young men devised an ingenious method of choreography in which they linked their bodies together to form sculptural configurations that, they said, danced for them.

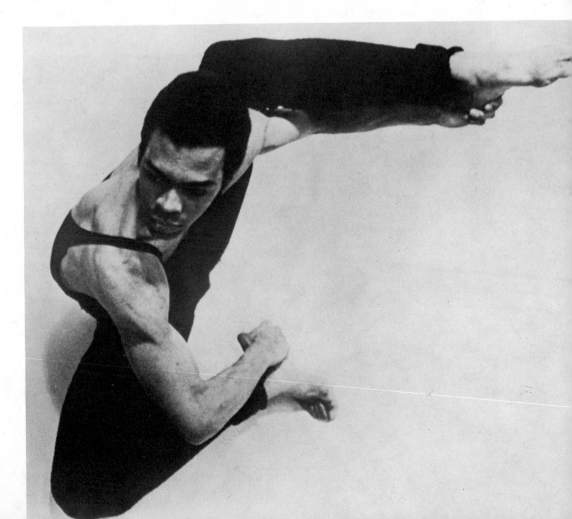

If the incomparable Agnes de Mille had been able to fit neatly into the classical mold, she might never have enriched ballet choreography by her use of indiginous American dance forms, or raised musical comedy dance beyond the level of simple entertainment to that of sophisticated dramatic characterization. "I had no real body line, because my legs were too short for my torso," she says, ". . . and I never had a feeling for the classic ballet approach."[*] But de Mille combined her classical training with a bent for storytelling and a love of folk and modern dance, and came up with a new brand of American ballet. *Rodeo*, *Three Virgins and a Devil*, *Fall River Legend* and the dances for *Oklahoma!*, *Carousel* and *Brigadoon* are a few of the masterworks that resulted. At the same time she created the perfect performing vehicles for herself and starred in several of her own ballets.

As we grapple with the physical standards and requirements for dancing, we should keep in mind that in many instances those who are making the rules and setting the trends today were the exceptions of yesterday. The physical equipment needed to master a given dance technique or style is as different as the choreographers and teachers who originate these styles from the needs of their own bodies. And what is considered to be the ideal dancer's body changes from year to year, dance form to dance form, and company to company.

[*]From Cynthia Lyle, *Dancers on Dancing*.

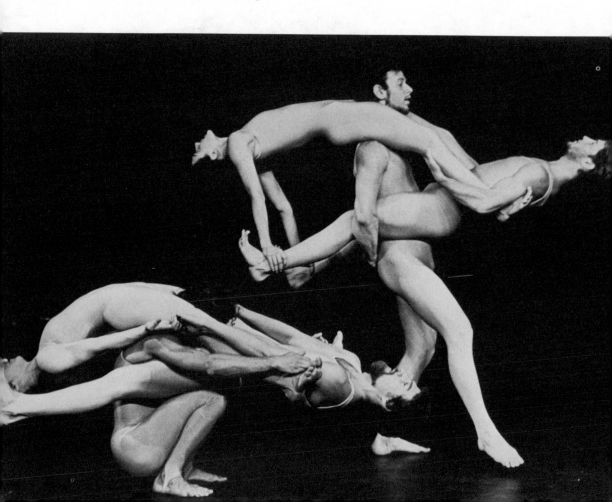

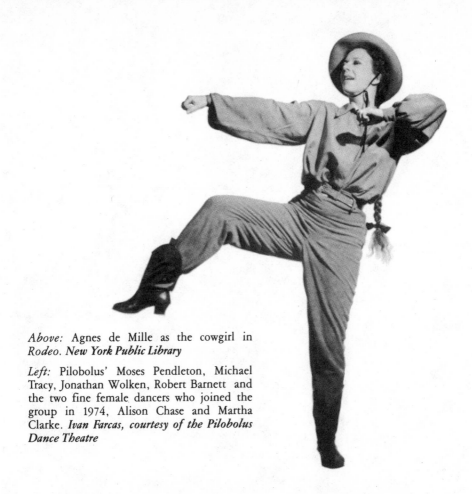

Above: Agnes de Mille as the cowgirl in *Rodeo. New York Public Library*

Left: Pilobolus' Moses Pendleton, Michael Tracy, Jonathan Wolken, Robert Barnett and the two fine female dancers who joined the group in 1974, Alison Chase and Martha Clarke. *Ivan Farcas, courtesy of the Pilobolus Dance Theatre*

"I've really tried to vary my choices to try to get rid of whatever it is that people call my style," he [Fosse] said. "And when you think about it, what are they talking about? Characteristics. I use a lot of hats, I suppose. But I started wearing hats because I started losing my hair. I'd wear one to a rehearsal and start doing tricks with it — so that became part of my 'style.'

"Also, I have bad posture. Look," he said, standing up to demonstrate. "A lot of my stuff comes out rounded over this way. And I don't have a natural turn-out," he added, pointing down at his booted feet. "In fact, I'm slightly turned in, so a lot of the steps I do are that way too." He did a quick pigeon-toed shuffle. "See? And the jerkiness of what they call my style is . . . well, I guess the jerkiness is just me." Then the famous Fosse style is just a simple translation of the Fosse physique? "You mean Fosse's handicaps," he said, laughing. "Given what I am, I guess I had no other way to go, did I?"

—From an interview with Broadway choreographer BOB FOSSE by Robert Berkvist in The New York Times, *March 26, 1978.*

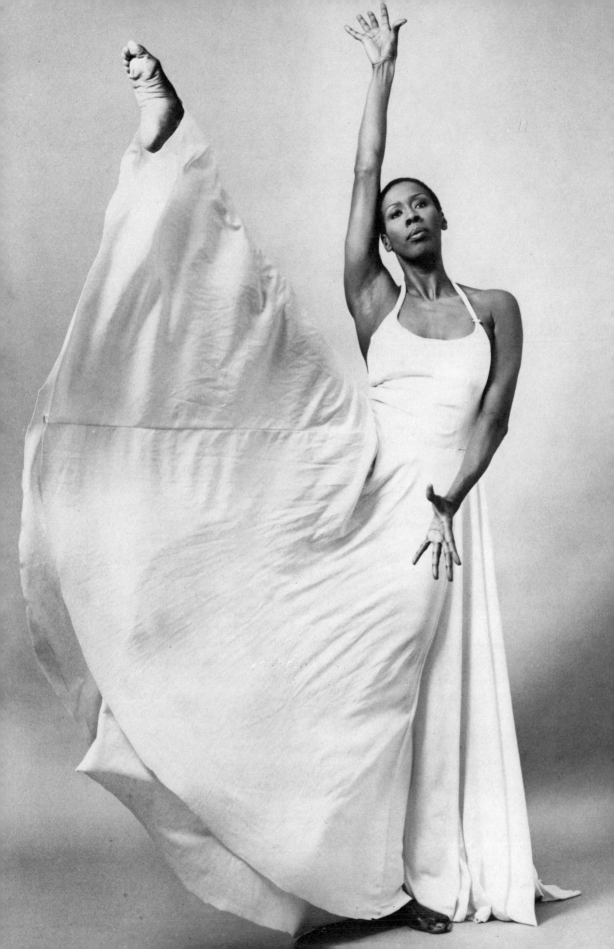

Time and again we see how choreographers select dancers according to their individual way of moving and personal taste. Martha Graham likes to use Japanese dancers because their compact build is similar to her's and very compatible with her movement; George Balanchine's dancers are tall and sinuous, while Robert Joffrey's are predominately small and incisive; and Paul Taylor is interested in working with diverse physical types. Five foot seven ballerina Martine van Hamel complains of missing out on roles and lacking suitable partners because she is so tall, while five foot ten modern dancer Judith Jamison claims she gets roles because of her height. A talented dancer like Marianna Tcherkassky couldn't get into the New York City Ballet, but today she is enchanting audiences as a member of American Ballet Theatre, where her shorter, more rounded figure is welcome.

If you wish to make the most of your dancing ability, you cannot afford to sacrifice your personal style by slavishly pursuing an ideal body form or a movement idiom that happens to be prized by current fashion. Of course, if you are seeking a job with a particular choreographer, you will have to consider whether you have the right equipment for him; but if you want to dance, and dance well, whatever you've got is all you need. Indeed, it is the greatest thing you have to offer. "Style is character," exclaims novelist Joan Didion. Style is an act of courage.

This doesn't mean that you don't also need skill and technique. The emergence of a dancer is a reward which cannot be come by in an easy way. As any veteran performer will tell you, learning to dance is a never-ending process of struggle and growth. But whether you are training primarily for your own pleasure or to achieve excellence, personal expression is the foundation of all dancing that is enjoyable and good (you can't have one without the other). If you start out with what you know about yourself, building on this as you develop, you'll get the best possible results from your efforts. Self-knowledge is also the key to choosing classes and teachers wisely, and the most reliable yardstick for evaluating whether they are working for you. This book begins, therefore, with an exploration of those tangible and intangible aspects of dancing which comprise individual style and make every dancer unique and interesting: your self-image, age, physique, movement preferences and sex.

Judith Jamison. *Jack Mitchell*

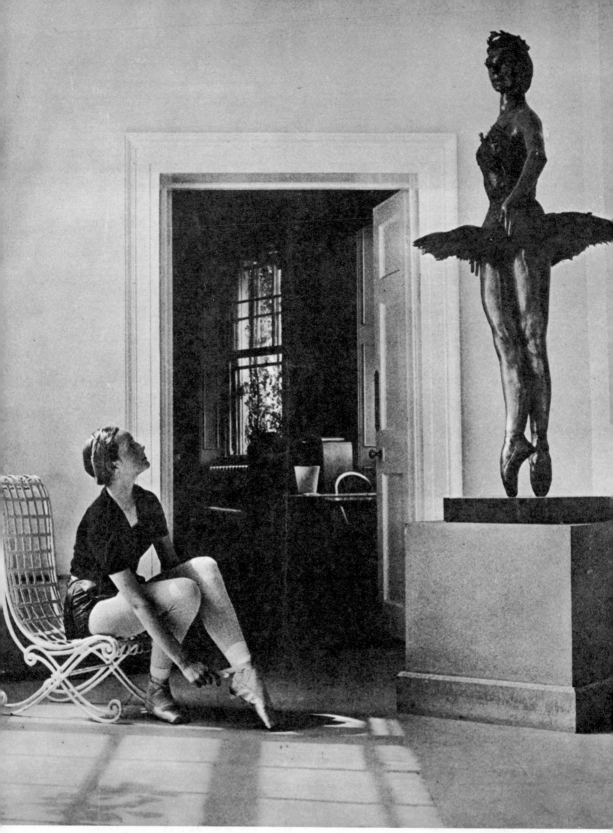

24

2

Your Image of Yourself Dancing

how you see yourself

as a dancer

One's real life is often the life one does not lead.

—OSCAR WILDE

One day after rehearsal in my second year with the Cliff Keuter Dance Company, I flopped down on the studio floor with some of the other dancers to pass around a Coke and share the usual motley assortment of snacks left at the end of the day. (Like most dancers, we were always hungry.) Weary from a long work-out, but not quite ready to pack up and start home, we rambled into one of those heartfelt talks that make dancing with a small company so much like growing up in a close family.

One by one we confided the reasons why each of us had become a dancer. "When I was a baby my feet just pointed naturally," offered the first. Another said he liked the attention he got. "I felt special when I danced," was a third response. I told the others that whenever I was afraid in the night as a child I would imagine a beautiful lady who danced the spooks away. Someone else said she thought she had become a dancer because she loved to sweat.

I recall thinking at the time how very ordinary our explanations were: because it comes naturally; to win love and admiration; to feel special; to escape pain or fear or the mundaneness of life; for the pure sweat and release of it; to look poised and graceful like a dancer; to look like a particular dancer. Judith Jamison needed "to get all that energy out." Ted Kivitt got started on Fred Astaire and Gene Kelly movies. Violette Verdy and Sallie Wilson were hooked on the music. Ted Shawn called dancing "a prime satisfier, like food when one

25

is hungry, water when one is thirsty, and sleep when one is tired." And Peter Martins said it was the only way he could express "everything that's inside of me." People dance because it is totally absorbing and makes them forget everything else. They dance for exercise, to control weight or to overcome a physical problem. In fact, people dance for all sorts of reasons, including some that are not fully conscious.

Whatever your motives for dancing may be, they are the first stirrings of the dancer within waiting to break out, and they are central to that powerful constellation of expectations and feelings which I call *your image of yourself dancing*. This is partly body image — your day-to-day picture of what your body looks and feels like, its powers and boundaries — and partly an idealized fantasy of yourself, a dream of what you hope to become. As such, your image of yourself dancing is part of the everyday world and part of some other world, but the two do have something important in common: They live together in the same person.

The way you feel inside your skin is the basis of your body image, and that in turn contributes greatly to how you see yourself. Through dancing, your body image becomes clearer. Testing and expanding the limits of what you can do makes you aware of your potential. As a matter of fact, your body image is in a constant state of flux and you have the power to alter it drastically for better or worse. To prove it, try this experiment: Change your own image by "getting into" other bodies. Concentrate on another person and try to feel what that body feels. Walk behind an old person. Do you feel tight, stiff, brittle? Get behind someone you admire in dance class; take his or her energy and muscle rhythms. See if imagining you are in that body opens you to new sensations and brings your own body image into sharper focus.

This mind-body connection, which is very important in dancing, works two ways. As you will see if you try the experiment, changing your mental image can affect your physical performance, and changing your physical performance can also alter your mental picture of yourself. Sometimes a negative body image creates problems where there is no physical cause. In Cynthia Lyle's book *Dancers on Dancing*, ballerina Martine van Hamel describes a typical experience:

> *It's very hard to dance when I'm depressed. It gets to be a real struggle. Physically, my body has a reaction. Suddenly it doesn't work; it doesn't feel like a dancer's body. I feel very thick. I feel like I've gained weight overnight. I feel like a blob. And it's not really got much to do with gaining weight. It's got to do with how I feel about myself.*

Probably every dancer has felt that way at one time or another, but by giving you feedback, instilling confidence and demonstrating the correct way of working, a good dance teacher can help you replace a negative or restricting body image with a stronger, freer one (see chapter 15 on dealing with physical limitations).

The late Dr. Lulu E. Sweigard actually documented this process in her book *Human Movement Potential*. Sweigard, who was a student of movement analyst Mabel Elsworth Todd, developed a technique for improving posture and range of movement based on the use of mental imagery. "Movement occurs in response to ideas," she wrote. We move because the nerves stimulate the muscles and the muscles move the bones. Since ideas excite the nerves into action, reasoned Sweigard, if we change our way of thinking about movement, we will automatically change our neuromuscular response. She called her muscle reeducation method *ideokinesis* (*ideo* for thought, *kinesis* for motion). Dr. Sweigard arrived at many of her theories while working with the students of Antony Tudor and José Limón at the Juilliard School, where she taught for eighteen years. During that time she helped hundreds of dancers overcome postural distortions and other physical problems such as chronic muscle strain and tightness, solely by having them visualize the skeleton inside their bodies and imagine movement when they were at rest or performing simple, slow actions. To get students to free the head and lengthen the neck, for example, she would ask them to "imagine your neck growing like an Alice-in-Wonderland neck to raise the head higher and higher." By keeping careful records of their progress in such areas as joint flexibility and energy expenditure, Sweigard proved that the right mental image can trigger freer, better coordinated and more efficient muscular action.

> *Plasticity of mind is what makes movement possible at all. If you can conceive of the human body doing a particular movement, then you can learn to do it. The miracle is when you don't fall down in shock when you find yourself doing it, every cell moving in perfect harmony, no room for a tiny knot that says, "I can't."*

> —*IRENE DOWD*

The fantasy side of your image of yourself dancing is just as important as the more realistic body image. We all need to have a dream of ourselves. All growth and achievement starts with a yearning, a reaching beyond what we are. Fantasy is one of the purely pleasurable aspects of dancing, and at the same time

*From "Visualizing Movement Potential," in *Dance Scope*, Fall 1978. Dowd teaches Sweigard technique at the Dance Notation Bureau and Columbia University's Teachers College in New York.

we can grow through our fantasies. The inner dancer can only develop an identity through your willingness to allow your fantasies full play. Just as a child playing doctor or cowboy discovers hidden interests and potentials which may later be realized in adult life, so everyone comes to know him or herself better by exercising the imaginative freedom to be other things than what reality dictates. An actress who plays Queen Elizabeth one day and a prostitute the next uses parts of herself she is probably not encouraged to express in ordinary social life. By the same token, a few imagined moments as Fred Astaire, or Ginger Rogers, or Isadora Duncan, or Mikhail Baryshnikov can allow you to get in touch with sides of yourself previously unknown and unexperienced.

It doesn't matter very much if you never quite fulfill your ideal vision of yourself. On the contrary, this vision would no longer serve its liberating purpose if you had already attained it. You can be sure that Isadora didn't dream that she was Isadora; she probably lived with other images more interesting to her. But your ideal image may well be what makes you work so hard that you do come to resemble what was once only a fantasy.

Your dreams should fuel your efforts and spur you on to achievement. But remember, they may be unreachable, or you may surpass them. You may become something very different from your fantasies, in which case they must change with you. Clinging too long to an inappropriate dream may very well interfere with the ability to develop your actual potential, or cause you to miss real opportunities.

Some dancers defeat themselves by holding to an unrealistic notion of their expertise. They insist on sticking it out in a technique class that is far too advanced for them, never showing any substantial improvement and getting in everyone else's way. Those same dancers would achieve greater skill by starting off in an elementary class where they could get a solid foundation in the basics and progress from there to attain a true, rather than pretend, mastery.

One young woman told me how for years her burning ambition had been to dance with the Alvin Ailey company. She moved to New York, won a scholarship at the Ailey school, advanced through her classes, went to the company auditions, but never got past the first cut. There were opportunities to audition for other groups while she was in New York, and to dance with promising but lesser-known choreographers. Yet she had grown so single-minded that she never took notice of the other possibilities around her. When it became clear that she wasn't going to get into Ailey's group, she concluded that she just didn't have the stuff, and packed her bags to go home. What a pity she had given herself only this one chance, and a slim one at that, considering how many other talented young hopefuls there were and how few new members were taken into the company.

Your image of yourself dancing, part real, part dream, is what gets you dancing and keeps you going, but it must adapt as you change. Keep your feet on the ground by asking yourself some questions. Why do I want to dance? What are my expectations based on — fantasy? experience? feedback from others? What do I tell my friends about my dancing? When I picture myself dancing what do I see — where am I, what am I wearing, how am I moving? Am I dancing alone, or with others? Why am I dancing — for myself? someone else? Is it my dream? my parents'? my friends'? In my fantasy, do I look like myself, or someone else?

There are no correct answers to these questions. Your answers will be unique, but they will be useful clues to help you find our why and how you want to dance. As time goes on you may want to ask them again.

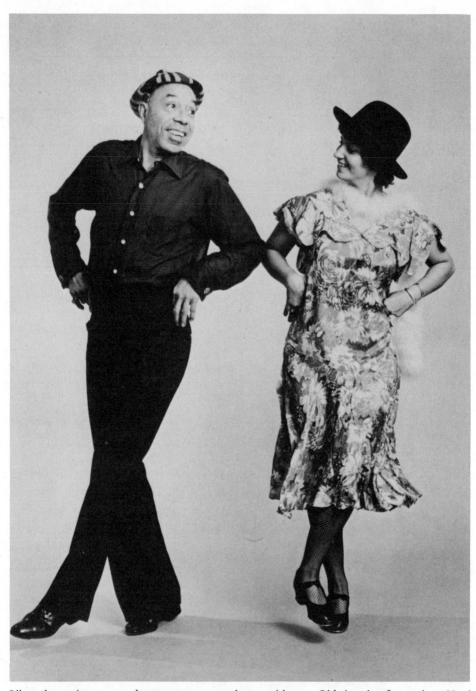

Like cabaret singers, tap dancers seem to get better with age. Old-time hoofers such as Honi Coles, Sandman Sims and Charles Cook still perform with exhilarating virtuosity. Here Cook and his former student Jane Goldberg do a number from Goldberg's jazz tap review "Shoot Me While I'm Happy." © *Lois Greenfield*

3

Making Your Age Work for You

it's never too late
or too early
to dance

Most children can't wait to be grown-ups, and most grown-ups look back with at least a little regret at the passage of their youth. No matter how old or young you are, another age always seems better — for something. Because the dance world is even more youth-oriented than the rest of our society, many older dancers feel compelled to remain twenty-one forever and rue the fact that they cannot. The truth is, however, that you can dance well at any age. It's just a matter of making the best use of the powers you have. Years alone do not determine a dancer's quality; they only affect the mental and physical resources he or she has to work with. Mother Nature is a democrat; she doesn't give any age group a monopoly on assets, but mixes her favors among all her children.

Heavyweight boxing champ Muhammad Ali is a supreme example of an athlete who made his age work for him. At the beginning of his career he used his youthful vigor and quick reflexes to confuse opponents in the ring. He would expend two or three times the energy they did to "float like a butterfly, sting like a bee," as he danced around and around and made it difficult for anyone to land a solid blow. When he grew older, Ali used his stronger body to absorb punches and his strategy and experience to outsmart adversaries who were younger and in better physical condition than he.

Like the athlete, the dancer has to respect the things he gains as well as loses with age. To a great extent age determines how much you can expect to change your body through conditioning and the kind of care and preparation it needs for dancing. There are certain periods of growth during which training yields the best results. For instance, the optimal time to learn languages is between the ages of two and five, when the speech center of the brain is developing. After that it is certainly possible to learn, but never with quite the same facility.

Similarly, most overall bone and muscle growth takes place during puberty. Experts disagree on the exact time, but it ranges between the ages of eight and fifteen for girls, and slightly later — from eleven to eighteen — for boys. Dance training undertaken at this age, while the body is still malleable, can effect the most dramatic changes in joint flexibility and muscle stretch. The capacity for turn-out, or outward leg rotation in the hip socket, can be improved the greatest amount between the ages of eight and ten, while the pelvic bones are undergoing a period of rapid growth. After the mid-teens, training will help you make maximal use of your given physical equipment, but it will not drastically alter it.

Although your basic body structure is well determined by the time you are twenty-one, muscle strength, control and coordination peak after growth stops. Therefore the dancer's physical prime is usually between the ages of twenty-five and thirty, when the largest strides in these areas are made. Here again, authorities differ on the precise year, some putting it as high as thirty-two for women and thirty-five for men.

After about thirty the aging process gradually reduces suppleness and resilience in the joints and muscle tissue. After forty the muscles start to lose strength. But over thirty isn't over the hill, not by a longshot. The key word here is *gradually*. The rate of aging is highly individual and depends on a number of factors, such as heredity, body type, whether or not you've stayed in good physical condition, and how long you've been dancing. Many of the degenerative changes that come with age can be retarded with regular exercise, and dancing is ideal for this purpose because, unlike most athletics, it helps maintain both strength and stretch. It is interesting to note that many dancers feel and perform better *after* their physical powers have supposedly started to wane. By that time they've learned to use their bodies more efficiently and with greater depth. I've seen fifty-year-old teachers who work eight hours a day and still dance circles around their students.

As the body ages, though, it requires more care. With less elasticity, the muscles tend to stiffen when inactive, and they don't retain tone as easily or react as quickly as they used to. It takes more time for an older dancer to bounce back from injury, fatigue and absences from dancing. Hence, the older you get the more conscientious you must be about warming up and proper physical conditioning (see chapter 18 on keeping fit). Dancers over thirty generally need a longer warm-up, and as the system grows more delicate, fewer liberties can be taken with diet and rest.

Some things don't change with age, however. Muscle growth (in bulk, as opposed to length) never stops. At any age, muscle size increases with activity and atrophies through disuse. Bone strength is also directly related to exercise rather than age. Did you know that astronauts returning from space flight suffer from weakened bones due to reduced physical activity?

Because dancing builds up the muscles and bones, it is a long term investment in your body. The longer you dance, the better condition your body keeps and the better it will wear. If you want to continue in your sixties, the time to start is earlier in life — in your thirties or twenties or before. Modern dance pioneer Ruth St. Denis was still performing in her eighties, Martha Graham was a knockout in her fifties, and Jacques d'Amboise has been a principal with the New York City Ballet for nearly thirty years — long enough to see his grown son Christopher become a member of the company; but St. Denis had been dancing since childhood, Graham and d'Amboise since their teens.

It's important to remember that dancing is a total activity involving the mind and personality as well as the body. What often matters most is not the physical condition of the body alone, but how the mind and body develop together in the same person. In this respect, each age brings typical potentialities and limitations to dancing. Ironically many of the factors which contribute most to a dancer's performance, such as experience, body knowledge and sense of self, come only with age, while his physical equipment grows more limited in time. Dancers sometimes hit their athletic prime before their personality and skill have fully matured. But good training can extend your physical powers so that they continue to serve you well while other sides of your dancing are progressing.

Children (ages 4-14). Youngsters are still forming mentally and physically, and while this constitutes their greatest asset as dancers, it also makes them vulnerable to certain problems. They are open and receptive to new experiences. They are spontaneous and nonjudgmental, and they carry none of the affectations and fears adults do. Their movements are simple and direct — what we work all the rest of our dancing lives to achieve.

At the same time children are particularly impressionable, and care must be taken to give them dance experiences that challenge them in ways which benefit their bodies and minds most (for specific recommendations, see chapter 8). Young bodies have yet to develop strength and coordination but they are quite resilient and flexible. As most parents know, children are also very energetic. They usually have good muscle tone. But because they are still growing as they learn to dance, and precisely because they are so supple, youngsters must not be pushed or strained beyond their capacities by overstrict training or too-early pointe work.* Children under ten, for example, can easily overstretch their ligaments and risk weakness in the joints for life. Little ones often don't know when they are hurting themselves. They like to please, and they'll do almost anything to win approval. Since they are used to obeying adults and being told to do things they don't like to do, young dancers cannot be relied on

---

*Toe dancing.

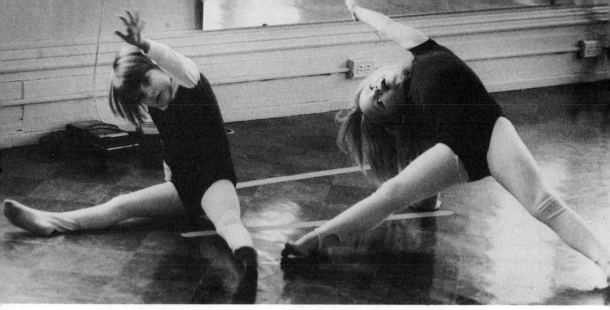

Mimi Fuller, courtesy of the Contemporary Dance Theater, Cincinnati, Ohio

to report discomfort or pain. "No amount of applause at age six is worth the possibility of chronically sore ankles, knees and lower backs later on," reflects Paul Draper in his book *On Tap Dancing*.

The preadolescent and early teenager have to contend with bodies that are changing with bewildering speed and eccentricity. Suddenly, they're tripping over feet that are much too large for them. Legs shoot out from under them, backs become longer or shorter in proportion, waistlines blow up. Steps that used to be manageable are now all out of control. Understanding parents and teachers can help keep things in perspective with a sense of humor and reassurances that this awkward period is only temporary and the new body is well worth waiting for.

Young adults (ages 15-25). Dancers in this category have the physical maturity to make rapid progress, and should take advantage of this optimal time for dance training to push ahead. They have energy to burn, but it is usually divided among the myriad demands of growing up and grappling with the vast physical and emotional upheavals that come with approaching adulthood. Even though it may be difficult at times for them to concentrate on classes, other things can and should come before dancing.

If anything, there is a danger that dancers in such top physical condition may spend too much time building their bodies and not enough seeking out experiences that will further their emotional and mental development. At this point there should be plenty of room for the emerging self to grow and change. Young people should try not to lock themselves prematurely into any one teacher's approach or way of thinking. It's better to explore and experiment, and to get out and see what all kinds of dance have to offer. Time is on their side, and they can afford to be a little indiscriminate with it.

34

Adults (over 25). As the beloved entertainer Maurice Chevalier once quipped, "Aging isn't so bad when you consider the alternative." Anyone who has been a member of this group for a long time will be the first to tell you that the chief advantages of maturity are greater self-knowledge and clearer goals. Although this may sound like a rationalization, it's not. Older dancers are physically and emotionally more settled than their youthful counterparts. They focus their concentration and energy better, have fuller, more sensitive knowledge of their bodies and bring greater life experience to dancing. As a result, their dancing has a depth, style and sophistication which the young cannot hope to match.

Adults probably have the greatest capacity to enjoy dance, but they are also the most self-conscious, self-critical dancers. Because dancers over thirty cannot alter their bodies structurally, they must accept what they've got and learn to capitalize on it with good technique and an astute choice of movement styles (see chapter 10). You may have noticed that the dancers who stay around the longest are those who have learned to adapt their dancing to their age. They are selective about what and how they dance. It's a mistake for a mature dancer to wear herself out trying to master a slam-bang, bone-crushing dance style, when she can be kinder to her body and use the assets that age has given her to better advantage. Margot Fonteyn, for example, didn't try to tackle all the rugged modern ballet choreography in the Royal Ballet repertory; she wisely returned to the classical roles that showed off her still wonderous talents. The limits imposed by his age have made Merce Cunningham all the more fascinating to watch because he has chosen to go with them rather than fight them. Cunningham, who used to have a spectacular jump, doesn't jump much anymore. His solos have grown more and more earthbound. But they push on to uncharted terrain — dark, primordial recesses to which he seems to have gained access only by virtue of age.

As they get older, dancers should concentrate on the quality of their dancing rather than compete with the quantity of youth. Hopefully wisdom comes with age, and, like athletes, dancers learn to set priorities for themselves. One ballet superstar observed that age had improved his dancing by forcing him to accept both his stongest and his weakest points: "I always have trouble with pirouettes," he said, "it's my biggest hangup. But since I passed thirty I look at it a different way. . . . Instead of trying to do eight pirouettes I do three, but I try to make them very clean and very definite. I work on my weak points, but I don't take chances and I don't get mad."*

> *I don't think anyone really starts shining until they're in their thirties. It's a shame, because you've lost those supposedly great years in your twenties, which ballet dancers have as their great years. But a modern dancer works a decade later, because it just*

*From Cynthia Lyle, *Dancers on Dancing*.

*takes that long to grow up, to get through all the hassles of pull-
ing yourself together. When you're a teenager, you fight the
hassles of your body. It takes ten years to acclimate yourself to
your growth. Then in your twenties, you have social and
emotional acclimations to make. By the time you're thirty, you
should have hit your balance, and life can be much more
pleasant when you do.*

*. . . A modern dancer works on the qualitative meaning of
his movement. How much more can a lifted arm say than
throwing a rose to somebody? In ballet, you get a twenty-five-
year-old playing Juliet, being coached to the teeth by a former
great Juliet. But how meaningless is it until she is about thirty-
two, has mellowed, and has had experiences of her own that
have given her a particular insight or a glint in the eye or a tilt of
the head that comes out of her own conviction. As you get
older, you also become more discriminating. Instead of shaking
an apple tree to get one apple, you must pluck one apple and
eat it. Why shake off a lot of apples you can't eat? That's what
maturation is all about. And that's why one sees a lot of kids
doing dances with ninety movements every ten seconds; they
have an insatiable urge just to move.**

—MURRAY LOUIS
modern dancer and choreographer

Age restrictions in professional dancing

The only categorical age restraints in dancing apply to professional
dancers. Whether they are truly warranted by the demands of the art or merely
reflect the current public taste for youth and high-powered athleticism is the
subject of continuing debate. Should an exceptional performer be forced into
premature retirement because so few roles today are created for mature talents?
Is it absolutely necessary for young children to commit themselves to a rigorous
training regimen before most are old enough to choose a dance career for themselves? Perhaps the rules will shift, but for the time being there are certain age
restrictions which career dancers have to live with.

Ballet. The tightest constraints on age are found in ballet dancing, where, at
least in a physical sense, they are the most justified. Eventually the sheer wear
and tear on the body which results from the quest for perfection gets to be too
great. The muscles and tendons start to go, timing becomes erratic, jumps lose
their bouyancy, hip and toe joints turn arthritic. An older ballet dancer may

---

*Ibid.

36

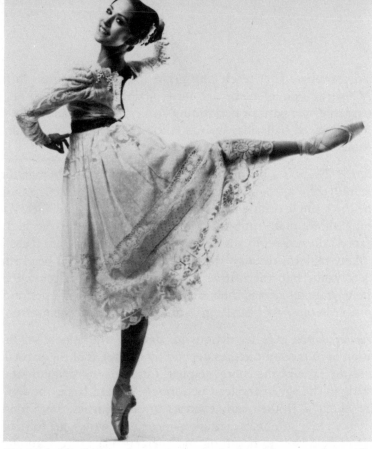

This kind of flexibility and strength must be developed from an early age. The dancer is Marianna Tcherkassky. *courtesy of the Stars of American Ballet*

look fine in class but simply be unable to keep up with the heightened energy demands and physical strains of performing.

Due to the mounting competition for work and the ever-increasing technical requirements, ballet dancers must start preparing for their careers when very young. In order to acquire the extreme flexibility and capacity for hip rotation needed for classical dance, a child should begin lessons when his or her muscles are the most supple and the ligaments and pelvic bones are not yet set. The ideal range is eight to ten years old, but it can extend to twelve years old for girls and up to fifteen or so for boys.

Cruelly, training must begin before it can be determined whether the child will grow up with the desirable body proportions and physical features for a ballet career (see chapter 4). Nonetheless, there are some major consolations: A solid ballet technique will serve as an invaluable foundation for almost any other kind of dancing, or, at the very least, will leave the young person with a strong and graceful body with which to start out life.

Because of their relative scarcity and later maturation, boys are often admitted into scholarship programs and ballet companies at a later age than girls, but for the most part ballet dancers' careers are well underway by the late teens or early twenties. They reach their prime in the early- to mid-thirties and are usually nearing retirement by age forty. Male dancers may go on a while longer, doing character parts or performing on a curtailed schedule. At present, however, middle-aged ballerinas such as Alicia Alonso and Zizi Jeanmaire are rare exceptions.

Modern dance. There is a bit more leeway for modern dancers regarding age, perhaps because the choreography is geared toward individual expression and is not confined to a single codified vocabulary of steps as it is in ballet. Although early training allows more time to develop and is better for the body, some modern dancers do not begin studying seriously until their late teens or early twenties. Many perform through their forties, and those who head their own companies continue into their fifties and sixties. A good percentage of them become choreographers later in their careers, and their extended performing life is often possible because they can keep creating new roles for themselves.

Musical-theater dance. Age restrictions for dancers who appear on Broadway and television or in motion pictures depend on the needs of the particular production and the taste of the choreographer. Casting is normally done by type and according to the age of the lead performers. By and large, though, chorus dancers are young — in their early twenties to early thirties. Since most entertainment dance today combines jazz or tap movement with some form of ballet, dancers in this field have to be strong and energetic. The successful ones don't stay in the chorus forever. By their mid-thirties or sooner they move up into featured parts and lead roles, assist the choreographer or become choreographers themselves.

4

Is Anatomy Destiny?

*how body type
affects the way you move
and how movement
looks on you*

*. . . a good archer can shoot further with a medium-strong bow
than an unspiritual archer can with the strongest. It does not
depend on the bow, but on the presence of mind, on the vitality
and awareness with which you shoot.*

—*EUGENE HERRIGEL,*
Zen in the Art of Archery

Despite basic structural similarities, there are remarkable differences
between one human body and another. Every medical student learns, for
example, that the heart is on the right rather than on the left side in a certain
percentage of the population. Other vital organs, and more frequently main ar-
teries, veins, and nerves are irregularly placed in many normal individuals.
Human beings have different numbers of vertebrae and ribs; they mature and
age at different rates; they are constitutionally stronger or weaker than one
another. The dancer who forgets that he or she is physically unique is a little like
the surgeon who plunges into every operation as if it were a textbook case.

You don't need a perfect body to dance well; you need a feeling for
movement and music, a sense of rhythm and good coordination. There are ex-
traordinarily talented dancers with bowed legs, curvatures of the spine and ec-
centric proportions. In most instances — the exception is discussed at the end of
this chapter — anatomy is not destiny, but understanding your individual body

and how to work with it is. Almost everyone can learn to turn, jump and balance adequately, if not brilliantly. Beautiful line can be attained without 180-degree turn-out in the hips or sky-high extensions. Few people fully realize that all body types are good for dancing, provided you choose a complementary dance style and get competent training. As with age, what matters most is not so much what you start out with in the way of physical equipment, but what you do with it.

Besides, there really is no preordained formula for the perfect dancer's body. We are all slaves of fashion to some degree. Pictures of performers through the ages testify that standards of beauty and excellence change over time. Dancers of the past appear stocky, if not downright plump, when judged by our present norms. Isadora Duncan was no sylph. Even Maria Taglioni, the consummate Romantic ballerina who danced the original *La Sylphide* in 1832, would not look the part in 1980. The great Auguste Vestris would be dwarfed today by male dancers of average size. For that matter, these three giants of dance history might easily be overlooked at a modern-day audition, where on top of everything else, their technique would probably be found quite lacking.

In *The Book of the Dance* Agnes de Mille reminds us that one reason for this alteration in the dancer's physique is the constant innovation in training methods. She observes, for instance, that by shifting the order of the barre exercises,* Russian training changed the muscular development and thus the look of ballet dancers in the first half of this century. ''We owe our slender legs to the Russians,'' de Mille proclaims, because they put the grands battements at the end instead of the beginning of the warm-up.† As we enter the 1980s, the frail, elfin body type that prevailed in the 1960s and early 70s is gradually being superseded by a crop of taller, more robust looking dancers. (There seems to be little choice in the matter, since it's a well-documented fact that the human skeleton has been steadily growing larger over the past two centuries, and particularly in the last fifty years.) Physical and technical standards are likely to go on changing in every area of dance. The point is that despite all sorts of fluctuations in taste and technique, every age has produced dancers who were considered great. They were the ones who knew how to make their bodies work for them, regardless of type.

Your body type determines the way you are inclined to move and how movement looks on you. It makes some things in dancing easier to do and some things harder. A knowledge of your physical make-up — information that unfolds little by little through feedback from teachers, self-observation and experience — should therefore help direct you to a compatible style of dancing,

---

*Ballet warm-up exercises performed while holding on to a wooden railing (also called the barre) that is attached to the wall, usually at waist height.
†Grands battements is the term for high, strenuous leg kicks. They are easiest to do at the end of the barre when the muscles are warm and stretched. When the exercise comes early in the warm-up (as it does in the older Italian system), the dancer often has to strain or grip the muscles because they aren't sufficiently warm. This practice has a tendency to produce bulging thighs.

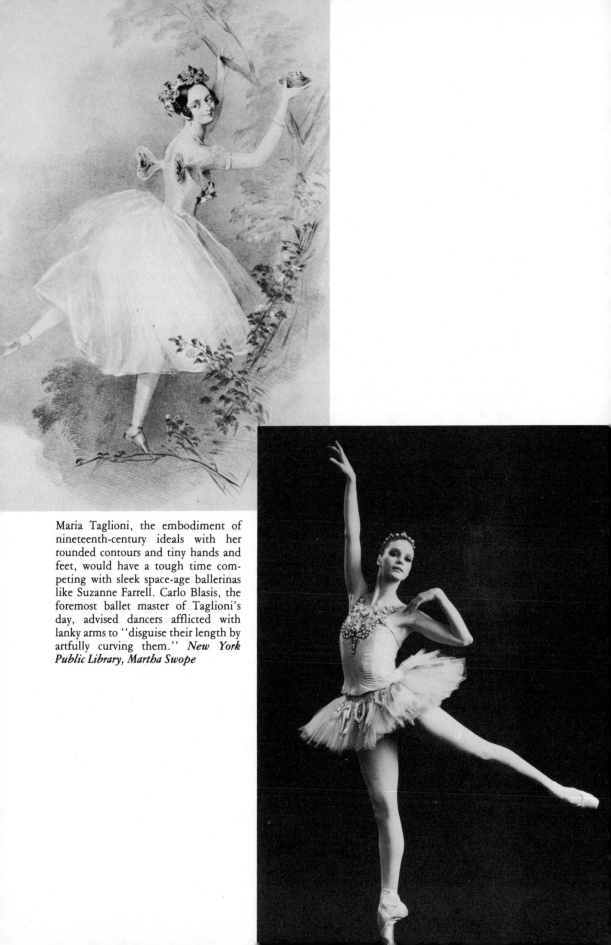

Maria Taglioni, the embodiment of nineteenth-century ideals with her rounded contours and tiny hands and feet, would have a tough time competing with sleek space-age ballerinas like Suzanne Farrell. Carlo Blasis, the foremost ballet master of Taglioni's day, advised dancers afflicted with lanky arms to "disguise their length by artfully curving them." *New York Public Library, Martha Swope*

as well as the teacher and training method that are best suited to you.

The whole idea behind dance training is to discover and develop your own unique capacity for movement. To be truly useful, any technique must be built upon your *actual* capabilities and body construction — not on what you wish they were or what your teacher's are. Training based on unrealistic goals is a waste of time. It will produce weak or inconsistent results and, worse, may ultimately cause injury by forcing the body too far. Probably every ambitious new ballet student, for example, has tried cementing his feet to the floor with a heavy coating of rosin* on his shoes in hopes of achieving the perfect first position — only to learn, sometimes years later, that this is an exercise in futility. No matter how much you'd like it to be, an overly turned-out foot position is unusable because you'll never be able to stand up securely on your legs if you haven't got the flexibility and strength to support the stance from the hips. Moreover, you'll have to distort your back and strain your knees and ankles (turning out from the knees or "screwing the knees," as it is called in classroom jargon, and rolling over on the arches are two dangerous ways of compensating for poor turn-out), and they can't sustain that kind of punishment indefinitely. It is far better to start out with the feet open comfortably to a ninety- or one-hundred-degree angle. Once you've established good postural alignment (see chapter 18) and are strong enough to hold that amount of rotation firmly from the top of the legs, you can gradually extend it to your maximum capacity. If you're like most people, you still may not end up with a 180-degree turn-out, but what you do attain will be sturdy and functional.

Before you start complaining about your bad luck, remember that there is usually a strength related to every physical weakness and a weakness tied to every strength. One of the most unnerving—and inspiring—things about studying dance is watching others work in class. The less you know about your own body the more likely you are to be impressed by your neighbor's real or imagined physical endowments. Don't be so quick to envy dancers who can flop to the floor in a split. They have to work harder than their tight-jointed classmates to control those rubbery limbs. Nature often compensates a weak characteristic with another stronger one. For instance, a short Achilles tendon (which runs down the back of the heel and facilitates jumping) is often paired with extra stretch in the thighs and feet. People with tight hips frequently have supple backs. Many dancers with meager extensions have good turn-out.

Remember too that good training will help you make the fullest use of your particular body build. Once you know what they are and how to work with them, your given physical features can be improved. As we'll see in this chapter, strength and stretch can be dramatically increased with regular work. Speed, coordination and overall motor efficiency come with the right kind of practice, and good technique evens out body contours by correcting muscular imbalances.

---

* An amber colored powder which is applied to the soles of ballet shoes to prevent slippage.

The idiosyncracies of body design

It's risky to generalize about body types because every body is put together—and thus works—differently. Most people are a mixture of physical traits. Not only are we loose in some places and tight in others, or strong in some ways and weak in others, but our skeletal proportions can vary from one part of the body to another. We can have a long trunk and short legs, or vice versa. Hence, the analysis that follows is meant only as a point of departure for your odyssey into the inner workings and capabilities of your body.

Flexibility. The range of movement at the joints of the body (shoulders, spinal vertebrae, hips, ankles, feet) is determined by three things: the bony architecture of the joints; the length of the ligaments, those wiry bonds of connective tissue between our bones which stabilize joints by limiting their movement; and the amount of stretch in the muscles and tendons (tendons are extensions of our muscles — tough, fibrous cords that connect muscle to bone). Although dancers who are loose in one joint tend to be loose in others, flexibility can vary throughout the body. It is possible, to be able to kick your legs high and yet have limited back mobility, or to have loose ankles and tight hips.

Tendons and, to a slightly lesser degree, ligaments are relatively inelastic in adults, and thus can be stretched very little through training. But muscle tissue is highly adaptive to exercise. Muscles can be gradually lengthened up to *one and a half times* their former size with regular stretching. Dancers often don't know how much joint flexibility they have until they are able to stretch their muscles fully. Many people have more plié, better leg extensions and looser backs than they're aware of, but can't utilize these capabilities because stiff muscles interfere. A foot that looks hopelessly rigid can be improved by a systematic program of stretching combined with exercises which strengthen the muscles of the instep and forefoot; and even bowed legs can be corrected somewhat by releasing the tense muscles along the outer portion of the lower legs that pull them out of line with the thighs. Stretch is so crucial to most forms of dancing that many dance schools offer special "stretch classes" where there is concentrated work on limbering the body.

Flexibility has a great deal to do with the ability to let go in the body. Excess muscular tension always inhibits movement and emotional tension adds to the physical kind. If you are tight, breathing deeply and making a conscious effort to relax are terribly important when you're trying to stretch. This permits your muscles and joints to open to their maximum range. Gritting your teeth and attacking the problem with force only makes matters worse by causing the muscles to grab and tighten up even more. Correct posture also facilitates stretch by taking the strain off overworked muscles and freeing them to extend fully (see illusrations in chapter 18).

Turn-out, the capacity to rotate the legs outward in the hip socket, is, like most joint actions, dependent on the individual skeletal construction (in

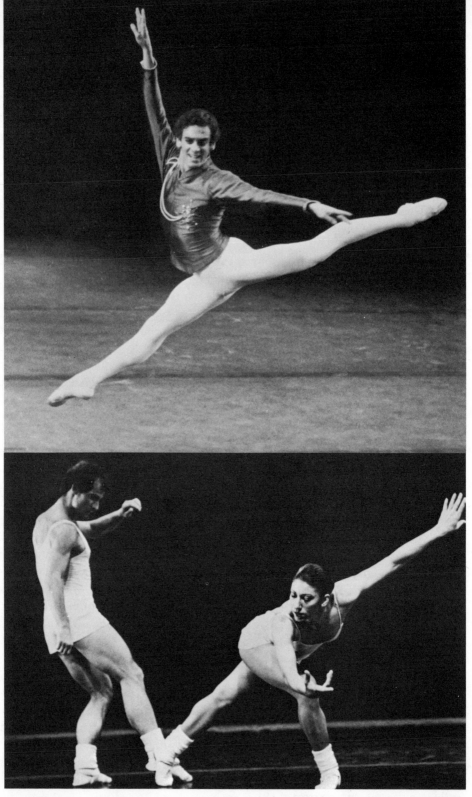

Fernando Bujones' leap is spectacular because his long, slender limbs seem to extend endlessly into space *(top left)*. By contrast, one is struck by the power and muscularity of Valery Panov's leap *(top right)*. Rose Marie Wright's physical stature gives her dancing a great deal of weight and

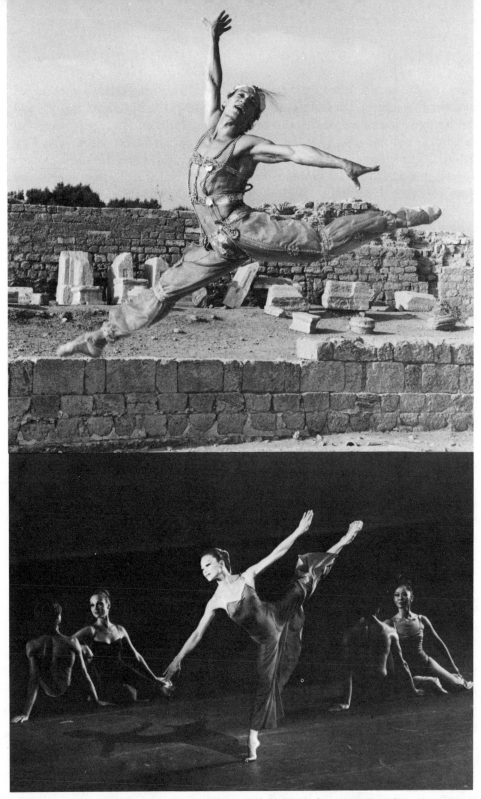

authority in Twyla Tharp's work *(bottom left)*, while Graham dancer Yuriko Kimura's compact and delicate build enables her to move with explosive speed and brilliance *(bottom right)*. *Fred Fehl, Jennie Walton, Barth Falkenberg, Martha Swope* this case, the architecture of the pelvis and the way in which the thighbone fits into the hip socket), the length of the ligaments in the hip joint capsule, and the strength and power of the outward rotator muscles of the legs. "It runs in families," remarks Dr. William Hamilton, physician to the New York City Ballet. "Some people are born to be pigeon-toed and others are duck-footed. Toeing-in is much more common than turn-out, which in the extreme comes close to being a deformity." Though adults cannot significantly alter their native turn-out, skill in using the amount of rotation they have can be vastly improved with good technique.

A loose body, one that is generally flexible in the joints and muscles, has greater suppleness and freedom of movement and requires less warming up than a stiff one. Beautiful line comes easily to this physical type. Yet the loose-jointed dancer has to work harder for control and strength, and is more injury prone because it is easy for her to distort body positions. A body with limited muscle stretch and play in the joints, on the other hand, has natural strength and control. It is also less susceptible to injury, provided it is always properly warmed up and not forced beyond its structural limits. However, a tight-jointed dancer has to acquire enough muscular stretch and elasticity to prevent his movements from becoming brittle or his range overly restricted. Stretching is also important to protect against muscle pulls, since stiff muscles are easily overstretched.

Strength. Technically speaking, it is the ability of certain muscles (called agonists) to contract or shorten and certain other muscle groups (antagonists) to relax or lengthen in opposition to them that enables us to produce movement. Strength, the power of a muscle to contract, is half the battle. It allows our muscles to move the skeleton smoothly and efficiently without overtaxing the bones and joints. It helps us sustain such strenuous actions as jumps and leg lifts without succumbing to fatigue. It gives our dancing security and ease. Strength makes a fragile-looking slip of a swan queen able to do thirty-two fouetté turns at the end of a grueling three-act ballet. Good muscle tone, a constant slight contraction in the muscles that keeps them firm and ready for action, is part of the attribute of strength.

Although most of the population is average with regard to strength, some people have a particularly high capacity for muscle building and retention. These are *mesomorphs,* husky types who are large boned and usually short to medium in height. Other extremes—*ectomorphs,* tall, slender, willowy types who have long, underdeveloped muscles, and *endomorphs,* people whose bodies are inherently soft, round and buoyant—have to work harder to acquire strength and maintain satisfactory muscle tone.

If you don't have it naturally, strength can be developed by progressively overloading the muscles beyond their present work capacity. With steady training over a period of months, muscular strength can be boosted to *more than three times its former amount*. There are several ways to do this: increasing the number of repetitions of a movement; increasing the time for which a given position is held; increasing the speed of the performance; increasing the muscle load with the use of weights; and increasing the length and frequency of the exercise sessions. Some dancers work out in gyms to build up weak muscles; but in most instances regular attendance at a good technique class ought to provide adequate strength conditioning.

Body proportion. The size and weight of your bones and muscles affect your dancing too. There is little you can do about your basic build except exploit its best features and where possible try to mitigate its shortcomings through good training. Most people are varying degrees of these two extremes:

Long, slender proportions in a dancer emphasize the line and design of movement and are therefore preferred for ballet dancing. The ectomorph also happens to be the body type that is currently in vogue. But it does present some problems. The farther the limbs extend from the center of the body, the less power and control the dancer has over them; and unless there is also strong muscle development, it is usually harder for long-legged, long-torsoed dancers to pull themselves together to move fast.

A compact build, with a short trunk and limbs, has other advantages. Strength and speed come more naturally to dancers with this kind of physique. Because of their close-knit body construction, these types hold themselves together well and thus can turn and jump with ease; but they may have a tendency to develop bulky muscles. People with short, powerful muscles need to be especially careful to maintain stretch along with strength.

Frame. A delicately built dancer with a light frame is generally more sensitive and supple, with quick reactions rather than powerful ones (many basketball players fall into this category). A heavily-muscled, large-framed dancer with a thick skeleton has strength and power, but frequently lacks quickness and flexibility.

What makes a jump? Some say one essential element in jumping is the desire to fly and argue that this can be even more important to a dancer than physical make-up. From a purely nuts-and-bolts standpoint, though, the size and buoyancy of a jump depends on the length of the dancer's Achilles tendon; the amount of flexion (ability to bend or fold) in the hip, knee and ankle joints; and the elasticity and power of the muscles of the legs and feet. The quicker the dancer's muscular reactions, the more brilliant the jump, and, as was already mentioned, a compact build also facilitates jumping.

Dancers with a short Achilles tendon, and consequently a limited demi-plié,* will have a harder time jumping. But they can get around this difficulty

---

*A leg bend done with the body erect and the entire foot resting on the floor. This movement is used to take off and land from jumps.

by strengthening the muscles of the legs and feet and learning to use them properly. Strong, articulate feet will cushion landings and help you spring from the floor. Relaxing the feet and ankles when rebounding from the floor—instead of gripping them with tension—will give you more bounce and save your ankle joints from taking a beating. Rhythm, coordination and correct body alignment are an enormous help too (see illustrations in chapter 18). If you have a short Achilles, be sure to get your heels completely down on the floor in all preparations and landings from jumps (this rests the tendon by stretching it); otherwise you may be an unwitting candidate for Achilles tendinitis, a painful inflammation of the Achilles tendon.

The Achilles is one of the toughest tendons in the body. It cannot be substantially lengthened by training, but the muscles that operate it can. The best exercise for stretching a tight Achilles and the surrounding ankle and calf muscles that may be hindering its movement is the good old demi-plié. Easy bouncing and stretching in this position is an excellent pre-class warm-up—again, be scrupulous about planting your entire foot on the floor every time you do it. My first ballet teacher showed me another useful limbering exercise: Stand on the edge of a step facing toward the top of the staircase, with the balls of your feet resting on the step and the heels hanging off the edge. Hold on to the handrail for support. Slowly press your heels down as far as they will go, and then come back up to the starting position with the weight on the balls of your feet again. After repeating this motion several times, take it into a controlled bounce. By the way, you can stretch out your plié every time you climb stairs simply by being conscious of getting your heels down with every step you take.

The limits of liberation: sex-linked physical features

Despite the controversy over sex roles that has erupted in our times, for hundreds of thousands of years in most human societies the men have traditionally been the hunters and warriors and the women have been the cultivators and homemakers. Both sexes have evolved certain adaptive biological features. Thus far in our evolution at least, the male physique is built for strength, speed and maximum force, while the female body is primarily equipped for the flexibility and steady, slow-burning energy needed for childbearing and caring for a household.

"Nowhere is this process of natural selection more striking," says Dr. Hamilton, "than in the differences between the male and female pelvis." The male pelvis is cone shaped, broader at the top and narrow toward the bottom where the legs attach. It is what Hamilton terms "a biomechanically more efficient construction," compact and powerful, and made for running and jumping. The female version is bowl shaped—wider and shallower—to ac-

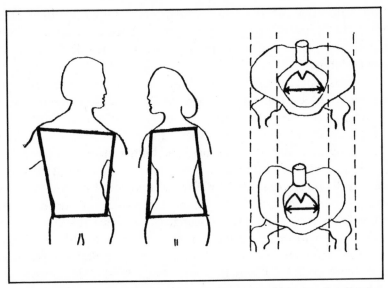

The drawings on the left show how relative shoulder and hip size gives females a lower center of gravity than males. The size and shape of the female *(top)* and male pelvis are compared at right. **Joan Jacob**

comodate a fetus, and inherent in its structure is more freedom of movement in the legs and hips.

Such design motifs repeat themselves throughout the body. Except for a brief interval before puberty when girls mature faster than boys and surpass them in strength, men have larger, tighter skeletons and bulkier muscles, due in part to male hormones called androgens. Men have considerably more muscle cells at their disposal than women. All this gives male dancers added power in jumping and turning. Another contributing factor is their higher center of gravity. Being broad shouldered and narrow hipped, the bulk of their weight is concentrated in the upper body. Since jumping entails lifting the center of gravity, men have a head-start when it comes to elevation. Broad shoulders afford them more leverage for turning, too. Most of the force in turning comes from shoulder and arm action, so male dancers have an advantage from both the strength and breadth of their upper bodies. For that reason, you rarely see women doing more than three multiple turns unsupported, but it's not an uncommon feat for men.

The female body has its own structural advantages for dancing. The hip size is closer to that of the shoulders, which puts the center of the body weight closer to the ground and gives women an edge in balancing. When they start to train, most men discover that they are stiffer in the hips and feet than their female classmates, who overall have lighter bones, looser joints and more supple muscles. It is not surprising, then, that women, with their built-in pliancy and facility for balancing, became the toe dancers. The so-called weaker sex is stronger in other ways. Women have more stable knee joints and, when equally well trained, ten percent more body fat than men. The latter aides them in long-term endurance.

Of course there is a great deal of individual variation in both sexes, and there are plenty of exceptions to prove the rule. Some women have narrow pelvises and a miserable time with turn-out, and others can jump as though they had springs in their legs. Some men can sit quite comfortably in a split, have gorgeously arched feet, and can kick higher than any of the women. Nagging doubts remain as to just how many of our reputedly sex-linked anatomical differences are caused by physical and social conditioning. The influence of exercise on muscle development, for example, is still not clear. Exercise has been shown by at least one researcher to increase the DNA and protein content of muscles in experimental animals. As female athletes compete and develop, they challenge the old definitions of their physical potential, and women are now taking on jobs that were once considered too strenuous for them: telephone linespersons, construction workers, truckdrivers, police and military personnel. Similarly, the tendency that male dancers have toward weak knee ligaments and stiff hips may be due in part to the late start that many of them get in training. This makes it harder to acquire joint flexibility and may cause them to compensate for scant turn-out by straining at the knee.

When anatomy is destiny: the physical requirements for professional ballet dancing

Although there are always dancers with such outstanding determination, talent and personal qualities that they manage to slip by the physical barriers with less than ideal features, most ballet masters believe that professional ballet dancing is too difficult and competitive unless you have the perfect build for it. They feel that dancers who aren't born with the right body end up frustrated in their careers, or else are doomed to early retirement by chronic injuries or premature degeneration of the joints from years of forcing themselves beyond capacity. Most orthopedic surgeons who are experienced in treating dance-related injuries support this opinion. Some ballet schools, such as the Royal Ballet School in England, are so wary of training dancers with physical imperfections that they take the precaution of having an orthopedist examine students at auditions. Not only European academies, but many prominent American schools select the dancers in their professional and scholarship programs largely on the basis of body type.

The physical requirements for ballet are based both on aesthetic and functional considerations, that is, how the body looks as well as its fitness for performing the specialized skills needed for the technique.

Well-balanced proportions. This is of utmost importance to the ballet dancer, who relies very heavily on the beauty of the lines created by the body. Long, slender arms and legs, which accentuate line and look graceful, are a great asset, particularly for women. Short legs and a long torso cut the arabesque line, as they do all extensions, and the burden of carrying the extra torso weight often poses added problems by producing tight hamstring and back muscles. The opposite proportion—the short back on long legs—is aesthetically acceptable but may be a handicap in the extreme, since it provides smaller and weaker back muscles with which to hold the arabesque position.

Flexibility. Ballet dancers need to be loose jointed and have ample stretch in the muscles. A flexible back, one that arches easily, is essential for girls because it is used a great deal in arabesque and port de bras,* and it gives the movements of the upper body suppleness and fluidity. Loose hips are needed for the wide turn-out and high extensions required by the choreography. A limber plié and flexible, well-arched feet and ankles are necessary for the soft, nimble footwork that is central to good ballet dancing.

Straight legs. Minor deviations can be overcome with careful training, though anything other than a slight degree of bowleg is aesthetically unacceptable and makes it difficult for the dancer to maintain correct leg alignment in balletic positions. Hyperextended or swaybacked knees are common among loose-jointed ballet dancers, and many people feel that the extra stretch enhances the line of the leg. However, swaybacked knees require special attention because they are weak.

Sloped shoulders. These are an advantage, especially for girls, but not a necessity. Sloped shoulders make the neck look long and lend freedom of movement to the head, arms and upper torso. Broad, square shoulders are the most difficult for ballet dancing (though not prohibitively so) because the shoulder girdle and upper back muscles are usually tight, limiting mobility in the arms.

Good feet for pointe work (girls only). The ideal foot for toe dancing is closely knit, with short toes that are even in length. Other foot types are certainly adaptable to toe work but require careful training. A big toe that is longer than the rest, or a long second toe, has to support all the dancer's weight on pointe and thus is extremely vulnerable to strain and injury. The dancer whose toes are long must build great strength in the arches in order to support herself well. The most beautiful foot, but the weakest for pointe work, is the too flexible, highly arched one with long, loose ligaments and weak muscles. Because this kind of construction makes it easy to roll over on the arches, the foot with a high instep needs a great deal of preparation before it can be used safely on pointe.

---

*Movements of the arms and upper body.

5

Your Movement Preferences

exploring your natural way of moving

We all like to move in ways that seem natural and comfortable to us. Everything we've talked about so far—your body type, age, self-image, your total personality—will lead you to prefer some actions over others and enjoy some ways of moving more than others. In this sense, movement preferences are the crowning expression of your individual style as a dancer.

It is interesting to watch social dancers at a party or discotheque, where everyone is improvising to the same music. Some dancers remain in one spot, while others travel around the dance floor. Some make large, powerful motions, while others play with small, subtle gestures. One dancer punches the space with a fist or stomps the floor aggressively; another glides smoothly by. This one likes to use her hips, that one his shoulders and arms.

A choreographer composes dances—entire repertories—from the way he likes to move (and, if he's good, from the way his dancers move). In class, a teacher repeatedly stresses the movements she is interested in or partial to. Whether a particular teacher is right for you partly depends on whether her way of moving is compatible with yours. Similarly, the style of dancing you do should use and complement your movement preferences. Some types of dancing that are exciting to watch can be frustrating to do because they don't exploit your innate facility for movement.

Even great dancers look bad when performing choreography that clashes with their personal movement style. Not long ago an internationally renowned ballerina made a guest appearance on a television special. She did a funky jazz number—bare midriff, high-heeled gold lamé boots and all. It was probably fun for her, but she was too soft and demure to bring the dance off.

To begin exploring your native movement qualities, examine the way you move outside the dance studio, at parties or while doing sports. You'll notice there are certain actions which always feel good, and which you consistently fall back on when left to your own devices.

For example, do you enjoy sustained, smooth-flowing motions? Sharp, abrupt motions? Fast or slow tempos? Are your movements heavy and forceful, or are you a light, delicate mover? Do you stay rooted to the ground, or are you happier flying through the space? Do you like to make broad, sweeping gestures, or is it more satisfying to move on a smaller, more contained scale? Are tricky movements with complex rhythms fun to do? Or do you find simple shapes and patterns more pleasing? Do you move in one place, or tend to isolate different body parts and move them separately? Do you enjoy an all-out, strenuous workout? Or do you prefer to move calmly and economically? Are you a long-distance runner or a sprinter? Your body will tell you soon enough. People often favor certain parts of their bodies over others. Good dancing always involves using the whole body; but some dance forms, such as tap and ballet, emphasize the limbs, while modern and jazz styles entail more varied torso movements.

These questions are not only good ones for beginning dancers to ask themselves; they should also be reconsidered from time to time by experienced dancers, who frequently lose track of their natural instincts for movement in the process of training. Like your image of yourself dancing and your physical features, your movement tastes will change as you broaden your range of experience and competence. The more you study and the better you understand your own body, the greater the variety of movement you can digest and assimilate. As you advance, you can and should take on the challenge of learning to perform dance styles that come less easily to you; you don't want to become limited by developing only your strengths. But your movement preferences should be a solid home base on which to build. If you are interested in exploring them in a structured way, try taking improvisation or dance composition classes (see chapter 12). It's a good idea for all of us to keep in touch with those urges which drew us to dance in the first place.

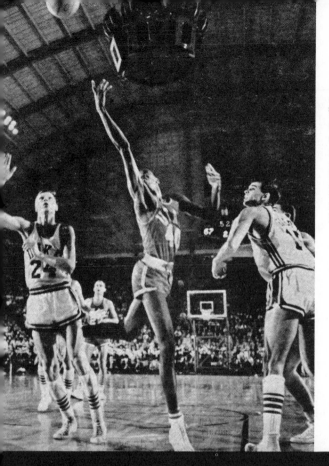

"Line" in dancing is the design made by the outline of the body in space. Striking line, such as that etched by the basketball player scoring a field goal *(top left)*, can occur spontaneously as the result of functional movement. But the choreographer, like the painter or sculptor, deliberately manipulates body line for its visual effect and dramatic impact. There are as many ways to do this as there are dancers' bodies. The classical line of Margot Fonteyn's arabesque in Frederick

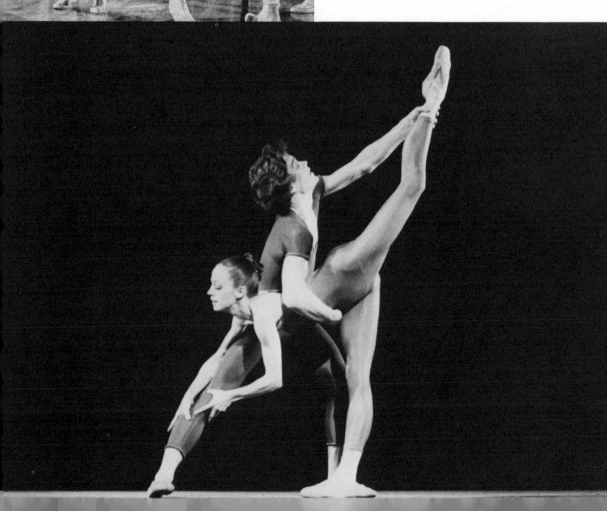

Ashton's ballet *Ondine (top right)* recalls the harmonious proportions and dignified grace of classical Greek architecture; Heather Watts and Daniel Duell go to an acrobatic extreme in Peter Martins' *Calcium Light Night (bottom left)*; and the poignant moment from Alvin Ailey's *Revelations* is derived from yet another movement approach *(bottom right)*. The dancers are James Truitte and Minnie Marshall. **New York Public Library, Martha Swope, Jack Mitchell**

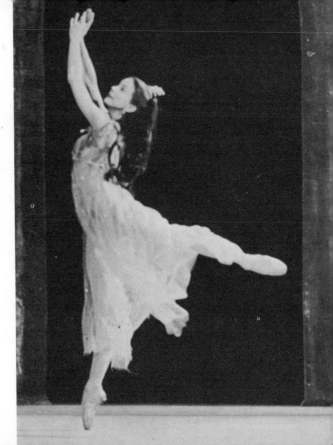

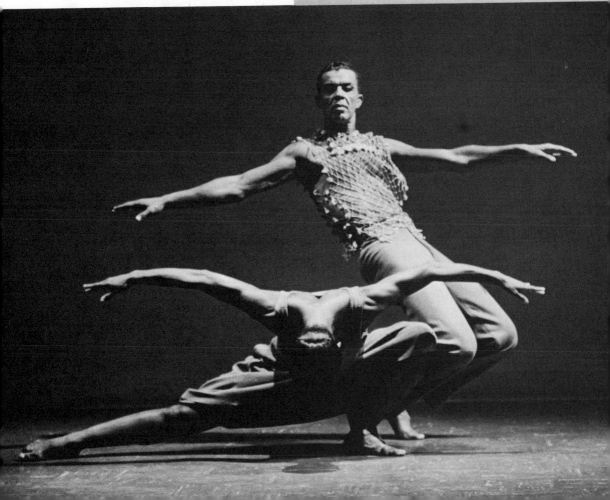

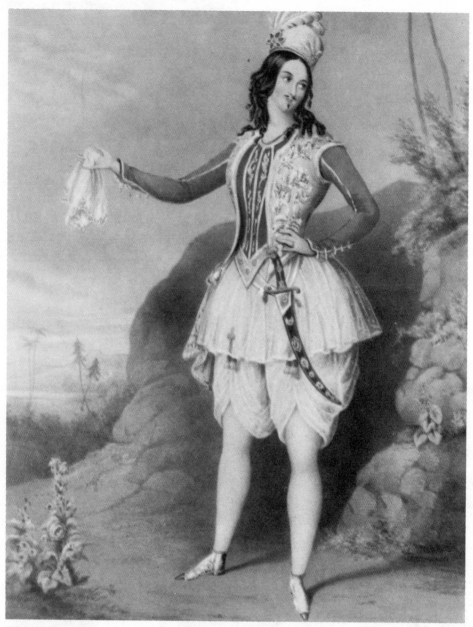

With mustachioed women usurping their roles, small wonder it took male dancers over a century to regain the respect of the American public. In 1838 Therese Elssler got rave notices for partnering her ballerina sister, Fanny, en travestie. In this lithograph a Miss Fairbrother portrays Aladdin in the nineteenth-century ballet *The Forty Thieves. **New York Public Library.***

6

The Sexual Revolution in Dance

dancing for men

Ever since the introduction of serious dance training to America in the early years of this century, the overwhelming image of the male dancer has been as a homosexual. Most parents refused to let their sons have anything to do with dance for fear of seeing them branded as sissies. Those boys who did take classes were constantly challenged, often physically, to prove their doubtful masculinity. Other countries, such as Russia and Denmark, have traditionally held the male dancer in high esteem, but until recently in America, a man had to fight not only for his personal identity but for his place in the dance world. Few men had the courage or determination to overcome the stigma attached to the profession. Only now, after a long and difficult period of evolution, is dance in America becoming something other than an activity for women and a few gay men.

A complex assortment of factors has been responsible for the unfortunate stereotyping of the male dancer. In the first place, by the time ballet came to America from Europe at the beginning of the Romantic Era, it had become essentially a female art. This was due in part to the startling invention of toe dancing, and partly because of the elevated role in which Romanticism cast women. In the 1830s the ballerina on pointe was the international rage—so much so that fans of Maria Taglioni were ecstatic to drink broth made from her toe shoes—and the male was reduced to less than second-class status. Some male roles in romantic ballets were even performed by women. When men *were* involved, their parts were frequently limited to supporting women in spectacular lifts and simulations of flying. The earliest American modern dance pioneers were women too, and although their innovations did invite greater participation by males, it wasn't until the 1930s and 1940s that male choreographers emerged to create dance styles which fully employed the male body and presence. To make matters worse, a dancer's wages in the early days of ballet and modern dance were completely inadequate to support a wife and family—something any real man was supposed to be able to do. In light of all this, it is not surprising that almost no men were willing to pursue careers in dance, and that those who did were often homosexuals without extensive financial burdens, and for whom the social stigma was largely irrelevant. Indeed gay men probably found greater freedom of expression in the dance world than they could have anywhere else in society, and this alone might have encouraged them to put up with the female-centeredness of the art. So in the end, and with good reason, there was more than a little truth to the stereotype of the effeminate male dancer.

The exception could be found in vaudeville, Broadway musicals and Hollywood films. Here tap, jazz, and later ballet dancers projected conventionally masculine images, while, incidentally, making decent money. Show business dancers were therefore much closer to the mainstream of American life than their counterparts in ballet and modern dance.

A number of artistic, social and cultural forces have contributed to the gradually but steadily improving image of the male dancer. Michel Fokine's reforms were certainly an important factor. They first reached America through the companies he choreographed for: Serge Diaghilev's Ballets Russes and the company of Anna Pavlova. These troupes were composed largely of Russian expatriates like Fokine himself, and they toured the United States triumphantly—the Diaghilev company in 1916; its spin-off troupes, the Ballet Russe de Monte Carlo and the Original Ballet Russe, from 1933 to 1950; and Pavlova's group from 1910 to 1925. After emigrating to this country in 1923, Fokine staged several of his ballets on American companies, among them *Les Sylphides, Le Spectre de la Rose, Firebird* and *Petrouchka.*

The Russian choreographer was strongly influenced by the American modern dancer Isadora Duncan. He strove to eliminate from his work the fussiness, artificiality and ornamentation that had encumbered late nineteenth-century ballet. Instead of using empty gestures and the overabundance of mime that were fashionable with his predecessors, Fokine insisted that dancers express themselves with their entire bodies and use only those gestures warranted by the dramatic action. He put to good advantage the male capacity for strength and elevation by cultivating the virtuoso technique developed by Marius Petipa before him, which was characterized by the spectacular leaps and turns we admire in Russian dancers today.

The physical daring and expansiveness of Fokine's time was epitomized by the great Ballets Russes dancer Vaslav Nijinsky, against whom probably every prominent male dancer since has been measured. Nijinsky's technical brilliance and magnetic stage personality created a stir wherever he performed, yet his was hardly the likeness of everyman dancing. He stood only five foot four inches tall

Fred Astaire and Ginger Rogers doing the Carioca tango in the 1933 film *Flying Down to Rio. Museum of Modern Art*

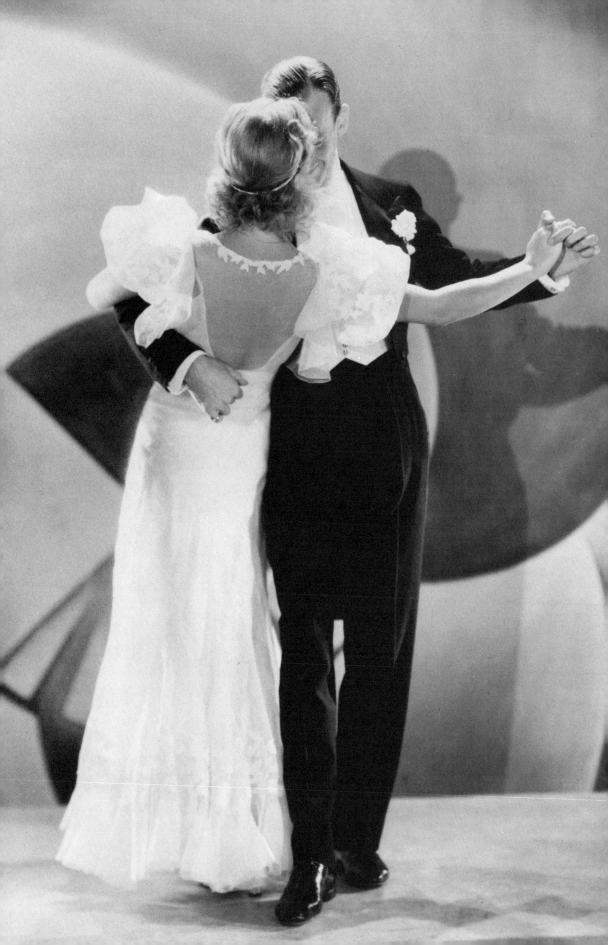

and excelled in portrayals of androgynous creatures: fauns, birds, dolls and spirits.

Although Michel Fokine found an appreciative audience for his work in America, the woman who inspired him wasn't so fortunate. Isadora Duncan was better received in Europe than at home. But she set up a school here, and performed in the United States several times until 1922. Duncan was a revolutionary in her taste for serious music and heroic themes. She rooted her dances in deeply felt emotions and personal experiences, which she expressed with such simple, natural movements as running, jumping, skipping and lying down on the floor. Such a physical vocabulary was one potentially suited to men as well as to women.

Ruth St. Denis was another modern dance pioneer, and her partner, Ted Shawn, became the first American male modern dance choreographer. Feeling that his six-foot, 175-pound frame was ill suited to ballet technique, Shawn devised a training system expressly for the American male body. In 1933 he established an all-male company called Ted Shawn and His Men Dancers, in

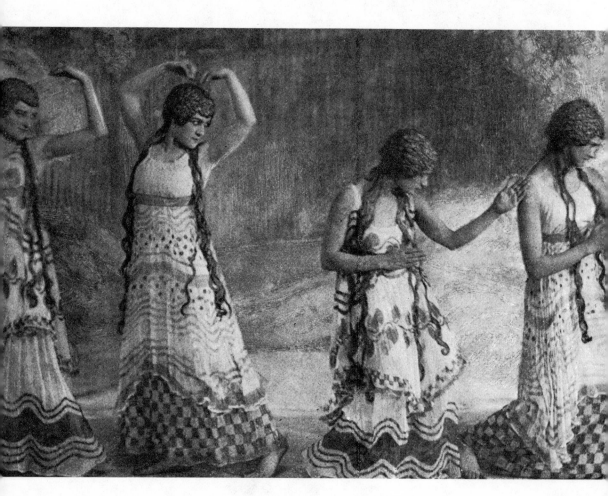

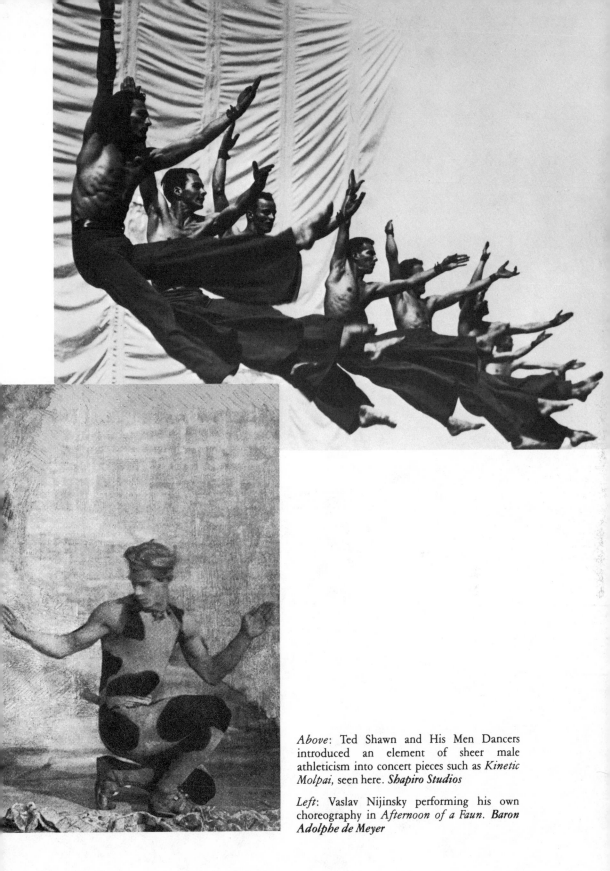

Above: Ted Shawn and His Men Dancers introduced an element of sheer male athleticism into concert pieces such as *Kinetic Molpai*, seen here. **Shapiro Studios**

Left: Vaslav Nijinsky performing his own choreography in *Afternoon of a Faun*. **Baron Adolphe de Meyer**

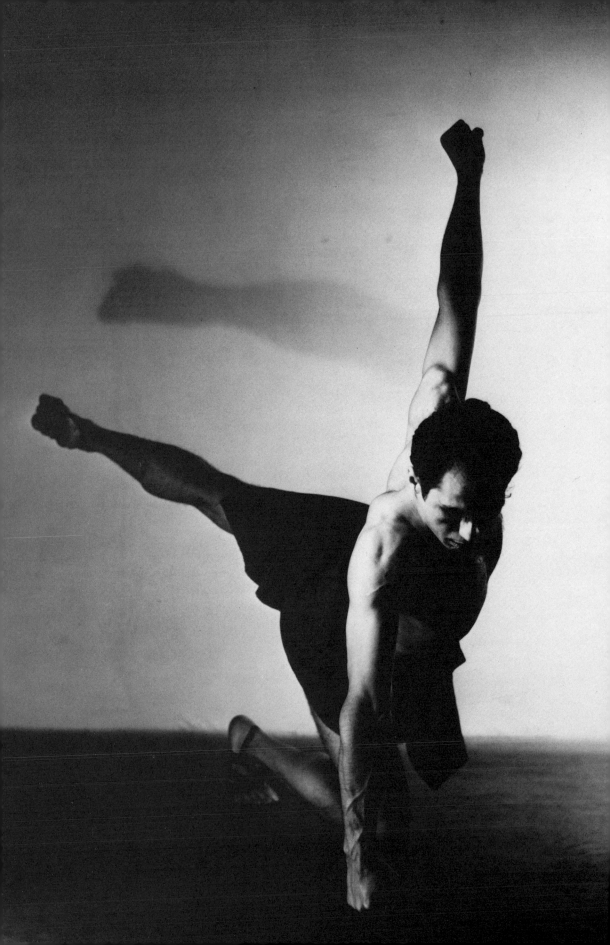

expression of his belief that men and women had separate and distinct styles of dancing which should be respected and preserved. For Shawn the proper female mode was tender, protective and contained, while the male style was forceful, aggressive and spatially extended. Shawn even identified dance themes and styles of music that were fitting for each of the sexes. If he overstated his case a bit, it was because he was determined to make dancing a respectable male occupation.

Still another important influence on male dancing was Martha Graham, who founded her company in 1926. Though she invented a technique that in some respects was female oriented, and many of her pieces were centered around women, she provided a dance vocabulary that men could identify with. Previously unexpressed dimensions of movement, such as effort, resistance and sheer physical strength, were incorporated into her choreography. Graham liked to use tall, imposing-looking men. In her work they portrayed substantial characters from Hebrew and Greek mythology and American history. It is no co-incidence that in the 1940s and 1950s three major male choreographers emerged from the Graham company: Merce Cunningham, Erick Hawkins and Paul Taylor. In California, Lester Horton established the first racially integrated dance troupe in 1932. Male protégés of other female teachers also became successful choreographers. Alwin Nikolais was a student of Hanya Holm and the German Expressionist school of Mary Wigman; Daniel Nagrin codirected a company in the 1940s with his teacher Helen Tamiris; and José Limón formed his company in the 1950s after studying and performing with Doris Humphrey.

As more men became dancers, choreographers and teachers, more dance styles and techniques were created for them, and more roles were generated to express the masculine point of view. Choreographers Eugene Loring, Agnes de Mille, Jerome Robbins, Antony Tudor, George Balanchine and Robert Joffrey have given the American male ballet dancer new substance and legitimacy on-stage. We are now approaching a time of virtual equality between the sexes in both modern dance and ballet.

This artistic development has been spurred on by accompanying shifts in the social and cultural climate of the country. In fact, it is probably safe to say that the emergence of male dancing as an accepted activity has done as much to advance the cause of sexual equality in general as changing sexual values have done to remove the stigma from male dancing. International superstars such as Rudolf Nureyev, Mikhail Baryshnikov and Peter Martins, who combine thrilling virtuosity with charismatic appeal, reach broad, enthusiastic audiences. These men and others like them have been instrumental in changing the image of the male dancer, but the American public has also been prepared for this change by

José Limón in his first major choreographic effort, *Danzas Mexicanas*. With his formidable appearance and noble bearing, Limón set a supreme example of what a man dancing could become. © *1972 Barbara Morgan* a softening of many old, rigid puritanical attitudes and a growing appreciation and enjoyment of the physical. Nowadays it isn't considered vain or effete for men to care about their bodies or the way they look. Male schoolteachers and female politicians are commonplace. There are men working as telephone operators and women as repairpersons. There are female bus drivers and male flight attendants. Although the male dancer is still a minority, he is no longer the oddity he once was.

As a reflection of this liberal trend, major ballet schools report that enrollment of young boys has tripled over the past fifteen years. Men come to dance through related interests such as painting, music, theater and sports. Lately single men have been going to dance class to meet women. The influx of more and better male dancers has raised the standards of male dancing in America across the board. Men are expected to be stronger technically and more polished than in the past.

But as long as women continue to outnumber men in the dance world, being a male will have decided advantages. Since they are in short supply, men are often given more attention and encouragement in class. Even the amateur taking lessons twice a week is someone special. A male with professional ambitions is apt to encounter many more opportunities and considerably less competition than a female. Men are sometimes accepted into scholarship programs and professional dance companies at older ages and with weaker techniques than women. Consequently, there have been several outstanding male dancers who were able to develop their talents later in life. Choreographers Antony Tudor and Paul Taylor began dancing in their early twenties. José Limón was twenty when he took his first dance class at the Humphrey-Weidman school. Paul Russell of the Dance Theatre of Harlem was Arthur Ashe's tennis partner at UCLA before he turned to dance. The great Russian premier danseur Igor Youskevitch was also a former athlete who started dance training at age twenty-one.

Owing to their anatomical differences, men and women have different needs as dance students. As was explained in chapter 4, men usually have to work harder than women for flexibility and suppleness, though they have natural strength and stamina. Their muscular bulk and heavy skeletons give men a more athletic, less refined movement quality than women, and this should be respected and encouraged. Yet despite these dissimilarities, little or no distinction is made in training male and female dancers. Both sexes practice essentially the same skills and identical steps, and for the most part it is up to the teachers and the dancers themselves to adapt.

Ballet is the only dance form which assigns specific movements to each sex. Following the successful example of the European academies, those few American ballet schools that can afford such a luxury hold separate classes for boys and girls. The boys work on a variety of multiple turns, leaps, jumps and beats. Girls work on balances, leg extensions, refinement of line and, as they advance, various steps on toe. In most ballet classes, however, everyone studies

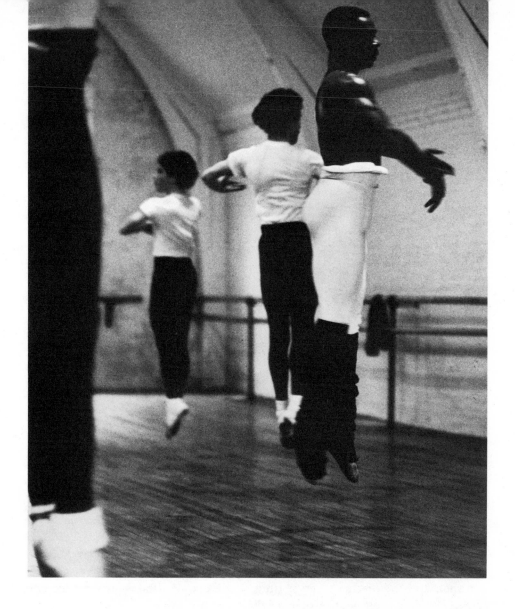

Above: Ballet students practicing air turns, a step performed exclusively by men. ***Frank Gimpaya***

Right: Jacques d'Amboise, shown in George Balanchine's *Apollo*, has been called the first American ballet star to look like an American. Six foot two, brawny and extraverted, he quickly won the admiration of the American press. During the 1950s and 60s making ballet "a manly art" became d'Amboise's personal crusade. ***New York Public Library***

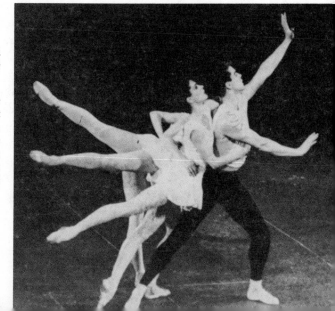

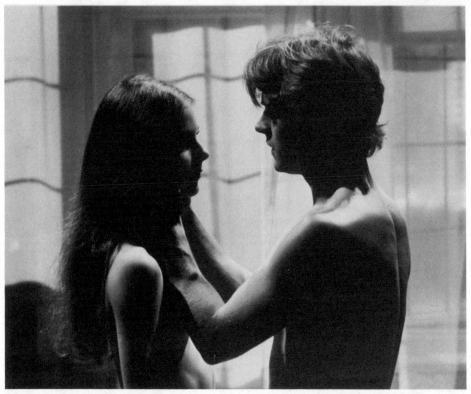

A turning point for the male image in America. In recent years the male dancer has become not only socially acceptable but something of a sex symbol. In *The Turning Point*, a 1977 remake of the old film classic *The Red Shoes*, Mikhail Baryshnikov played the romantic lead opposite Leslie Browne *(above)*. Soon after, John Travolta hustled his way into the hearts of millions in the box office smash *Saturday Night Fever*, and Broadway choreographer Bob Fosse emblazoned the screen with his heterosexual adventures in *All That Jazz*. *Museum of Modern Art*

together, and the teacher reserves time at the end of the lesson for male and female students to alternately practice their specialized steps.

For an eight-year-old boy, there is something more important than technique about being in a class with other males. A child learns largely by imitation, and boys need other males to model themselves after. They also need to move in a bigger, more aggressive way than girls. While a twenty-five-year-old may enjoy being the only man in a class full of women, a young boy will probably feel ill at ease surrounded by girls. A parent enrolling his or her son in dance class should therefore try to find one that is either taught by a male or attended by other male students—ideally, both. Large, well-established schools affiliated with professional dance companies are the most likely to have this. A boy needs to know that dancing is something men do. As Erick Hawkins has said, "A man dancing somehow will have to stand for what a man can become." For a great many reasons, more and more men in America are becoming dancers.

Part II

Dance
is
for
everyone

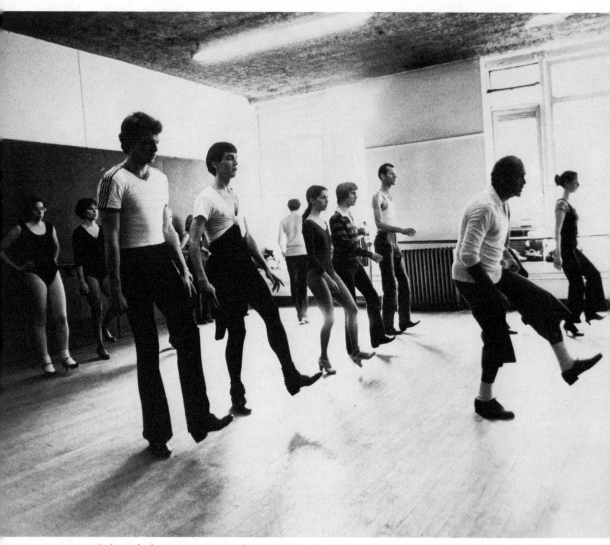

Bob Audy demonstrates a step for beginning tap students in New York. *Frank Gimpaya*

The Amateur Dancer: A New Breed

*nonprofessionals
may actually get more
out of dancing*

Amateurs are the newest, fastest-growing group of dancers in the country. They dance primarily for enjoyment—to relax, keep in shape, improve body awareness, to make new friends or impress old ones. Some amateurs are seeking fresh means of self-expression, or want to gain firsthand experience of a performing art. Many—and perhaps this is the real reason—have long harbored secret desires to dance. Whatever their motives, recreational dancers are usually people with other responsibilities and interests besides dancing. They can't devote all their time to classes, but they dance because they love it.

The benefits: dance as exercise plus

Dance is becoming a national pastime because it is uniquely beneficial to our modern American lives. Everybody comes to it with slightly different intentions and interests, but the wonderful thing about dancing is that it provides so many varied benefits. The beginner arrives with a narrow purpose but quickly finds that he or she has stirred a great passion.

Tom spends his whole day sitting with his shoulders hunched over a desk. He is beginning to develop a stoop, and for some reason his hands and feet are always cold. Unless he is reminded by these minor annoyances, he often forgets he has a body at all. A friend persuades Tom to try dancing. He is not

69

entirely convinced, but curiosity gets the best of him, and after a few lessons he is hooked on the fun he's having. It's a great way to clear his head at the end of the day. Pretty soon Tom is standing taller, his circulation has improved, and—something he never expected—he's feeling sexier than he has in years.

Dancing is the ideal way to stay in shape, since it conditions the body several ways at once by developing strength and endurance as well as stretch and flexibility. Dancers have better rhythm, balance and agility than many other athletes. While calisthenics and athletics work the body alone, dance training awakens the senses and attunes the mind to the body. The dancer learns how to control his body by becoming sensitized to it. Even the rank beginner is taught to cultivate the sensuous side of his being. In this respect, dancing can change your life because the very process of learning is a way to self-discovery and personal growth.

Liz has just had a baby. She is overweight, lethargic and is feeling like a middle-aged matron. Worst of all, she remembers how slinky she used to look in an evening gown. As much as she loves Junior, she just has to get out of the house a few hours a week away from his squalling. Liz would like to do something nice for herself, but jogging bores her, and she quit her exercise class because she couldn't face another sit-up. Months ago she clipped an ad from the local newspaper for an adult beginner class in ballet. But it's been yellowing on her kitchen bulletin board, buried under shopping lists and phone messages. How can she put on a pair of leotards and tights in the condition she's in?

Finally, out of desperation, Liz musters the nerve to go. When she walks into the dance studio she is immediately consoled by the sight of several other ladies standing at the barre—some in much worse shape than she—pulling tight leotards over their protruding bellies and nervously glancing around the room. She picks a spot next to a woman with a friendly, open face. They share their misgivings, laugh and make friends. The women go to class faithfully. Not only do they find themselves doing steps they never dreamed possible, but the progress is starting to show on their bodies. Liz sees a return to a more youthful, energetic self, one she likes a lot better. Dancing is invigorating. It improves appearance by correcting posture and body proportion. It tones the muscles and gives them definition (you'll notice a difference even after the first lesson). It puts roses in your cheeks and a smile on your face. Weight loss is often dramatic, and the grace and stage presence instilled in dance training carry over to everyday life.

Dancing is also a relatively inexpensive recreation. At an average of $4.50 for a ninety-minute class, dance lessons cost considerably less than tennis, golf or music lessons—or, for that matter, some exercise classes. The equipment is minimal; you don't have expensive skis, rackets or clubs to pay for. It is cheaper to dance than to go to the theater or a football game, and you can do it regardless of the weather, time of day or season. In some classes the music alone is so good that it's worth the price of admission.

All dancing girls are seventeen.

—*BALINESE PROVERB*

Sandy has been closeted away in a small real estate office for three years, and to tell the truth she wouldn't mind meeting some new people for a change. Come to think of it, her life has been altogether too routine lately. Every night on the way home from work she passes the neighborhood dance school. A barrage of conga rhythms bursts out of a partially opened studio window, its seductive beat quickening the pace of her walk. But until now, she has never thought of stopping by and taking a look around. Why not?

For Sandy, it's love at first sight. Dancing is entertainment, escape and a good workout rolled into one. Once she slips into her dance clothes and the music starts, she's a different person—freer, looser, bolder than before. The sheer energy of so many moving bodies is electrifying. After jazz class some of the dancers have been getting together for dinner and a few beers. Instead of the end, it feels like the beginning of Sandy's day.

Americans are flocking to dance classes in unprecedented numbers for more than just fitness. Dance is one of the most fundamental forms of self-expression. It satisfies the body and soul in a total way by providing an emotional outlet over and above the physical release of hard exercise. Dancing affords a rare chance for adults to play, to enjoy their fantasies and grow through them. The colorful costumes, the music and the atmosphere create an aura of romance that makes every lesson special and exciting. Where else but in dance class can you wear a garish shirt or pink tights and not feel silly? Dancing has always been an inherently social activity, and today it offers people a wonderful opportunity to meet others who share a common interest. Lifelong friendships have begun in dance class—and lately even romances are blossoming there.

What you bring to dancing

Even if you have never taken a dance class in your life, you probably have some useful experience with which to begin. You may have done some social dancing or experimented with your favorite music in the privacy of your living room. Maybe you've flicked a Frisbee around the park or played softball with the kids on Sundays. If so, you already know something about timing and coordination. If you've had athletic training, you have acquired the ability to work deeply physically.

If you are in good shape, so much the better. But no matter how well conditioned you are, don't be distressed by the soreness and weakness you may feel after the first dance class. Remember how you ached after your first tennis lesson? Dancing requires a different kind of stamina and suppleness from most sports and it employs a different distribution of muscle work. A swimmer, for instance, has strong back and leg muscles, powerful arms, a flexible shoulder girdle, and plenty of heart-lung endurance. This is a fine start, but he may discover that his neck and trapezius muscles are a bit overdeveloped for dancing and need to be stretched. Most people in our society take the path of least resistance when exercising. They do only what is pleasurable, increasing their strengths and doing little about their shortcomings. It is very important in dance training to work the entire body systematically, and one of the gratifying results is that this enables you to develop your whole range of physicality.

The pacing and atmosphere of a dance class are also very different from sports training. Take time to adjust to the new format and the unaccustomed demands on your body. Depending upon your physical type and the amount of activity you're used to, you may lack energy and stamina at first. Don't worry, strength will come with regular work. Women may be particularly unused to strenuous activity, but partly as a result, and partly because of their anatomical structure, they generally have looser joints and muscles than men. Each sex has to develop what the other possesses naturally. You should attend dance classes at least twice a week in order to accomplish anything of value. Of course, the more frequently you go the more fun it will be and the faster you'll progress, but if you can only go twice a week, do so with consistency.

Like all beginners, you may feel a little awkward or self-conscious, but look at it this way: You won't have any bad habits to overcome from prior training. You may even adapt to the classroom situation more quickly, since you won't feel the pressures of a professional dancer and you'll have fewer expectations based on past experiences. It may take a little extra determination to haul your body to dance class after a full day's work, but you'll always be glad you did.

Health factors

For most people, dancing is a boon to health. It improves circulation, relieves tension and headaches, builds up weak muscles and regulates breathing. It can even ease or correct minor back problems. You'll sleep more soundly when you dance, and the rigorous workout will help purge your system of lingering colds—not to mention hangovers. Diabetics and hypoglycemics will find that dancing regularly aides in stabilizing the blood sugar level, and many expectant mothers who have been dancing for a while continue in moderation throughout their pregnancy—with their obstetrician's approval, of course. They feel better and have easier deliveries and shorter postnatal recovery

Dancers warm up their backs in a beginning modern class at the Alvin Ailey American Dance Center. *Frank Gimpaya* periods. But like dancers of advanced age, pregnant dancers must have started earlier and stayed in shape if they hope to continue. To be beneficial, dancing must be something your body is already used to doing.

Don't make the mistake of regarding dance as a cure for everything. People over thirty-five who are out of condition or who have back problems, high blood pressure or heart disease should have a full medical checkup before embarking on any dance program. A stress test is advisable after the age of forty. Dancing is a healthy outlet for basically sound bodies, but if trouble does arise in the course of study, be sure to see your physician.

What kinds of dance are best for you?

Bear in mind when choosing a class that each dance form presents unique challenges and generates a different class ambience (see chapter 10 on ways of dancing). Although all types of dancing furnish good exercise, each one works the body a different way:

Tap and jazz are familiar dance modes because they are frequently seen on television and in other popular entertainments. The music is lively—show tunes for tap, and disco, popular music or live jazz for jazz classes. Tap dancing primarily works the legs and feet, while jazz stresses torso movement. Although they'll challenge you rhythmically, you can master the basics of tap and jazz in less time than you would need for ballet or modern dance, and you'll feel like you're dancing after only a few lessons.

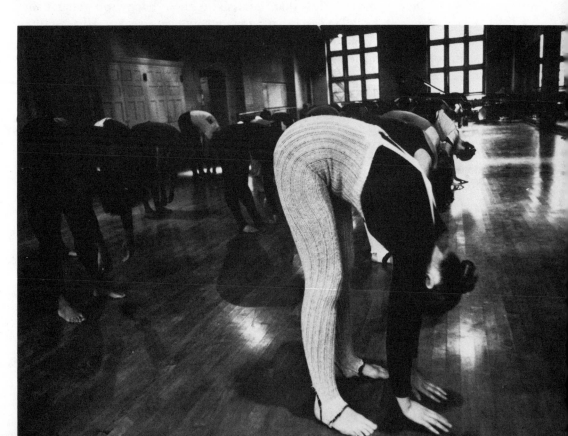

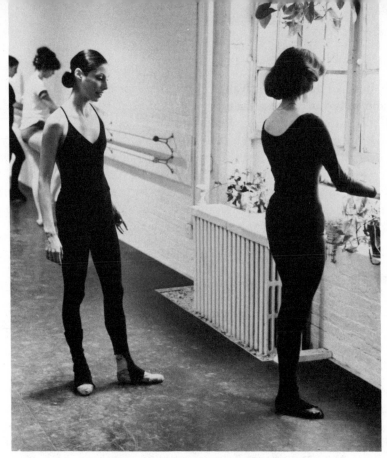

Jerry Mundy, courtesy of the Dance Movement School, New York

There is more action than analysis in these happy, outgoing dance forms. You learn by doing and can progress at your own rate. Since dress is often left up to the individual in jazz and tap classes, you may feel less vulnerable than you would in the standard leotards and tights. Tap dancers have an added advantage in that they can practice profitably at home—if the neighbors don't object—because they can *hear* their mistakes.

Ballet and most styles of modern dance provide thorough training for the entire body. They build strength and give the dancer an overall understanding of body mechanics. But they are also the most serious and demanding in terms of technique, and therefore they devote the most class time to warm-up and conditioning exercises. Both ballet and modern dance require a good deal of perseverance to learn properly.

There are some major differences between the two methods of training, however. Modern dance is easier on the body than ballet, because it uses natural movement and is generally adaptable to the quirks of individual physique. Ballet technique, on the other hand, was evolved on the bodies of dancers who were physically perfect for it and molded from childhood to its specialized demands. When competently taught, ballet is probably the best head-to-toe training system there is, but at the same time it is the most difficult for the raw beginner to attempt. For one thing, it requires a considerable amount of stretch, and for another, students are obliged to learn the names of the steps in French. If you don't want to get discouraged, you should take a minimum of three ballet lessons a week. Most ballet exercises focus on developing the legs, feet and arms, as well as a strong, vertical spine. Most modern dance movement comes from the trunk, so there is more work on the midsection and the back in modern classes. As a rule, modern dance is rhythmically and dynamically more varied than ballet.

Dance exercise classes, or dancercize classes as they are sometimes called, are for people who are primarily interested in body conditioning. Taught by dancers, these classes incorporate dance movement (usually ballet or jazz) and music, and as one enthusiast told me, "their approach to exercise is so much more positive than fighting fat—it's inspiring." Not only are dancercize classes more fun than regular exercise classes, they may also be less intimidating than dance classes for the beginner and thus a good way to ease into dancing.

What to look for when choosing a class

Special adult beginner classes. Today, because of the rising amateur enrollment, many dance schools schedule dance fundamentals or prebeginner classes for adults with no previous training. At the very least, most schools have evening beginner classes which are heavily attended by working women and men (these normally attract a mixture of absolute beginners and more advanced dancers). Adult beginner classes provide a relaxed, informal setting in which you can feel comfortable and unselfconscious. They move slowly, include a prudent warm-up, and they are especially geared to mature bodies and minds. Since the dance terms and exercises are explained in detail, you cannot get irretrievably lost or disheartened.

Chances to get moving. If, like most recreational dancers, you aren't interested in a lot of theory and technical analysis, try to find classes that are well paced and that give you a chance to move; but be sure you get enough explanation from the teacher to know what you are doing and avoid injury. Everyone has slightly different warm-up requirements. Choose a teacher who gets *your* body warmed up adequately (see chapters 15 and 18 on warming up).

Convenience. Class times, the location of the dance school, and school facilities (showers, change rooms, locker space) are generally important to amateur dancers because they have to fit dancing into already full lives. Parents might ask if they can bring a young child to class with them (some schools allow this), or whether there are children's classes available at the same time they are dancing.

Deeper involvement with dance

What begins as a recreational interest in dance sometimes grows into a deeper involvement. Many serious amateurs have danced earlier in their lives or are former professionals, now out of practice, who return to dancing purely for their own enjoyment. Others are people who have been dancing for a while, have progressed beyond the beginner stage and wish to strive for greater mastery. This is no mere casual sideline—after all, Olympic athletes aren't professionals either—and it calls for a much stronger commitment to training. Three lessons a week is the minimum for amateurs who choose to study in depth and achieve a satisfying degree of proficiency. Once you reach the intermediate level, you will probably be taking class with full-time dancers in an environment where the students expect a great deal from themselves and the teacher is more demanding. If you decide to pursue dance seriously, don't be intimidated. Take time to get used to your new, more challenging classes. You will eventually find them very stimulating, and they will inspire you to new heights of achievement. Just like playing tennis with a superior partner, dancing with superior dancers improves your own performance.

Those who are prepared to devote the necessary time and energy will be able to study any dance form profitably, including ballet. With the right supervision, amateurs who have always longed to wear satin toe shoes and dance on pointe can—provided they are strong enough and sufficiently advanced in ballet technique. Ask your teacher's advice. Some dance schools even offer elementary toe classes for adults.

Tap Dancing Has Changed My Life

In my twenty-seventh year I began to tap dance in earnest. It started rather slowly. I had taken a tap class briefly at the YMCA with a friend, mostly out of homage to Busby Berkeley, Eleanor Powell, et al. When the class was over, we were so enthralled that we moved on to a real dance school. It was sort of a sleazy one, up a flight of stairs from a storefront, but it was nevertheless a dance school with wooden floors and mirrors, and classes from hula to modern jazz. It was really quite thrilling, and I looked forward to putting on my dancing shoes each week. Then I moved into another phase in my life and thought I didn't have time for dancing anymore. I quit, and immediately regretted it.

Two years later, on an impulse, I went to a tap class at Al Gilbert's studio in Hollywood. It is the kind of place that aspiring show-biz kids start out in, but it also has classes for adults (because of the location and reputation, a lot of TV and movie people come for lessons as well). We did lots of foot exercises to strengthen our feet and to build up our ability to move quickly but surely. We also worked on an ongoing routine, adding a few new steps each week. During the two years I was at Al Gilbert's I was in two recitals. Each year the students are given an opportunity to display their talents. Most of them are under twelve years old, so there is a plethora of lacy tutus and glitter and plump, rouged cheeks. Everyone takes the shows very seriously; we could easily have been opening on Broadway.

I must say, in all honesty, that tap dancing has changed my life. I tap during every available moment: on street corners, at the grocery store, in front of the elevator at work, and wherever else I can find a surface with good sound. I have found that one of the best places is in courthouses, because they generally have long, wide corridors and marble floors. I am a lawyer, and it gives me great pleasure to sneak in a few steps here and there as I go about my daily business.

After a brief vacation and some more changes in my life, I am now taking an intermediate-level tap class at the Danny Daniels Dance America School in Santa Monica. The format is similar to that at Al Gilbert's, about half exercise and half dancing, but the style is quite different. Danny Daniels is much more oriented toward moving across the floor than toward perfecting a few intricate steps, and he is very conscious of how things look from a distance. Whereas it used to take all my concentration to get my feet to move on cue, I find that I am now able to notice such stylistic differences and to make a few more choices in the way I dance. I am also beginning to take ballet, hoping to become stronger and more graceful and to incorporate some of the ballet arm movements into my tap.

I think that there is probably a dancer in everyone, and that one doesn't have to have a lot of ability or training in order to enjoy dancing. Even more importantly, I think people ought to realize that one doesn't have to have lofty goals for their dancing, such as becoming a professional or becoming a performer per se. One can dance for the sheer pleasure of it, for the discipline it engenders, for the opportunities it presents for self-expression, for the strength it builds or for the fantasies it fulfills.

—SUE BURRELL
Venice, California

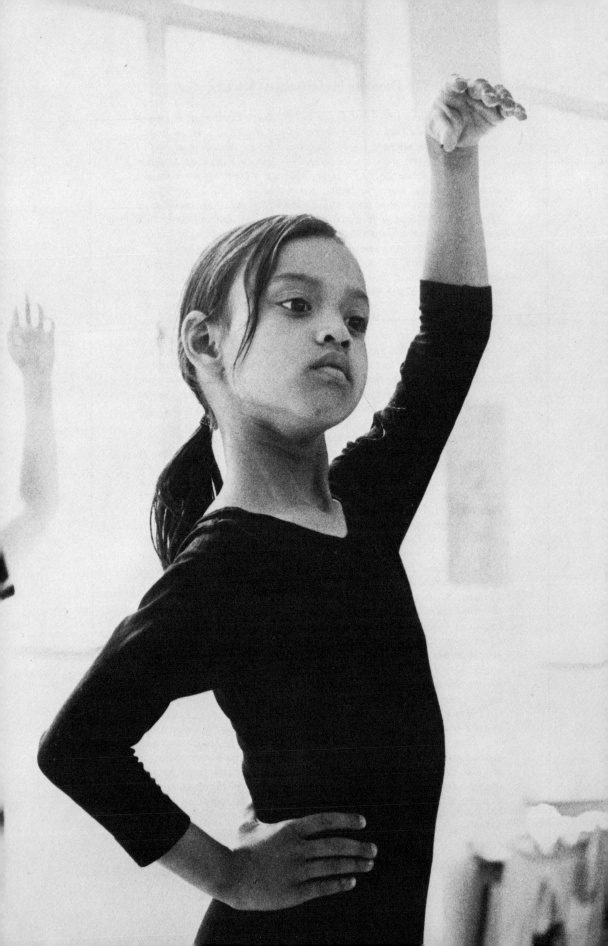

8

Dancing for Children

they're born dancers,
and not just
on rainy days

Do you have an itchy child on your hands who seems to have more energy than he knows what to do with? Who is always bumping into lamps and crashing into furniture? Are his childhood pranks getting on your nerves? There are many things you can do with a rambunctious youngster, but few activities allow him to burn up youthful energy and give his active imagination free reign the way dancing does. And what about the child who already knows she wants to dance, who flits about the house jumping and spinning? What's the best way to start her off?

Children are born dancers. If you find the right teacher and class environment for them, most will thrive. For many reasons childhood is a prime time to introduce young people to dance. Isadora Duncan, who revolutionized theatrical dancing with her childlike naturalness and integrity, knew that dancing came most easily to the very young who were still utterly instinctive and spontaneous. She saw in children all of mankind's innate and essential impulses to express itself in movement.

From birth, a child communicates with his body, and physical movement is therefore his most mature medium of expression. He can dance out feelings that he is unable or even afraid to communicate in words. If children have limited means of expression, they often compensate with an overabundance of energy. This is welcome in dancing, which provides a creative outlet for both physical and emotional spirit. The dance class is one place where a frisky child will not be mistakenly treated as a victim of hyperactivity. There is mounting evidence that movement training, which entails learning about spatial relations, can help young children learn reading, writing and mathematics. Toward this end, the United States Commissioner of Education has urged that dance be permanently incorporated into the public school curriculum.

Childhood is a time of optimal physical and mental growth. Most children are very receptive to new ideas, and it is during the early years of their lives that they can develop confidence and joy in the possibilities of their own bodies. Dancing helps youngsters establish a good body image, while it builds strong, straight spines and aids in regulating weight. Dance classes offer children a chance to make new friends in a shared activity; they teach social skills, and they bring parents together, too.

What parents should know

One of the first, most important obligations of the parent who is enrolling a child in dance class is to be clear about which goals are yours and which are your child's. You probably want to give your offspring an introduction to dance, music and artistic expression. You may even be hoping that she or he will have a career in dance. But for your daughter or son, the fun of dancing must come first, for without this there can be nothing else. It is imperative that you give your child time to come to her own conclusions about dancing. Often children who begin ''working'' toward a career at the age of four or five don't ever have the opportunity to make a conscious choice for dance because of the love they feel for it.

Though it is true that professional ballet dancing requires an early start, this doesn't mean that the child should learn to dance before she can walk. Most reputable ballet schools will not admit children for formal study under the age of eight, and a ballet career for your youngster is by no means out of reach if she starts at ten or twelve (see chapter 3 on age restrictions in professional dancing). Even then, parents should remember that each child develops at her own rate and cannot be rushed.

The kind of early dance training that a young person receives will shape her attitudes toward dancing for the rest of her life, so it should be carefully chosen. After your child expresses an interest in dance, it is up to you to find the appropriate class and teacher for her, and to follow her learning experience as it evolves. Parents are generally discouraged from dropping in casually to watch lessons, but most dance schools hold open-house days or year-end student demonstrations to which family and friends are cordially invited. Teachers are usually available to talk informally before or after class, or at prearranged conferences.

Above all else, watch for those exciting first signs of your child's emergence as an individual, in dance as in everything else. The eccentricities which may at times drive you mad as a parent can produce a distinguished style or character in your girl or boy's dancing. As that individual emerges, you should be sure that the class and the teacher continue to serve well. Keep in touch with your youngster's feelings about her dance class. She will probably make them clear to you one way or another. Is she interested, responding, having a good time? Does she like her teacher and feel comfortable with the other students? A child's progress should not be judged in terms of technical expertise, but in terms of her growing enjoyment, range of movement and confidence.

Children's special needs as dancers

Just as a child's needs should determine his diet, so his stage of physical development should determine the kind of dance encounter he gets in class. As with all learning, certain things come only with age, and for dancing to be a positive experience, your child should be challenged in areas where his growing body and mind can benefit most. Children are stimulated by projects just a bit past their present capacities; but when these tasks are too far beyond them they fall back and retreat into a shell.

As dance therapist Blanche Evan has observed, a child's body becomes capable of different movements at different ages. First he rolls, then crawls, then walks awkwardly by age two, and finally he learns to walk more gracefully by age three. An average three-and-a-half-year-old won't spontaneously skip to lively music because he hasn't yet got the balance and coordination to do so.*

Not only must the child be allowed to acquire motor skills in his own good time, he must be given the freedom to move in his own way, whether or not this seems awkward or graceful to the adult eye. A young dancer must be permitted, as Evan puts it, "to do a wild dance as well as a pretty or a sad one." This is necessary in order to establish dancing as a means of expression. Each child has an individual movement style based on his particular personality and body type. Very simply, a heavy child will move differently from a light one, an extravert will dance differently from an introvert, and these differences have to be respected. If children are molded too early by rules of technique, or encouraged to imitate rather than to create, they lose the invaluable sense of themselves in their movement. For children, enjoyment and discovery ought to come first; technique should certainly not be seriously introduced before the age of eight or nine.

Children up to the age of seven should be given simple, natural movements to do—rolling, walking, skipping, running, jumping; moving forward, backward, and sideways, and turning around in space. Circle and line dances offer a further opportunity to develop spatial awareness. Young children may be introduced to basic rhythms but shouldn't be held too strictly to these. They must be allowed to find their own body timing. Improvisational play,

*From Blanche Evan, "The Child's World," Parts I & III, in *Dancemagazine*, January 1949 and February 1951.

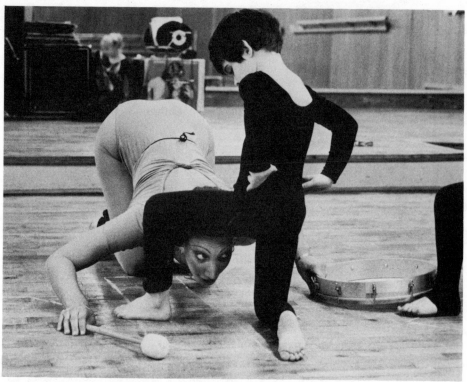

Movement games teach spatial relations. *Robert McLeroy, courtesy of the Studio of Creative Arts, Longview, Texas*

movement games, exercises using props such as scarves and balls, and dancing out stories or images of birds and animals are good ways for children to find their own expression in movement while relating to others in a group.

Older children of eight or nine are ready to begin working on the rudiments of technique and rhythm, but even at this age spontaneity should not be dampened by too many restrictions or an overly dogmatic teaching approach. There should be some point in class where free-form or natural movement is given so that the youngsters can enjoy themselves without having to think about rules. This might include runs, skips, jumps, gallops or chassés in ballet (sliding steps done across the floor).

Any dance class for the young must protect the child's developing anatomy. Particularly in ballet, overstrict training that forces the body too far can cause real damage by overstretching the ligaments that stabilize the joints. Dr. William Liebler, an orthopedic surgeon in New York who specializes in treating dancers' injuries, cautions: ''Once a dancer has stretched his ligaments they remain that way for life. That's why a dancer's muscular development is so important. It really holds him together.''* Insisting on extremely turned-out or

*From David Lindner, ''Dancer's Pain,'' in *Dance Life in New York*, Spring 1975.

crossed positions from children will distort the spine, weaken the joints, twist the legs and strain the knees. Because of the stringent demands that ballet dancing makes on the body, it is absolutely essential for young students to learn good postural alignment (see illustrations in chapter 18). Deep-breathing and tension-relieving exercises should also be incorporated into each lesson to reduce strain.

One of the worst things you can do is allow a little girl to dance on her toes before she is ready. A child who is too young simply does not have sufficient muscular development or training to withstand the rigors of pointe work.* Children's eagerness to perform tricks on their toes, backed up by incompetent teachers, unfortunately makes premature pointe work all too common. Under these circumstances toe dancing can be awfully risky. The strain on the body can damage the soft tissue around the bones of the feet and knees, resulting in painfully enlarged joints, or it can cause injury to the lower spine.

To make matters worse, the stiffened blocks and large supporting boxes of modern-day pointe shoes enable virtually anyone to stand on her toes. In the past it was the dancer, and not the shoe, that had to do it. The dancer ought to be able to lift her body out of the pointe shoes by the use of strong stomach,

*As a public service, Capezio issues a free pamphlet on the dangers and prevention of too-early pointe work entitled "Why Can't I Go on My Toes?" Write to Capezio Ballet Makers, 1860 Broadway, New York, New York 10023.

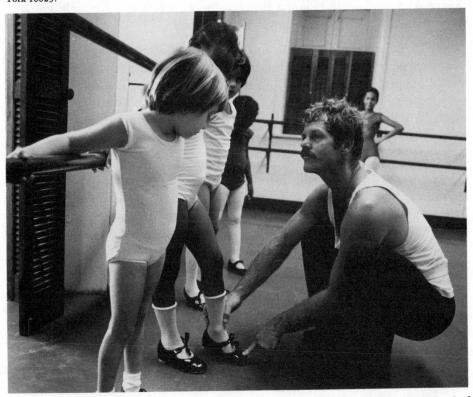

Teacher Day Power shows small fry how to make clear tap sounds at the St. Thomas School of Dance in the Virgin Islands.

groin, leg and foot muscles; she shouldn't be leaning on them for support. Authorities such as Dame Margot Fonteyn maintain that beginning toe students should be strong enough to wear moderately flexible (not hard) shoes, so there is full articulation and maximum development of the entire foot. To discourage the practice of putting little girls on toe too early, Capezio Ballet Makers and other shoe manufacturers have stopped making children's pointe shoes under size thirteen. It is generally agreed that toe dancing should begin no earlier than the age of ten, and only after two full years of prior daily training. Children new to pointe work should be carefully supervised, and they should hold on to the barre for support for at least a year.

Which kinds of dance are best for children?

Regardless of the dance style they are studying, all children should take special classes designed for their age group and level of experience. Adult classes are neither expressive for them nor well suited to their bodies. You and your child may wish to experiment with different types of dance before settling on one (see chapter 10 on ways of dancing). This won't hurt, since exposure to a variety of styles early in life will allow a youngster to select the one that fits her best as an individual when the time comes. Although it lies outside the scope of this book, folk dancing makes a fine introduction to dance for children. It is fun, informal, highly musical and widely available.

Young children ages 4-7. Preschool creative movement classes or preballet classes are best for young children. In these the emphasis is on natural movement (running, skipping, jumping, rolling, etc.), free expression, learning to participate in a group, and improvisational games in which the children are encouraged to make up their own dances. Preballet classes introduce some simple ballet steps, but here again, in an atmosphere of play.

Children ages 8-12. Not all modern dance studios offer children's classes, but modern dance, which is predicated on creativity and self-expression, is probably the most appropriate form for children. There is also a broad range of modern styles and teaching methods to choose from.

Tap is another good dance mode for children of this age because it does not overtax the body and it has a relaxed, outgoing air. However, the rhythms and physical coordinations are a bit advanced for some young people, and they should learn at their own pace.

Children's ballet chasses should be taught with great care. Otherwise they can be terribly repressive. "You can't expect all children to like ballet classes," says George Balanchine, whose School of American Ballet has been dubbed the "West Point of dance." "I certainly did not like them at first, and I think this is more or less true of most young pupils. Only gradually do they learn to like it. They like the music the pianist plays for them to move to. Slowly they become trained to move well and to listen, and from a few steps and exercises they are able to do simple dance sequences. They watch grown-up dancers in other classes, admire them, and want to move beautifully too."* Inasmuch as ballet dancing requires a good deal of concentration and physical effort, young students need to be in small classes where they can get lots of individual attention and motivation from the teacher. The work must not be unreasonably demanding, and there should be some time allocated in every class for the children to cut loose and dance for pure enjoyment.

Jazz dance is seldom taught to youngsters, perhaps because it calls for rather sophisticated coordinations which come with later development, but mostly because it has a sexual undercurrent which is peculiarly adult.

Backtalk

Interview of five- and six-year-olds coming out of ballet class:

Do you want to be a ballerina when you grow up?
—Yes, 'cause if I am my mommy will buy me a tutu.

What's your favorite part of class?
—Well, I like to lean on the barre.

What do you like best about ballet?
—Nothing!

Why do you take ballet?
—I don't know. My mother signed me up because my sister took it.

Do you take ballet classes because they're fun?
—It isn't fun.

Do you think you're pretty good at it?
—No. We don't do it enough to get good at it.

Do you want to do it more?
—No!

Don't you think dancing is fun?
—No! I hate it.

Mom: Oh, I think you like it very much.
—No! I *hate* it.

---

*From George Balachine, "Ballet for Your Children," in *Dancemagazine*, June 1954.

Teenagers. Adolescents can study any form of dance—ideally in a special class for them or one attended by other young people. Depending on the individual child, a thirteen- or fourteen-year-old may be ready for a standard beginner class for adults.

What to look for when choosing a class for your child

The class should be well paced for your child's attention span and endurance. This is important because there is a great deal of difference in development between a five-year-old and an eight-year-old, or an eight-year-old and a twelve-year-old. These days most dance schools offer children's classes that are graded according to age and experience. As was pointed out in chapter 6, it is best for boys to be in a class with other boys, so that they are not alone in a world of females. It is also preferable for them to study with male teachers who can serve as appropriate models. You are most likely to find this at a large, established dance school that is affiliated with a professional company.

The teacher should be someone your child likes to be around. More than anything else, children seem to respond to the warmth of the person and his or her love of dancing. You'll want a relaxed individual who has a good time with kids and sees to it that they enjoy themselves too. (Some people who teach children shouldn't. They don't have the temperament and they get shrill and irritable.) Your child's instructor ought to be experienced in teaching youngsters and able to communicate with them on their own level. It's a good idea to ask about her prior training and teaching background. She should be sensitive to the needs of the individual child, as well as to the group as a whole. The teacher should demonstrate good postural habits, never allowing young children to twist or distort the spine (see illustrations in chapter 18), and she shouldn't be insistent on perfect results. Children should certainly never be encouraged to force or strain physically.

Convenience for you. Young children, of course, will have to be accompanied to and from classes, so you'll want to make sure they are held at a convenient time and location for you. If you find a situation in which your child prospers, you don't want logistical snafus to interfere. After all, you deserve a break too. Parents often get together to share car pools or take turns escorting children to dance school. You may even want to look for dance classes for yourself, given at the same time as your child's, in the same school or close by. (Actress Joanne Woodward became an avid balletomane and amateur dancer as a result of taking her daughter to ballet lessons.)

Costs. Most children's dance classes are shorter—they are forty-five minutes to an hour—and therefore less expensive than adults' classes. Some schools offer lower tuition rates to families with more than one child enrolled.

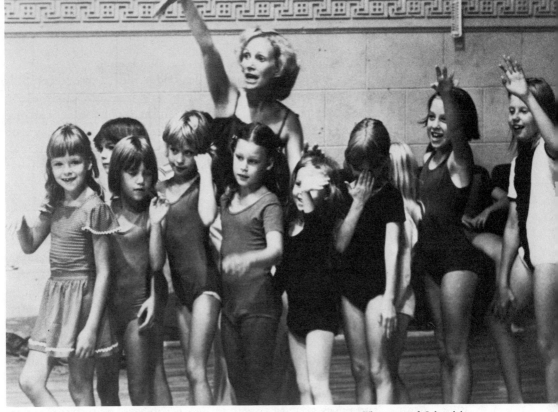

Marcia Chapman with her children's ballet class at the Minnesota Dance Theatre and School in Minneapolis.

How many classes to take

It is far better for children to look forward to one or two dance classes a week than to dread the prospect of going every day. Don't overload your child with classes at first. Even at the professionally-oriented School of American Ballet, eight-and nine-year-olds take only two weekly lessons. Young children cannot and should not devote too much time to dancing. They have school and other interests to pursue, and these are at least as important as dance class in making them full people and eventually complete dancers.

Discipline is a much overused word in dance, I think. It implies force or compulsion. Children are particularly vulnerable to injury if they are driven to perform beyond their capacities, and nothing kills the joy so essential to good dancing faster than too much discipline. Regardless of age, a person must dance because he loves it. Dedication and devotion are better words to use with respect to dancing, because they come from love.

Most kids hate to practice at home or to work during their school vacations. Happily these two activities are discouraged by most dance experts because they are of doubtful value and deprive children of a much needed respite from dancing. George Balanchine advises, "While practicing at home is not generally harmful, it actually does very little good; children should certainly not be made to do it. At home there is no teacher to watch and correct them; only in class can they practice with real profit." Even the serious student should have his vacations free, declares Balanchine, for he needs the rest and relaxation as much as anyone else.

Especially for children

Public school programs. You may not have to go any further than the local school district to give your child his or her first exposure to dance. The National Endowment for the Arts Artists-in-Schools program engages approved professional dance companies and instructors to conduct informal classes and lecture-demonstrations at elementary and secondary schools throughout the country. Artists are usually hired for two-week residencies which allow them to work with the children on a personal level.

Another public school program that may be available to your child is Young Audiences. This is sponsored by a nationwide nonprofit organization that brings professional performing arts presentations to schools in thirty-four states. Young Audiences activities include dance concerts, workshops, classes and lecture-demonstrations. By employing local companies this program also helps support the neighboring arts community, and it splits the cost with the host school.

If you are interested in working through your PTA to start an Artists-in-Schools or Young Audiences program in your school district, contact the following national offices:

> Charles Reinhart, National Coordinator
> NEA Artists-in-Schools Program
> 1860 Broadway
> New York, New York 10023
> (212) 586-1925

> Warren H. Yost, Executive Director
> Young Audiences
> 115 East 92nd Street
> New York, New York 10028
> (212) 831-8110

Children's dance books and records. Children's dance books are still slim pickings, but there are a few more good ones each year, such as Jill Krementz's excellent *A Very Young Dancer* and Camilla Jessel's *Life at the Royal Ballet School*. There is also a smattering of recordings of famous ballet scores, as well as folk and ethnic dance music for juveniles. You may be able to find some children's dance books and records at your public library or local bookseller.

If you are ever in New York City be sure to visit the Children's Library at the Lincoln Center Library and Museum for the Performing Arts, which has these materials available in a specially designed environment for young people. In the nearby Hecksher Oval, children's story hours, puppet shows and other programs are regularly scheduled.

Children's Library
Second Floor
Library and Museum of the Performing Arts
New York Public Library at Lincoln Center
111 Amsterdam Avenue at 65th Street
New York, New York 10023
(212) 799-2200

Here are some books that your young reader may enjoy:

Nonfiction

Ambrose, Kay. *The Ballet Student's Primer.* New York: Knopf, 1953.

Berger, Melvin. *The World of Dance.* New York: Phillips, Inc., 1978.

de Mille, Agnes. *To a Young Dancer.* Boston: Little Brown and Company, 1962.

Franks, A.H., ed. *Every Child's Book of Dance and Ballet.* London: Burke Publishing Company, 1976.

Gouldin, Shirley. *The Royal Book of Ballet.* Chicago: Follett Publishing Company, 1977.

Harnan, Terry. *African Rhythm — American Dance: A Biography of Katherine Dunham.* New York: Knopf, 1974.

Haskell, Arnold Lionel. *The Wonderful World of Dance.* New York: Doubleday, 1969.

Jessel, Camilla. *Life at the Royal Ballet School.* New York: Methuen, 1979.

Karsavina, Tamara. *Classical Ballet: The Flow of Movement.* London: A. and C. Black, 1962.

Krementz, Jill. *A Very Young Dancer.* New York: Knopf, 1977.

Kushida, Magoichi, ed. *P. I. Tchaikovsky's The Nutcracker.* Tokyo: Gakken Company, 1971.

Lemaitre, Odon-Jerome. *The Dance.* New York: Barron's, 1977.

Mara, Thalia. *First Steps in Ballet.* New York: Dance Horizons, 1976.

Martin, John. *John Martin's Book of the Dance.* New York: Tudor, 1963.

Moldon, Peter L. *Your Book of Ballet.* London: Faber & Faber, 1974.

Nelson, Esther. *Movement Games for Children.* New York: Sterling Publishing Company, 1976.

Sparger, Celia. *Beginning Ballet.* New York: Theatre Arts, 1973.

Streatfield, Noel. *A Young Person's Guide to Ballet.* London: Frederick Warne & Company, 1975.

Tennant, Veronica. *On Stage, Please*. Toronto: McClelland and Stewart, 1978.

Terry, Walter. *Frontiers of Dance: The Life of Martha Graham*. New York: Thomas Y. Crowell, 1975.

Tobias, Tobi. *Arthur Mitchell*. New York: Thomas Y. Crowell, 1975.

Warren, Lee. *The Dance of Africa*. Englewood Cliffs, New Jersey: Prentice-Hall, 1972.

Fiction

Behrman, Carol H. *Catch a Dancing Star*. Minneapolis: Dillon Press, 1975.

Lambie, Laurie Jo. *Daisy Discovers Dance*. New York: John Day (Harper & Row), 1973.

Myers, Walter Dean. *The Dancers*. New York: Parents Magazine Press, 1972.

Simon, Marcia L. *A Special Gift*. New York: Harcourt Brace Jovanovich, 1978.

Tallon, Robert. *Handella*. Indianapolis: Bobbs-Merrill Company, 1972.

Coloring books

The Nutcracker Ballet Coloring Book (from the designs of Alexander Benois). San Francisco: Bellerophon Books, 1977. Write to: 153 Steuart Street, San Francisco, California 94105.

The Sleeping Beauty Ballet Coloring Book (from the designs of Leon Bakst). San Francisco: Bellerophon Books, 1977. Write to address given above.

Tichenor, Kay, and Helen Kunic. *Ballet Coloring Book*. San Francisco: Troubador Press, 1976.

If you cannot locate any suitable children's dance books, try adapting a good adult book. Your child may have fun thumbing through some of the many wonderful photographic volumes on dance, such as Albert E. Kahn's *Days With Ulanova*, Barbara Morgan's *Martha Graham* and Mikhail Baryshnikov's *Baryshnikov at Work* (with photos by Martha Swope). She or he may love to hear excerpts from George Balanchine's *101 Stories of the Great Ballets*, or from the extraordinary lives of such dancers as Anna Pavlova, Vaslav Nijinsky and Isadora Duncan. As a young child I remember being read a biography of Pavlova at bedtime, and though I didn't understand very much of it, the parts about her childhood have stayed with me to this day.

Dance performances. The companies listed below specialize in children's dance theater. Some of them feature child performers, which makes them all the more appealing to young audiences. Most professional ballet companies present full-length story ballets, such as *The Nutcracker* and *Coppélia*, which also employ child dancers. Folk and ethnic dance concerts are another good choice for children because they are upbeat and colorful.

Baba-Yaga from Russia
Rita Toy, Director
219 East 88th Street
New York, New York 10028
(212) 427-6196

Bergen Junior Ballet Company
Betty H. Swenson, Artistic Director
121 New Bridge Road
Bergenfield, New Jersey 07621
(201) 385-7796

Cartoon Opera/Storytelling in Song,
Dance and Mime
Heather Forest, Director
P.O. Box 354
Huntington, New York 11743
(516) 271-2511

Children's Ballet Theatre
Christine Neubert, Artistic Director
Carnegie Hall, Studio 803
881 Seventh Avenue
New York, New York 10019
(212) MU5-7754

Children's Dance Theatre
Deanne Collins, Director
P.O. Box 5352
Huntsville, Alabama 35805
(205) 852-6842

Children's Dance Theatre
University of Utah Annex 1152
Salt Lake City, Utah 84112
(801) 581-7374

Children's Repertory Dance Theater
Jean Liebenberg, Artistic Director
Georgetown Day School
4530 MacArthur Boulevard, N.W.
Washington, D.C. 20007
(212) 483-8165

Lotte Goslar's Pantomime Circus
c/o Sheldon Soffer Management Agency
130 West 56th Street
New York, New York 10019
(212) 757-8060

The Paper Bag Players
Judith Martin, Artistic Director
50 Riverside Drive
New York, New York 10024
(212) EN2-0431

Pumpernickel Players
Lurie Horns, Director
223 East 5th Street, #14
New York, New York 10002
(212) 673-4880, 850-4065

Qwindo's Window
Anne Dunkin and Brad Willis
Artistic Directors
P.O. Box 6333
Washington, D.C. 20015
(703) 360-5922

The Turnabouts
Alma Bowden and Kathryn Shapinsky
Directors
305 East 6th Street
New York, New York 10003
(212) YU2-7360, BE3-3575

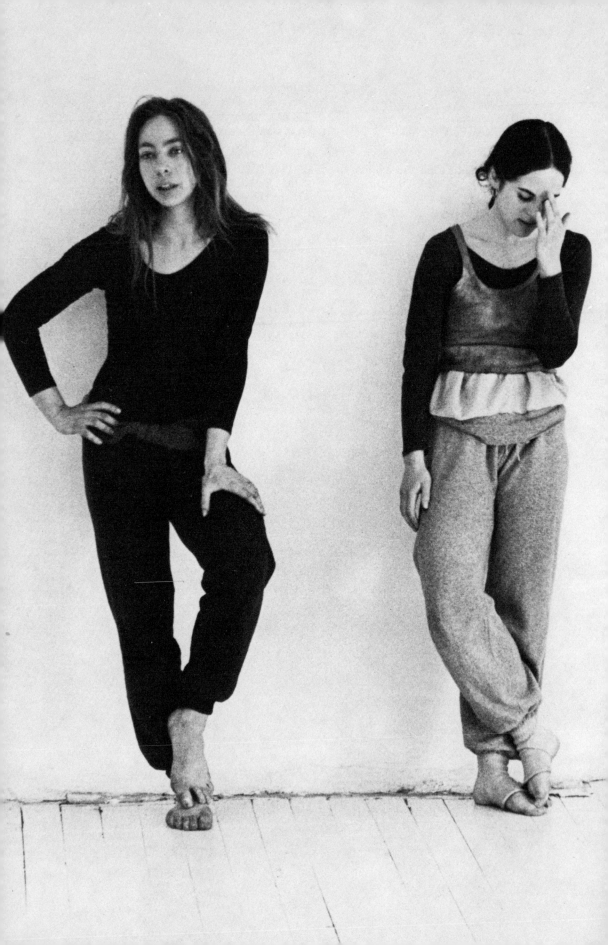

9

The Career-Minded Dancer

*what you should know
about dancing professionally
and training for a career*

A few realities

You must love to dance if you are going to dance professionally. Then, despite all that is said about a dancer's need for discipline and self-sacrifice, the work is actually the easiest and most satisfying part of your life. You spend most of your time doing what you love, and your performing career catapults you to heights of exhilaration no other occupation can match. In some ways, a professional dancer is like an astronaut who goes places and does things that most people cannot even imagine. Dancing gives you a beautiful body and a way of life that is fanciful, vigorous and exciting. And dancing is utterly absorbing because it exacts creativity from every fiber of your being. Like any profession chosen out of love, it gives you a sense of purpose. When you are working well professionally, you will find that dancing is more than a pleasure. It is a profound privilege.

But dancing professionally is not a nine-to-five occupation. Its rewards are rarely such conventional ones as stability and financial security, and it doesn't make ordinary demands on your talents and energies. Even after you've invested time, effort and money in training, there is no guarantee that you'll make it—though there are usually good indications along the way. It takes a rather special person to be a career dancer, and the decision to dance professionally must be grounded in a knowledge of the realities involved, as well as in a genuine need to dance.

Frank Gimpaya

Do you have what it takes? From the moment she sets her sights on a career to the day she retires, a dancer never really stops asking these questions:

Am I good?
Do I want to dance badly enough?
Is it worth it?

The answers come only with time. There is no set formula for success. A dancer needs different attributes for different styles of dancing: It takes a different set of qualities and ambitions to become a soloist with a ballet or modern dance company than it does to succeed on Broadway.

It may be several years before you can be certain that you have the makings of a professional. Everyone finds out at a different time and in a different way. There are always good days and bad days, but after studying intensively awhile, certain trends will emerge. You'll know whether you find happiness and expression in dancing as in nothing else, and whether you are making steady progress. Another indication is the feedback you get from your teachers and from other dancers you respect. I didn't know for sure until the first time I performed (in a student piece at college) and felt what it was like to move an audience. Some dancers don't discover they are performers until they become choreographers—that is, until they can make movement that truly expresses them.

"Talent is work," said Ulanova, the great Bolshoi ballerina. Many people have natural gifts for movement, but they don't have what it takes to build a career. The desire to dance, along with the conviction that you have something to give, is at least as important as inborn ability. Success also depends on how resourceful you are at finding opportunities, and taking advantage of the ones that come your way. A professional's drive to dance must be very strong, because only the most steadfast heart can take the competition in stride and overcome the inevitable disappointments.

I remember a beginner class that Paul Taylor taught at Adelphi University when I was there. He had us all do a développé in second position at the barre and look at the doubtful results in the mirror. Then he said, "Isn't that depressing?" It wasn't until many years later that I realized he wasn't being cruel; he was just trying to get us to be realistic. "I go into colleges and tell them all to forget it," Taylor says, "because I think a little discouragement is the most I can do to help them. They should know what they're getting into. And I've always believed that unless somebody really has a very big need to dance and feels absolutely driven and has some kind of real dream about it, he shouldn't take up people's time."*

The hardships. While some difficulties begin to make themselves felt at the onset of serious training, most of the hardships of professional dancing don't hit full force until the middle or end of a dancer's career. With luck, it's possible to

*From Cynthia Lyle, *Dancers on Dancing*.

work for several years before feeling the inevitable pinch and strain of a dancer's life.

Long training, short career. One fact of life that dancers must contend with is a long training period and a relatively short career. Martha Graham's famous contention that it takes ten years to make a dancer is true, although many people start to perform before their technique is fully developed. Most dancers are retiring at just about the time other professionals are approaching their prime, after a twelve- to twenty-year career on average. This is not only because youthful appearance and physicality are important in the dance world, but also because the nomadic, isolated and financially insecure lifestyle of performers—which may be exciting to the young—becomes more and more difficult to bear after the early thirties. By that age, many dancers begin to want what their contemporaries want—to settle down comfortably, have a stable social life and perhaps raise a family. The thrill of an all-consuming involvement with dance begins to fade. Someone once told me, "You can live a lifetime as a dancer before you're thirty-five. It's a very fast, very hard-riding life. As you get more experienced there's the feeling that you've done it all, gotten all you can from dancing." In short, professional dancing is work that most people cannot do all their lives—a reality that almost always necessitates a second career.

The nomadic life of touring. Most American dance companies must tour extensively to survive. The large ones travel as much as ten months of the year, while the smaller ones tour from one to three months. Broadway and musical-theater dancers move about in road companies, and generally go where the work is—to clubs and theaters around the country. Under these conditions it is hard enough to maintain an apartment, let alone keep up friendships and family ties. This is true no matter how successful you become. Before his retirement from the stage, American Ballet Theatre's Ivan Nagy complained, "I tour maybe six or seven months out of the year. Many times I sit in a posh hotel with my room service, but I'm by myself. I'll think to myself, 'I have a wife whom I love; I have two children, and I love them . . . and I'm sitting here by myself. I finished the performance and got curtain calls and flowers, but I'm lonely.' Many times I am so lonely. I am a guest, so nobody dares to invite me or to get close to me. They make all the arrangements so I can be comfortable, but I am left alone."*

Demands on your time and the ensuing social isolation. Daily classes, rehearsals and performances take up most of a professional dancer's days and nights. You may easily be working on Christmas, Passover or Saturday night. When you do come home, often you'll be so exhausted that you'll barely have the strength to wolf down a snack and collapse into the nearest chair. The demands on your time and energy make dancing an insular way of life. It takes a great deal of ef-

*Ibid.

fort to make friends outside the circle of people you work with. It's even hard to keep abreast of other dance performances.

> *I thought it would be a hell of a lot more glamorous. I'm find-*
> *ing out you're always beat, you're always bushed. You don't*
> *have time to feel glamorous. I thought, just a few years ago,*
> *that dancing the roles I'm doing now would be a lot of fun and*
> *games, and New York would be endlessly exciting, and there*
> *would be a lot of terrific parties. Now I've found out that when*
> *there are parties, I don't go because I'm too tired. **

> —*PATRICK BISSELL*
> *American Ballet Theatre*

The financial problems. Nobody goes into dancing for the money. Money troubles start to besiege some dancers when serious training begins, with the accelerating cost of several classes per week, transportation and equipment. Unfortunately, thus far in our nation's history, dance education is very much a private enterprise. You can't get state or federal loans to pay for your dance training the way you might for college. The answer most of the time is to seek scholarships and other tuition breaks (see chapter 12), family assistance or a part-time job.

To be fair, the situation has improved since the old days, when most modern dancers and many ballet dancers didn't get paid at all; many of them even stitched their own costumes. Today, thanks to the dance boom and the greater support of dance that it has generated through various arts-funding organizations, most American dancers earn enough money to live on. Still it's a modest living at best. Though a handful of superstars make over $100,000 a year, the rank and file make just about enough to meet expenses. The highest-paid concert dancers are those who work in the few unionized companies, but the vast majority of dancers in professional companies do *not* belong to the union.

AGMA (the Amercan Guild of Musical Artists) is the official union for concert dance companies. Every year, it publishes a minimum scale of wages which unionized companies must pay their dancers. AGMA groups include: the Alvin Ailey American Dance Theater (New York), American Ballet Theatre (New York), Ballet Spectacular (Miami), the Boston Ballet, the Chicago Ballet, Merce Cunningham and Dance Company (New York), the Dance Theatre of Harlem (New York), the Eliot Feld Ballet (New York), the Martha Graham

*From Lee Edward Stern, "How It Really Is in the Dance World," in *The New York Times*, November 18, 1979.

Dance Company (New York), the Houston Ballet, the Joffrey Ballet (New York), Lola Montes and Her Spanish Dancers (Los Angeles), the New York City Ballet, the New York Shakespeare Festival, the Pennsylvania Ballet Company (Philadelphia), and the San Francisco Ballet. Companies which are not unionized but which tour under the National Endowment for the Arts Dance Touring Program must also pay AGMA scale for each residency obtained through the program.

1980-81 AGMA SALARY SCALE*

New dancers $280/week
Corps dancers $330/week
Solo dancers $360/week
Principal dancers $390/week
Per diem (daily living allowance on tour) $40/day

But even unionized companies have layoff periods when there is no work; then even dancers from the New York City Ballet can be found on unemployment lines.

Unionized dance companies also provide standard benefits, such as major medical insurance, social security and retirement pensions. Other groups do without these, although they may offer workman's compensation insurance to cover dancers injured on the job. Small companies usually pay for performances only—not for rehearsals—unless there is grant money available. If they accrue twenty weeks of combined work from bookings and grants, members of these companies become eligible for unemployment benefits, and they can collect a tax-free weekly subsistence check from their state government when there is no other salary coming in. This meager arrangement is considered to be financial success for many dance troupes because it enables them to continue creating new works and rehearsing full time.

Musical-theater performers—in Broadway, summer stock, regional-theater and dinner-theater productions—make good money and receive standard union benefits. The current pay scale for dancers belonging to Actor's Equity starts at $400 per week.

There are varying degrees of job security in professional dancing. Members of ballet and modern dance companies who are happy with their circumstances often stay where they are for their entire careers. Musical-theater dancers, on the other hand, work only as long as any particular show runs. This

---

* These figures are for companies that employ under forty dancers. Larger AGMA companies, such as American Ballet Theatre and the New York City Ballet, negotiate separate contracts. In 1979 Ballet Theatre had a protracted labor dispute when management's offer of a $235 weekly starting salary for corps dancers was rejected. This, the dancers argued, was less than the stage hands and orchestra musicians were earning. They held out for more than six months and succeeded in winning a wage scale that was well above the AGMA minimum, plus the guarantee of a forty-week season.

can be as little as two weeks, but it is rarely longer than two years. As a result, they are constantly between jobs in a highly competitive field. As Actor's Equity Vice-President Gena Belkin points out, "At any given time eighty percent of us are out of work." Perhaps this explains why the entertainment field is more businesslike and less protected than the concert dance world.

Sometimes job security entails accepting the status quo in exchange for steady work. Even though most dancers have the need to move on to greater challenges, they may have to resist this impulse in order to be assured of receiving a weekly paycheck. For years one talented dancer I know stayed with a certain ballet company because he had a wife and family to support, in spite of the fact that he was bored with the repertory and no new roles were being created for him. Regardless of the personal sacrifices a dancer makes to work steadily, there are always the overriding uncertainties of company finances. The mortality rate is high in dance, and even the best troupes may fold when beset by economic woes.

Some solutions. The many imponderables of a dance career make it advisable for most dancers to cultivate an alternative means of earning a living or at least supplementing their income. Many have to find a way to pay for classes and support themselves while training. When they are getting their first experience, young performers are paid very little or not at all. And even when dancing has become self-supporting, there are always lean times during layoffs or in between jobs.

What kinds of things do dancers do to pay the rent when not working? Anything and everything. Anna Sokolow's parents didn't approve of her dancing, so she left home at age fifteen and got a job in a tea-bag factory. Although she is an established choreographer, Kei Takei must still take odd jobs now and then—baby-sitting, making clothes and teaching children's classes. Traditionally dancers have also worked as waiters and waitresses (though this is hard on the legs), taxi drivers, artists' models, receptionists, salespeople, exercise instructors, and theater ushers (not very lucrative but the fringe benefit is free admission).

But the best solution is to acquire a money-earning skill that can lead to part-time, temporary, or free-lance employment. This has several advantages. You can work around dance classes, auditions or rehearsals; you don't have to take poor quality work in dance just to make ends meet; and your expertise can be parlayed into a second career after retirement. Dancers with the necessary training have become part-time masseurs, seamstresses, graphic designers and computer programmers; some double as secretaries, proofreaders, free-lance editors or tutors. They also work as chefs, hairstylists and bank tellers. I even know one who is a lawyer. Not as many active performers teach as you might guess, because teaching is often a full-time, permanent occupation that conflicts with a stage career.

Although those with a college education are better prepared for survival outside the dance world, the usefulness of a college diploma as such is debatable

Actor's Equity Association
1500 Broadway
New York, New York 10036
(212) 869-8530
For actors, singers and dancers in live musical theater: Broadway, stock tents, regional theater and dinner theater. Also has offices in Los Angeles and Chicago.

American Federation of Television and Radio Artists (AFTRA)
1350 Avenue of the Americas
New York, New York 10019
(212) 265-7700
For television variety and musical performers.

American Guild of Musical Artists (AGMA)
1841 Broadway
New York, New York 10023
(212) 265-3687
For professional dance companies. Publishes an annual wage scale that is used for the National Endowment for the Arts Dance Touring Program.

American Guild of Variety Artists (AGVA)
1540 Broadway
New York, New York 10036
(212) 765-0800
For performers in live variety entertainment, at hotels, nightclubs, lounges and in circuses. Examples are Disney on Parade and the Ice Capades.

Screen Actors Guild (SAG)
551 Fifth Avenue
New York, New York 10036
(212) 687-4623
For performers in films, from industrial movies to major motion pictures.

for some professional dancers (see chapter 22). Therefore an increasing number of them are devoting their youths to their careers and going on to college afterwards. Several colleges now have general studies divisions expressly for older students with work experience.

After retirement, many dancers become teachers or coach younger dancers. Others turn to choreography or become ballet masters and mistresses, who rehearse pieces for a company. The rapidly growing related fields of dance management, criticism, history, notation and therapy also offer good second careers for retired performers.

A career in professional dance is both difficult and exhilarating. It promises some hardships, but even greater rewards, to people who are in earnest about their art. Now we'll look at what such a career entails purely in terms of dance.

The career-minded beginner

Rome wasn't built in a day and neither was a soaring leap or a clean turn or a beautiful arabesque. You can help yourself a great deal by realizing that as a beginner you are just setting out on a long road. Pace yourself by limiting your goals at first. Start by gaining a good basic foundation in technique. Your initial training should lay the groundwork for understanding and working deeply with your body, and for learning basic movement principles and vocabulary. It should give you an awareness of space and a feeling for music and rhythm. Your first task will be to find a teacher and a technique you will be able to stay with at least until you learn the basics, and perhaps beyond to intermediate training. You may not even know for sure what kind of dancing you want to do, or if a performing career is for you; but you should be able to commit yourself to one or two dance classes a day.

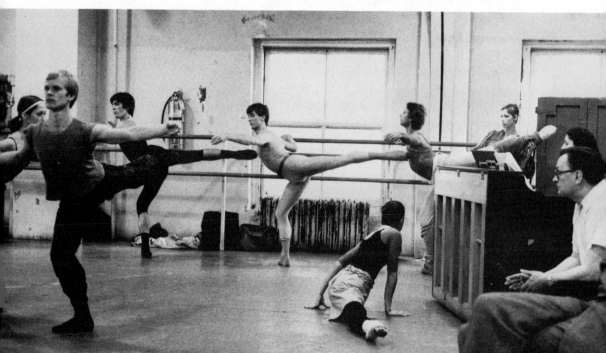

By the end of the first two years of serious study you will have a more realistic picture of professional training and know whether you are willing to make a long-term commitment to it. While some of your ideas about dancing may be romanticized, you will soon find out quite concretely what it means in terms of tenacity and courage and rewards—the excitement of learning and the growth of self-expression. The decision to dance based on the dream in your heart will have to be remade in the real world from day to day.

What to look for in a teacher and school. Select your first dance teacher and school with care. Because you are vulnerable in the beginning, bad experiences can be especially harmful or defeating. Poor training will only have to be unlearned later, sometimes at the cost of painful injury. Right from the start it is important for aspiring professionals to study with teachers who have reputable training and performing backgrounds. The advice that the Italian ballet master Carlo Blasis gave would-be dancers in his textbook *An Elementary Treatise upon the Theory and Practice of the Art of Dancing* holds as true today as when he wrote it in 1820: "...theoretical knowledge of the art alone can never produce an ideal teacher. Only one who has been a first-rate dancer himself makes a good master, because in the absence of practical experience instruction becomes a mechanical routine and both lessons and demonstrations lack authenticity." Indeed, you have every right to ask about your teacher's credentials. If you have any doubts about her competence, ask an experienced dancer's opinion or follow the recommendations in chapters 13 and 25.

Look for a teacher who can communicate simply and clearly, who can work with you as an individual and who above all loves to dance. Career beginners should study slowly and carefully with an analytic instructor who explains the movement step-by-step and gives students a chance to repeat exercises. You'll also need close personal supervision to establish good work habits and proper body placement (see illustrations in chapter 18). Acquiring a sound technique is an investment in your future. Not only does it give you the strength and consistency you'll need for a career, but it enables you to dance longer by protecting your body against stress and injury. At the same time, your teacher should make sure you have some chance in every class to move without analysis—just to dance—so that you can hold on to the enjoyment of dancing and develop your own movement qualities.

Your dance school ought to provide a comfortable atmosphere, yet one which stimulates growth. There should be talented students to inspire you and act as models. Good dancers at a school are an indication of its merit and they raise everyone's level of performance.

Even professional ballet dancers must work daily to stay in top form. Taking the company class shown above are members of the American Ballet Theatre, including, in the far right background, the now retired Hungarian danseur Ivan Nagy and ballerina Natalia Makarova, who was several months pregnant at the time. *David Lindner*

What kind and how many classes to take. In today's competitive dance marketplace, no matter what type of dancing you do, you need some solid ballet training behind you. The modern dance techniques of Martha Graham and Merce Cunningham develop overall strength and flexibility, but nothing builds bodies like ballet. It is generally agreed that modern dance, jazz or tap classes alone are not sufficient to produce a polished, well-rounded dancer. Good ballet training gives you a knowledge of movement principles and standard vocabulary that are used in all forms of theatrical dancing. It teaches essential skills needed for jumping, turning and balancing well, and it produces articulate feet and legs. A foundation in ballet gives dancers good line as well as an elegant carriage of the arms and upper body. Therefore, even if your career interests lie elsewhere, you should study ballet. If you can't take a ballet class every day (which is ideal), take at least three ballet lessons per week. The remaining three to six weekly classes may be devoted to any style of dancing that appeals to you and feels good to do. It is important as a beginner to build on your natural strengths and movement preferences (see chapter 5).

Dancers training for a ballet career should start by taking all their classes in ballet. Be especially careful to find a teacher who stresses good postural alignment and who has you working correctly. Remember that in the beginning proper functioning of the body is more important than achieving perfect positions or line. The teacher should not push for what is beautiful too soon. If she has you going for the external effect—i.e., extreme turn-out and high extensions—without any real understanding of how to achieve this according to what is functional for *your* body, you won't develop a strong or usable technique. Work correctly, do the movements the right way, and eventually they will be beautiful.

Musical-theater dancers have to learn to do everything—and sing, too. Not only a broad dance base, but also good voice and acting training are necessary for those who aspire to a Broadway career. In the old days Broadway musicals employed two separate choruses, one of singers and another of dancers, but lately show producers have been economizing by hiring single choruses of dancers who can sing. When I asked Gena Belkin of Actor's Equity in New York what kind of dance background one needed to get work these days, she replied emphatically, "First of all a good strong ballet technique. Then some modern dance, and of course jazz. Tap helps a lot, and acrobatics wouldn't hurt." Well, that just about covers all the bases, but as a beginner you might best start out with two years of ballet and jazz study, and then add tap or modern dance and whatever else there is time for.

Whatever your career aspirations, try to remember that the effects of dance training are cumulative; it is the day-to-day effort that yields appreciable results. Ambition is fine, but it can be your undoing if you don't also learn patience. You may feel the usual pressure to prove yourself. However, you have much to learn as a beginner, about yourself, about classroom procedure and about dancing in general (see chapter 14). All these new experiences must be assimilated a little at a time; otherwise you'll become unduly discouraged. Don't worry, progress will be faster than you might expect because you are taking daily classes. But learn to defer judgment. You'll be trying to match apples and oranges if you compare yourself with more advanced dancers. They had to start at the beginning too. Remember to give yourself time.

You may wish to experiment with different teachers and classes for a while, but once you've settled down stick with your decisions for at least a year; wandering around from class to class is confusing and counterproductive. Don't study more than two types of dancing for now. You need to let the new ways of moving seep through your muscles and bones. Start exploring dance on your own. Watch it live, on television or on film. Read about it. The more you know, the more meaningful your classes will be and the better informed your choices will be about what and where to study (see chapter 26 on finding out more about dance). Recalling his salad days as a dance student, choreographer Louis Falco says, "I hadn't even seen Martha Graham...although we were taught Graham technique. We sat on the floor and did contractions hour after hour. Only when I saw the Graham company in the premiere of *Clytemnestra* did I realize, 'Oh, this is what you end up doing.' "*

Intermediate and advanced dancers

By the time you have reached the intermediate level of training you ought to know what serious dancing is about and whether you have the love and determination to continue. You should be taking two classes a day. This is a good time to consolidate your gains and increase stamina by studying intensively. If you are young, strong and ambitious, you may be able to squeeze as many as three classes into one day. But quantity is meaningless unless you can work productively in each class, and if you dance when you can no longer concentrate or your body is exhausted, the lesson will be wasted.

By now the initial struggles with technique are over and dancing should be more satisfying than ever. You should understand how to work well in class, and have some appreciation of your strengths and weaknesses, likes and dislikes — in other words, a budding dance identity.

But this stage of growth can also be the most difficult, for thus far many of the challenges of dancing have been encountered, yet none of the rewards of performing. After three or four years of daily study many dancers feel frustrated with simply going to classes. They begin to feel, rightly, that technique is only one small part of dancing. These are healthy emotions but they may test your drive and faith in yourself. You have reached the time when you must start to make the transition from student to performer.

*From Anna Kisselgoff, " 'I Would Love to Create Earthquakes Onstage,' " in *The New York Times*, April 10, 1977.

103

This means you will probably need to shift gears or make some changes. Now that you have a foundation of knowledge and skill, you should strive to work more deeply physically, more consistently, and in a more musical and expressive way. Finding out where and how you would like to perform is equally pressing right now. It is imperative for the experienced dancer to develop her own personal performance style and to determine her tastes in choreography. This may necessitate trying new teachers and classes, investigating other schools, branching out to other ways of dancing or doing some experimentation on your own.

As soon as you have enough technique to begin putting it to use, find an outlet for performing. Many schools provide this for students (see chapter 12). But even before you are ready to step onstage, you can get your feet wet by using dance classes to prepare.

Reevaluate your present teachers and classes. It is easy in dancing to get ensconced, once you feel secure. Inertia takes over and you drift along comfortably. But especially now it is a mistake to let yourself get stuck in one place or cling to preconceived notions about how and where you should dance. If you feel you're in a rut, you may have outgrown your present classes and need fresh stimulation. You may need to be pushed in different ways than you were as a beginner. Broadway dancers, for instance, have to learn to pick up combinations and grasp diverse choreographic styles quickly, because in the entertainment field, time is money. At this point they may profit from taking fast-paced classes that expand their movement vocabulary and develop memory. Examine new ways of dancing. Sample other teachers, even if it is just to prove that your old stand-bys are still effective.

In some respects you will need more from your dance teacher than before. You should have an instructor who can help direct your career and guide your day-to-day growth as an artist, someone who can realistically appraise your good and bad points and help you make the most of your individual qualities as a dancer. Your teacher should be working with you on performance skills such as musical phrasing, the use of space, and the refinements of style. In *Baryshnikov at Work*, Mikhail Baryshnikov speaks about the traits of his beloved mentor at the Kirov School, Alexander Pushkin:

> He taught in such a way that the dancer began to know himself more completely, and that, I believe, is the first key to serious work, to becoming an artist — to know oneself, one's gifts, one's limitations, as fully as possible. Pushkin had this ability — to guide the dancer down the right path toward being realistic about his gifts, and then to inspire him to work, and work hard, at making the most artistically of those gifts...He taught me about the difference between technique — dancing in the classroom — and real dancing. Real dancing happens on

the space of a stage, and to be aware of that space — its flexibility, its rules, its relationship to the audience — was what he stressed.

Broaden your range. Even if you are happy with your present dance classes, it's a good idea to increase your stylistic range by working in some new areas. If your training has been primarily balletic, for example, you may want to study modern dance or jazz to explore how you can use your back. Tap and jazz dancers can improve their strength and line by taking a few extra ballet classes. Modern dancers may enjoy loosening up with some jazz. Because choreography is becoming more and more eclectic, dancers of all kinds are expected to be more versatile than in the past. Besides enriching your background, versatility broadens your job potential by preparing you to perform a variety of dance styles.

Another thing you can do to open up your dancing is change the way you are working in class. If you have been concentrating on certain technical problems, focus on new ones. Dance for pure enjoyment, or take more chances — go for higher jumps, longer balances, more turns, faster, sharper footwork. Or adopt the goal of making each exercise work smoothly and finish cleanly, as you would in a performance.

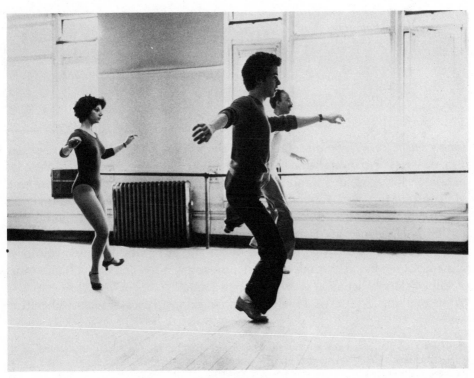

Running through an advanced tap routine. *Frank Gimpaya*

You don't think about performing when you're younger. They don't teach that, they really don't. And I think it's very important, especially if you're going to try to make money at dancing. You have to know what's going to sell. I had to figure out how I could get a job the fastest. So I worked on developing my own style. I studied with a jazz teacher who taught me how to pick up combinations because he wouldn't have a count, and so I would learn how to watch his feet and watch his body as opposed to knowing something by five, six, seven, eight. I would watch the person. It was a practical education. That's where my head has always been. When I was in front of a mirror the only thing that I was thinking about was what somebody on the other side was going to see. I was trying to produce a product that somebody wanted to use or would pay money to see, and it had to be something that was not like anybody else's. Before I was working steadily I was in a jazz dance company. It was directed by a choreographer who also ran a school. Most of the other kids were ballet dancers who came to the school for jazz. Out of the eight dancers in that company I think I was the only one who could put something across, because they were all into technique. When we did a number I don't think anybody ever thought about smiling. There were a hundred people in the audience watching them and all they could think about was where their arms were, does this look good.

— *ADAM GRAMMIS*
Broadway dancer

Take a break from technique. Don't lose the joy that first inspired your odyssey into dance. For dancers who have been plugging away at the discipline of technique for years, it is important to get out and take a class every once in a while just for fun. Jazz, tap, folk, ethnic, ballroom — any class is good that gets you away from the exacting routine you've been using to build your body. Folk and ballroom dance are especially helpful because they entail dancing with others. Dance in your living room, at discos and at parties, to music you love. Someday, even baton twirling can come in handy. Why, one of the high points of Eliot Feld's ballet *Half Time* is Helen Douglas' tongue-in-cheek solo as a baton-wielding Statue of Liberty. Improvisation classes are also liberating

The Cleveland Ballet is one of many professional companies whose dancers are trained in affiliated schools. Here Christopher Tabor and the corps perform Leonide Massine's *Gâité Parisienne. Louis Peres* because they allow you to find your own natural expression in movement without having to worry about technique.

Develop tastes and opinions of your own. Along with deepening your knowledge of technique and expanding your movement range, you should be thinking about where and how you want to perform. Begin by seeing all the dance you can. See historical pieces and works by both established and new choreographers. Look at all kinds of movement styles. Read up on dance. Dance periodicals will put you in touch with the rest of the dance world. You may want to attend a dance history or music course if there is one available near you. Develop your own tastes and opinions, and you will be well on your way to finding out who you are as a dancer.

Take classes that expose you to choreography. "Students can learn to dance well only by doing good dances," writes Agnes de Mille in *To a Young Dancer*. Ballet and modern dancers can take advantage of special classes that expose them to legitimate choreography — perhaps even great works of art — and sharpen their performance skills. Unlike technique lessons, these classes offer an opportunity to study complete dances and work together with other dancers.

In variations classes ballet students learn solos from classic works performed all over the world. Advanced dancers can also take pas de deux or part-

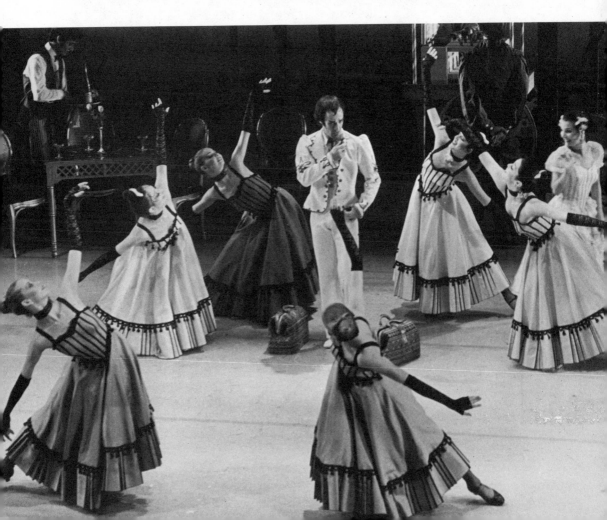

nering classes, where young men and women learn to do the spectacular lifts and supports that are staples of ballet choreography. Effective partnering is an art in itself, demanding strength, experience and rapport from both partners. If your ballet technique is adequate, pas de deux classes are helpful even if you are not a ballet dancer.

Repertory classes are usually held at modern dance schools that are affiliated with professional companies. Pieces from the company repertory are taught by dancers who have performed them onstage. Sometimes repertory classes end in informal workshop performances or grow into student dance companies.

You don't have to be an aspiring choreographer to benefit from taking choreography or dance composition courses. They will give you a clearer understanding of movement and its structure, and valuable insight into the process and materials out of which dances are made. You'll get a sneak preview of what it's like to work with a choreographer, and this will make you all the more useful to him or her when you do. In addition, creating your own movement and getting feedback from others help you know yourself better as a performer.

At the School of American Ballet they prepared you for performing in different ways. In variations class we wore pretty white leotards and tutus, and instead of dancing in groups we danced alone or in pairs, so we got used to being in the spotlight. We learned solos from well-known ballets; sometimes it would be the same one over and over for four or five weeks in a row. The first week I'd be huffing and puffing. I'd barely get through it. But after a while you knew the steps so well that you didn't have to think about them, and you could think about other things, you could perform. We also got to perform with the company in ballets like The Nutcracker *and* A Midsummer Night's Dream. *You could watch your favorite dancers work onstage or from the wings, and it's very different from watching them from the audience. You could see how they did things, the little tricks they used. That's how you learn. Then there's the student repertory workshop, for advanced students mostly, and some children, depending on the ballets they are doing. The workshop performances at the end of the year get reviewed by* The New York Times. *It's a big deal.*

— *VICTORIA BROMBERG*
New York City Ballet

Attend a company-affiliated school. If you haven't already done so, now is the time to investigate dance schools with professional company affiliations and other performing opportunities. Besides providing occasions to perform, these schools are career oriented and the focus of the training and the general atmosphere reflect this. They are also more likely to keep you informed of auditions, upcoming concerts and other dance events in your area.

Some schools connected with active dance companies offer opportunities to become involved in performances behind the scenes too. They frequently use student volunteers as ushers, stagehands, and assistants to the lighting and costume designers. Ballet companies mounting elaborate productions may ask students to participate as supernumeraries, or extras. While these jobs don't usually entail dancing (or getting paid), they give you a feeling for the stage and contact with professional dancers and choreographers.

Coping with competition

Some of us are natural born competitors, others shy away from competition, but eventually all career dancers have to find a way of dealing with it. Covert or overt, it is ever present in the dance world. Starting in the classroom, dancers vie for their teachers' attention; later they compete for scholarships and roles in student workshops and, after that, at company auditions. Even among established professionals there is contention for bigger and better roles. The pressure to compete is far greater in some dance schools and companies than others, and this should be taken into consideration; but it is as much of a mistake to ignore the competitive aspect of dancing as it is to let it get out of hand.

A certain amount of friendly rivalry is healthy. It pushes you to excel and it toughens you for professional life. As a young dancer with the New York City Ballet told me, "Learning to cope with competition at the school prepared me for life in the company. You have to pull yourself together and stay together if you want to remain in the school, and that's the way it is in the company."

An overly competitive attitude, on the other hand, creates a lot of unnecessary pressure. What is worse, if you always have your eye on the other dancers you can't devote full attention to yourself. We all get distracted or discouraged by competition at times, but the best antidote to too much comparing and competing is cultivating your own personal qualities and abilities. Only you can do what you do best, and in that sense competition among dancers is immaterial.

Another professional dancer put it this way: "When I left my hometown teacher, the late André Eglevsky, to begin study in New York, he gave me the best advice I have ever received about dancing. He said that wherever you go there will always be someone who dances better than you and someone who doesn't dance as well. If you spend your class time worrying and competing you'll never progress and your dance identity will become nebulous. A strong sense of self is important in class and in the dance world in general. In many ways you must be alone with your teacher — no matter how many people are in class.''

Probably the worst thing about overcompetitiveness is that it cuts you off from fellow dancers who can be a tremendous source of help and moral support. Franklin Stevens describes it well in *Dance as Life*:

> *After every class, if the studio is then unoccupied, there will be students who stay to practice, to struggle with, a turn, a beat, a jump, a combination that troubles or intrigues them.*
>
> *Other dancers, toweling themselves, massaging feet, or just sprawled out resting, will watch and comment, and the practicing students will comment upon each other when they aren't working themselves. Older dancers, moreover, can help the student not only with criticism ("You've really made progress since the last time I was here. But you — you haven't progressed at all. Have you forgotten how to work?") and bits of technical advice ("You're never going to do a double tour until you stop trying to jump up and then around, and just tell yourself to jump around") but with the kind of necessary miscellaneous information and personal support which can't all be acquired from the teacher, in class.*

Part III

The
choices

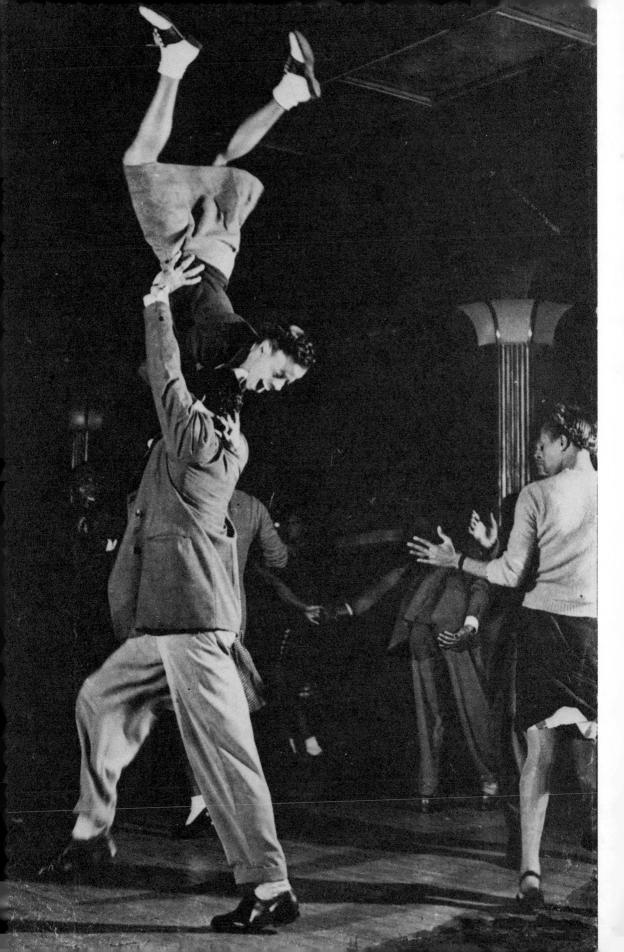

10

Ways of Dancing

ballet, modern, tap or jazz?

America's theatrical dance forms are still young and evolving. They have grown up together and have influenced each other's development, both onstage and in the classroom. Just as exposure to modern dance has expanded the scope of ballet choreographers, ballet training has given modern dancers a stronger technique* and awareness of line. Jazz, or popular dancing, continues to wash over all the American dance idioms like recurrent tidewaters.

By the same token, all dance classes share a common purpose and format. Whether you are studying ballet, modern, tap or jazz, the object of the training is to prepare you to perform a particular set of dance movements. Every dance class begins slowly with simple exercises to warm and condition the body, to focus the mind and to improve timing and coordination. At the same time, steps and gestures that will be used later on in the lesson are introduced, practiced and varied. Simple movements are then combined into more complex sequences, and finally these are built into longer dance combinations which travel through space.

But despite their overlapping interests, ballet, modern, tap and jazz remain separate and distinct dance forms. Each has a different historical perspective and a different way of working the body. Each has its own peculiar values and priorities, music and ambience. And each mode of dancing presents unique challenges, thus requiring specialized training. An advanced tap dancer taking her first ballet class, for example, is nonetheless a beginner in ballet, and an experienced ballet dancer still has to start with the basics if he wants to understand modern dance.

As we'll see in this chapter, though all the dance forms employ warm-

---

*The word *technique* is a confusing one. It can mean either the method or the vocabulary used for performing an established choreographic system(as in "Graham is a demanding technique"); or it can refer to skill in execution (as in "I need to improve my ballet technique").

ups, ballet training places the greatest emphasis on a thorough and systematic warm-up. This is because classical dancing demands a great deal of physical preparation and because the standard movements that comprise a ballet warm-up are also used in the actual choreography, so practicing them serves a double purpose. Since tap and jazz dancing depend on invention and style more than on technique, classes usually devote the greatest amount of time to teaching and practicing routines. Modern dance classes vary tremendously in structure and content, as befits an art form which values, above all, creativity and individual expression. There are many ways to dance well, and your choice of dance style should excite and inspire you. Nothing less will do.

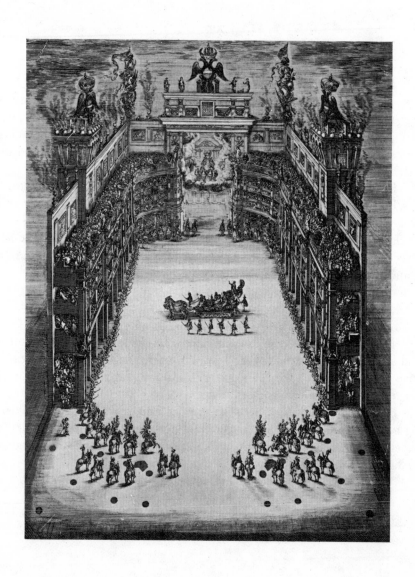

Ballet:
The Dance of Kings

When a ballet dancer anywhere in the world stands at the barre in first position ready to begin pliés, she places her feet in the same turned-out stance that was formulated more than three hundred years ago by the French dancing master Pierre Beauchamp. She strives for the same upright and noble carriage he taught his star pupil Louis XIV, the dancing king of France. And regardless of her nationality, she knows the ballet steps by the same French names Beauchamp used so long ago.

Of all the dance modes we are considering here, ballet has the longest, most widely documented history and the most highly codified training system. All ballet performed today descends from the five basic positions of the feet and principles of technique that were established by Beauchamp in the seventeenth century and set down in the 1820s in two textbooks by the Italian master Carlo Blasis. Blasis' seminal works, *An Elementary Treatise upon the Theory and Practice of the Art of Dancing* and *The Code of Terpsichore,* have endured to this day as the backbone of classical ballet technique.

From these beginnings ballet has grown to be the most widespread and predominant dance form in the world. There are more ballet schools and companies than any other kind, and balletic steps and positions have become integral to all other forms of theatrical dance. Because of the fluid interchange over the centuries of teachers, choreographers and dancers among countries on every continent, ballet is truly international. Although there are four distinct teaching methods—French, Danish, Russian and Italian/English—ballet dancing is essentially the same the world over, and a well-trained ballet dancer can usually adapt to different choreographic styles. That is why Rudolf Nureyev can perform with the National Ballet of Canada; and other Europeans such as Peter Martins, Anthony Dowell, Natalia Makarova and Mikhail Baryshnikov can feel at home in American companies. It is also why so many American dancers can find jobs with ballet troupes abroad.

The earliest ballets were lavish dance spectacles intended to display the wealth and generosity of the European courts. They began in fifteenth-century Italy, chiefly as entertainments at royal banquet fetes. Though the main attraction was the food, all the essential ingredients of ballet were there—music, storytelling, traditional dances, pantomime and resplendent decor. At first,

Explaining his lack of interest in ballet, New York's famous mayor Fiorello La Guardia said, "I'm the kind of guy who likes to keep score, and in ballet you can't tell who's winning." As this triumphal procession from a seventeenth-century horse ballet shows, he was just about two hundred years too late. *New York Public Library*

115

actual outdoor combats were choreographed to amuse the aristocratic guests, but by the end of the century these were toned down and staged indoors as mock battles that were performed by the noblemen themselves. Because of the martial origins of court entertainment and because dancing was considered morally questionable, for a long time only the men danced; indeed dance was thought to be an indispensable part of any true gentleman's education. It wasn't until 1681 that female performers appeared in ballets.

Extravagant dance pageants flourished in Renaissance Italy and France, but the first bona fide ballet was produced in 1581 at the behest of the Italian Catherine de Medici after she became the new queen of France. The *Ballet Comique de la Reine* was unique at the time, since it was the only one whose verses, music and dances were organized around a unified theme, the myth of Circe. It was performed before ten thousand guests, lasted five hours, and literally cost a fortune, nearly bankrupting the French monarchy. But the occasion achieved the prestige that Catherine had hoped for and it established France as the center of ballet for the next three hundred and fifty years.

Louis XIII was another avid balletomane. He constructed the first proscenium stage in Paris, starred in a number of ballets himself and even choreographed one in which he played the female lead. His son, Louis XIV, grew up dancing in court spectacles. Young Louis acquired the name by which history remembers him—the Sun King—from his role in the *Ballet de la Nuit*. In it he portrayed the ultimate star around which the entire civilized world revolved. Louis XIV put his father's proscenium stage to regular use, thus formalizing the previously blurred distinction between royal viewers and performers and paving the way for the professional status of ballet dancers. The proscenium stage placed greater importance on individual performances, and it necessitated the outward rotation of the legs, or turn-out, so that pleasing steps and body lines could be seen from the front. At age thirty the Sun King retired from dancing due to overweight, although he did attempt a comeback seventeen years later in the unlikely role of a nymph. In 1661 he founded a dancing school for his courtiers (the Académie Royale de Danse) so that the art of ballet would not suffer after his own departure from the stage.

Much about ballet dancing as we know it today has its origin in seventeenth-century court dress and decorum. Dancers then wore high feathered headdresses, high-heeled shoes and layered costumes so cumbersome that they restricted activity everywhere but in the extremities and upper body. The arms were held wide to avoid contact with the billowing skirts worn by both sexes, and the feet were carefully pointed to show off the ornate ribbons and jeweled buckles on the shoes. Present-day ballet dancers still retain the straight spine, the high-held chest, the elegantly carried head and arms and the scrupulously arched feet of the French courtier. Now, as then, the grace and beauty of the movement are paramount.

Remarkably, the basic hierarchical structure of the court ballet has also survived. In Louis XIV's time top billing naturally went to the ruler, who did most of the performing. Other major roles were assigned to the highest ranking nobility, backed up by a full supporting cast. Most contemporary ballet companies are similarly organized, with principal dancers ranked first, then soloists, followed by the corps de ballet or ensemble dancers. In the ballet class, too, the teacher—no matter how beloved he or she may be—is the undisputed authority behind whom the students arrange themselves or are arranged.

Yet another carry-over from the past is ballet etiquette. Ballet was originally taught hand in hand with manners and deportment, and modern-day ballet dancers are still imbued with a gracious regard for one another. Nowhere is this more apparent than in the classical pas de deux or love duet, which is always performed with an air of chivalrous attentiveness and mutual admiration. Even today, it is customary for ballet lessons to end with a respectful bow, or révérence, to the teacher.

The beginning ballet student struggling with them in class may wonder how such difficult body positions were ever invented, but believe it or not, balletic movement is fundamentally an exaggeration of natural movement. The first ballets were actually refined adaptations of popular peasant dances and consisted of simple steps done in elaborate spatial patterns. The five basic positions of the feet were derived from two gentlemen's arts of the time, horsemanship and fencing.

Toward the end of the seventeenth century, the new technical demands necessitated by the proscenium stage and by the pride of the European rulers in their dance spectacles paved the way for the first professional ballet dancers. Rising standards of performance required lengthy rehearsals and a skilled execution that was beyond the capacities of the part-time dancers of the court. With the establishment of an official ballet academy and Beauchamp's standardized rules of technique, professionals began to emerge. The technique grew more and more strenuous and the turned-out positions became more extreme. But the performance still had to look elegant, dignified and effortless. In order to execute the increasingly arduous steps with aplomb, ballet dancers had to be structurally well suited to the task and trained from childhood. Perfection became both an aesthetic ideal and a physical necessity.

Ballet in America. Even though ballet had been seen in this country since colonial times, most Americans considered it a fancy kind of circus act, and as a result no ballet schools or companies of consequence were founded here until the 1930s.

In the early nineteenth century teachers from the Paris Opéra Ballet began arriving in the United States, some of them refugees from the French Revolution. In the 1820s and 30s, French and Italian companies toured Philadelphia, Boston, New York and other prominent American cities. It seemed that our commercial theater offered greater profits and artistic freedom than did many of the European capitals. From the 1830s onward, opera ballet was performed in the United States. European-trained American dancers, such as Mary Ann Lee and George Washington Smith, restaged some of the popular romantic ballets and also choreographed their own works with some success. Then there was the hit theatrical extravaganza *The Black Crook,* a forerunner of the Broadway musical that owed much of its box-office appeal to a chorus of outstanding ballet dancers. The show enjoyed a two-year run in New York, followed by a string of revivals from 1868 to 1909. By the late 1800s vaudeville was employing ballet dancers too.

The most celebrated dance event of the nineteenth century was the extended visit to America of the Viennese star Fanny Elssler, from 1840 to 1841. Wherever she went, the fiery romantic ballerina from the Paris Opéra was greeted with wild acclaim. Congress was recessed on the evenings she appeared in Washington because nearly everyone was at the ballet. Yet even after Elssler's triumph there were no American ballet companies and very few native-born ballet dancers of distinction. Americans continued to depend on visiting Europeans for training. In 1883 the Metropolitan Opera House opened in New York, but it imported all its dancers from abroad and didn't operate a school until 1909.

To make matters worse, as the nineteenth century drew to a close ballet everywhere was suffering a serious decline. It had become overgrown with empty ornamentation that was often no more than a thin cover for girlie shows. The French Folies Bergères and its imitators in American saloons and nightclubs were direct descendants of this period; even the can-can is a bastardized version of the classical step *rond de jambe en l'air.* Only the steady trickle of itinerant masters from Europe kept legitimate ballet alive in America until the Russians came and established it as a permanent institution.

The Russians took this country by storm. They made a large American public want to see more ballet and inspired countless young people to go into the profession. The first to dance in the United States were Anna Pavlova and her partner Mikhail Mordkin, at the Metropolitan Opera House in New York in 1910. Pavlova played to adoring audiences throughout the nation frequently until 1925. In 1916, impresario Serge Diaghilev's Ballets Russes arrived, a veritable galaxy of the brightest young artists ever assembled in a single company. Under Diaghilev's audacious leadership and organizational ability, the dying art of ballet was revitalized. It took the great leap forward into modern times.

Through the Ballets Russes and its two offshoots, the Ballet Russe de Monte Carlo and the Original Ballet Russe, Americans were introduced to the innovative choreography of Michel Fokine, George Balanchine, Vaslav Nijinsky and Leonide Massine. Advanced composers such as Debussy, Ravel and Stravinsky contributed scores. Opulent sets and costumes—visual feasts in themselves—were designed by such modern artists as Picasso, Cocteau, Matisse, Bakst and Benois. Over the forty-one years during which the Ballet Russe companies toured the United States, the dancers included Anna Pavlova, Vaslav

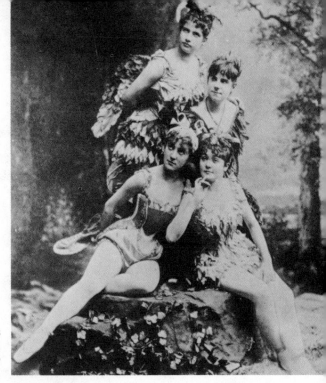

The Black Crook's main attraction was its chorus of well-endowed ballet dancers, who, among other things, introduced the can-can to the American stage. **New York Public Library**

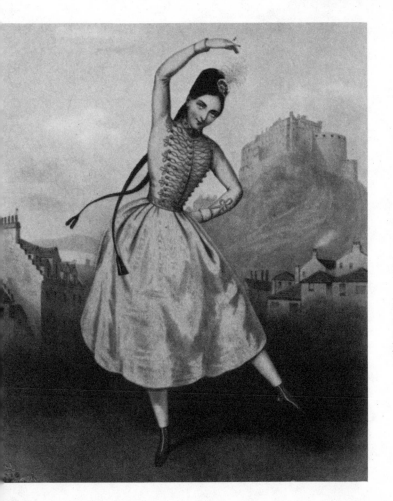

Earthy and voluptuous, Fanny Elssler was a flop in *La Sylphide*, but she quickened pulses with such fiery character dances as "La Cracovienne," from Mazilier's *La Gypsy*. **New York Public Library**

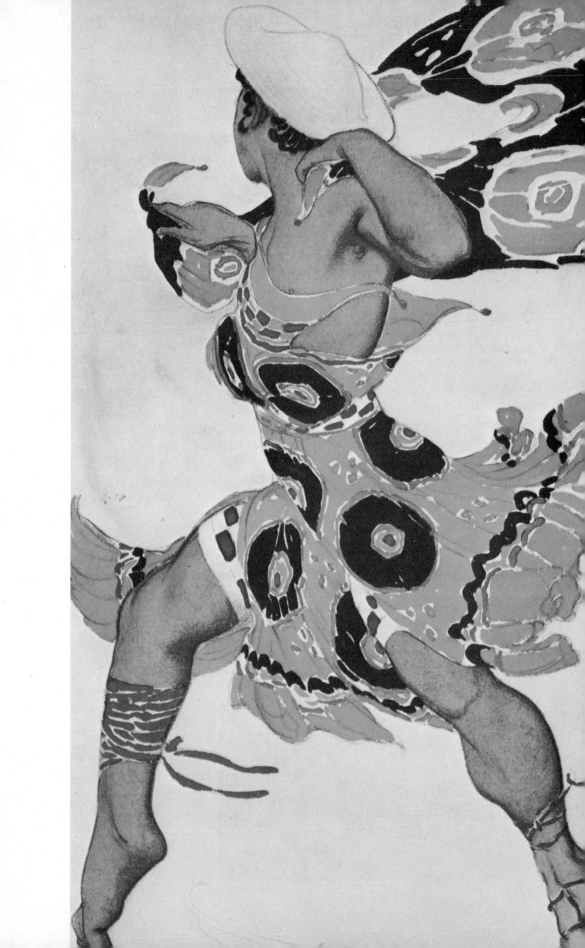

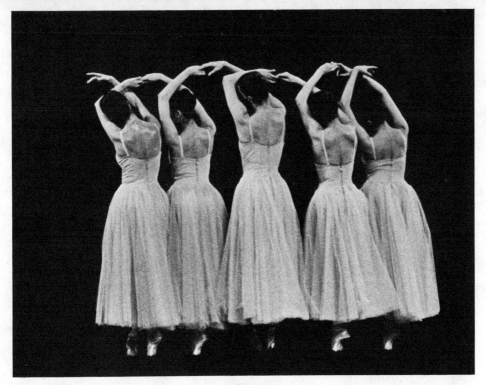

A jewel-like image from George Balanchine's beloved *Serenade*. *David Lindner*

Left: Leon Bakst's costume design for the Ballets Russes production of *Narcissus* in 1911. *New York Public Library*

Nijinsky, Tamara Karsavina, Adolf Bolm, Mikhail Mordkin, Olga Spessivtzeva, Lubov Egorova, Anton Dolin, Serge Lifar, Alexandra Danilova, Alicia Markova, Ruth Page, André Eglevsky, Frederic Franklin, Igor Youskevitch, Alicia Alonso, Mia Slavenska and Tamara Toumanova.

After the revolution of 1917, many expatriate Russians settled in the United States to teach or perform. America's first major ballet schools and companies were founded by Russian émigrés, and for the first half of the twentieth century American ballet was Russian ballet. As recently as 1972 Doris Hering, director of the National Association for Regional Ballet, wrote, "There are still plenty of communities in this country where only Russian names are accepted as symbols of balletic knowledge."

In 1934 George Balanchine, at the invitation of Lincoln Kirstein, founded the School of American Ballet and the American Ballet Company, which eventually became the New York City Ballet. Balanchine brought a Russian teaching staff with him. At his school he sought to recreate his own training at the Imperial Ballet School in St. Petersburg (now the Kirov School in Leningrad). When he grafted classical Russian technique onto the long-limbed, athletic American body, he created a new style of contemporary American ballet.

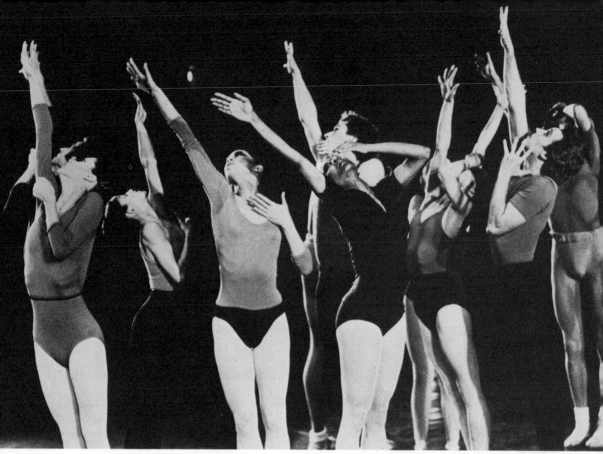

Above: The Joffrey Ballet in a performance of Jerome Robbins' *Moves. courtesy of the Joffrey Ballet*

Right: An adagio exercise in the center of the floor. *courtesy of the Youngstown Academy of Ballet, Youngstown, Ohio*

Below: Students at the Studio of Creative Arts in Longview, Texas, stretch while teacher Pat George Mitchell corrects their feet. *Margaret V. Estes*

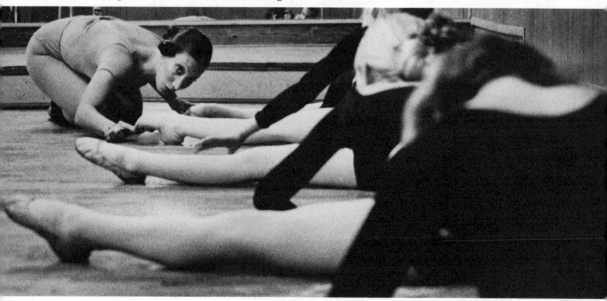

Other important companies, such as the American Ballet Theatre and the San Francisco Ballet, developed. By the 1940s and 50s the first generation of American choreographers came of age, among them Eugene Loring, Agnes de Mille and Jerome Robbins. American ballet now embraces the influences of the French, Russian, Danish, Italian and English schools, and many people believe that out of this mixture a truly American school is emerging.*

The ballet class. Ballet classes are highly structured and methodical. They have a formal atmosphere that is tinged with romanticism—an antique flavor due perhaps to the pink tights, the airiness and delicacy of the movements, the constant references in French and the lilting piano music of Chopin, Brahms and Tchaikovsky.

Every ballet class starts off with a warm-up at the *barre,* a wooden railing that runs along the wall and provides an external source of support for the dancers. Exercises begin with *pliés* (knee bends) and continue with a progression of *battements* (stretching, brushing and beating foot movements done close to

*The wave of Soviet defections in the past decade—Makarova and Baryshnikov in the early 1970s, Alexandr Godunov and Valentina and Leonid Koslov in 1979, and the renowned Bolshoi teacher Sulamif Messerer and her son Mikhail in 1980—has given Russian dancers renewed visibility in America, but it has not restored their former dominance. It is a sign of the changing times that even a consummate artist like Mikhail Baryshnikov could not completely adapt to George Balanchine's Americanized style.

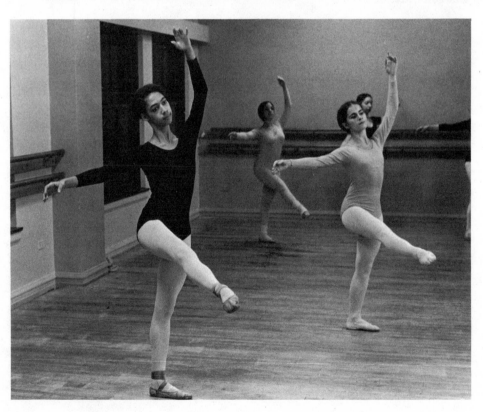

the floor or with a high leg extension). The barre warm-up also includes *ronds de jambe* (circular movements of the leg, on the floor and in the air), and *développés* (a drawing up and extension of the leg in the air). The *ports de bras* (movements of the arms and upper body) are coordinated with the leg and foot exercises. Cyril Beaumont, the English ballet scholar and publisher, has compared these preliminary exercises to the scales and arpeggios which musicians must practice daily. An average ballet barre lasts from thirty to forty-five minutes. Many teachers conclude the warm-up with stretches.

Afterwards students move to the center of the room, where they practice the *adagio,* the *allegro* and a variety of turns. The adagio is a sequence of fluid movements executed at a slow tempo, which incorporates ports de bras, balances and sustained leg extensions. The allegro is a fast movement combination composed of all sorts of fleet footwork and small jumps. Either type of exercise can be performed with simple or complex steps, according to the technical level of the students.

Finally, the teacher will string together big swooping, traveling movements—jumps, leaps, waltzes and turns—which the dancers perform one or two at a time, across the floor. A ballet class usually ends with a jumping combination or with grands battements (high kicks) in the center. Some instructors close with pliés or a simple port de bras to lower the class energy and relax charged muscles.

Modern Dance: The Voice of the Individual

In principle and heritage ballet and modern dance are at opposite poles. Whereas ballet is rooted in an aristocratic tradition, modern dance is truly a child of American democracy. It arose in direct opposition to ballet's rigid standards and codified technique, out of a need for meaningful personal expression. In modern dance there is no single answer or authority, only the many voices of separate artists. In order to find one's own voice it is often necessary to invent new ways of moving. For this reason, modern dance is closely allied with creative discovery. In the same way that the first modern dancer, Isadora Duncan, couldn't use ballet steps to communicate her artistic vision, Martha Graham couldn't use Duncan's movement vocabulary, and Merce Cunningham couldn't use Graham's.

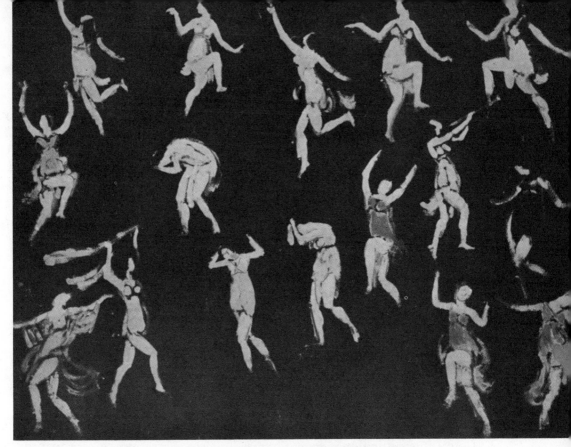

Studies of Isadora Duncan by painter Maurice Denis, 1913. *New York Public Library*

If the term "modern dance" sounds a bit dated, that's because it is. It was coined fifty years ago by critic John Martin to describe the pieces of a few pioneers, such as Martha Graham, Doris Humphrey, Charles Weidman and Helen Tamiris, which he linked to the "modern" music, art and literature of the time. Even today, the expression conjures up pictures of the gaunt-faced young men and women dressed in black who were typical of modern dance in the 1930s. Somehow the tag has stuck, although this form of dancing really began at the turn of the century and has grown to encompass a multitude of movement styles.

But as Martin recognized, more than a single set of beliefs or method of training, modern dance is a point of view. No matter how divergent their approaches, modern dancers are all bound by a common concern: *not to be bound* by any previously set rules or traditions. Contemporaneity is central to their way of dancing. From the first generation to the present, modern dancers have worked closely with innovative artists and musicians and have been interested in exploring current ideas. They have compelled audiences to see in new ways, and they have experimented with the materials of their art as no dancers had done before them.

American modern dance has at least three sources: the iconoclastic legacy of Isadora Duncan; the inspirational atmosphere and eclectic training

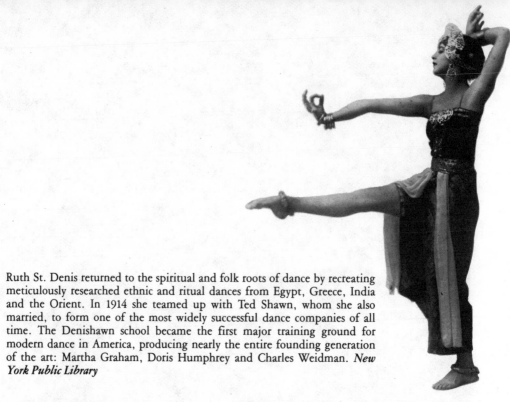

Ruth St. Denis returned to the spiritual and folk roots of dance by recreating meticulously researched ethnic and ritual dances from Egypt, Greece, India and the Orient. In 1914 she teamed up with Ted Shawn, whom she also married, to form one of the most widely successful dance companies of all time. The Denishawn school became the first major training ground for modern dance in America, producing nearly the entire founding generation of the art: Martha Graham, Doris Humphrey and Charles Weidman. *New York Public Library*

system fostered by the Denishawn* company and school during the 1920s, in which were blended ballet, ethnic and freestyle dance; and the principles of German Expressionism eloquently introduced to this country in the 1930s by Mary Wigman and her followers. In common with Duncan, the Expressionists believed that all movement came from emotional impulses and the natural body rhythms they produced, and that the physical space the dancer inhabited was a powerful psychological element of the dance. Wigman technique combined improvisation and the study of percussion accompaniment with a program of rigorous gymnastic exercises that were designed to make the body a fully expressive instrument.

Isadora Duncan burst upon the American dance scene in 1909, when ballet had grown corrupt and most theatrical dancing was, in the words of writer Walter Terry, "limited to acrobatic display and happy hoofing." She literally brought dancing back down to earth, back to the essentials of the art. There was no virtuosity when Isadora performed, yet she touched her audiences with the power of deeply felt emotions and simple, honest, natural movement. She sat, she walked, she ran, she skipped. She lay on the ground. Duncan used her own body timing, and those who saw her say that she moved with a slowness and quietness and fluidity that had been absent from dance a long while. She was not interested in making pretty dances, but gutsy ones; she was not interested in form, but in content; and though always dignified, her dances came from the depths of an unfettered Dionysian soul. Duncan insisted on total freedom of expression. An uncompromising feminist, she shocked all but her fellow artists by

*The group's name was a compound of the names of its directors, Ruth St. Denis and Ted Shawn.

dancing barefoot and uncorseted, clad only in a thin tunic. She dared to interpret great music—Chopin, Beethoven, Wagner—music that would certainly have dwarfed a lesser talent.

From Duncan, Denishawn and Wigman sprang the vanguard of American modern dance: Martha Graham, Doris Humphrey, Charles Weidman, Helen Tamiris, Hanya Holm and Lester Horton. They experimented further with music (including dancing to silence), stage decor and lighting. They read Freud and were intrigued by psychological motivation. They delved into American history and researched indigenous dance forms such as those of the American Indian and black man. Some of them made stinging social commentaries, and a few took up political causes. Many of the early modern dancers held that studying dance would make people into better human beings. Through their efforts, modern dance classes were taught at colleges, YMCAs and community centers at rates that factory workers and store clerks could afford.

Except for Tamiris, each of the artists in the first generation of modern dancers developed a training system based on his or her unique point of view, particular body and distinctive way of moving. For instance, Graham evolved a technique based on the contraction and release of the midsection. Humphrey concerned herself with what she called "the arc between two deaths,"—the range of possibilities between balance and unbalance, fall and recovery, perfect control and total surrender to the pull of gravity. Like Isadora, both used movement from everyday life, such as walking, running and jumping, and both based their movement dynamics on the natural rise and fall of the breath.

*It took nothing less than burning missionary zeal to be a modern dancer in the old days, as is demonstrated by the classic exchange between Ted Shawn and Doris Humphrey that took place while the latter was a member of the Denishawn company. At a staff meeting in 1928, the story goes, Humphrey told St. Denis and Shawn that she thought they had cheapened their repertory when they performed with the Ziegfeld Follies because the choreography had been revised to give it more commercial appeal. Shawn, who had been studying for the ministry before he chose dance as his life's work, was well prepared for that reprimand. He answered, "Do you mean to say that Jesus Christ was any the less great because he addressed the common people?" "No," snapped Humphrey, "but you're not Jesus Christ." To which Shawn retorted, "But I am, I am the Jesus Christ of the dance."**

*From *Dance*. New York: Newsweek Books, 1974.

The next generation of modern dance choreographers ventured out in different directions. Some, like José Limón and Alvin Ailey, chose to expand on the movement vocabularies and training systems of their teachers. But others invented their own styles, taking what they needed from their teachers, modifying and adding their own innovations. Former Graham dancer Erick Hawkins, for example, took the starch out of the Graham exercises and devised a gentle, free-flowing way of dancing that is reminiscent of Isadora Duncan.

Of all those who broke from the previous generation, Merce Cunningham's reforms have been the most influential and widespread. Cunningham fused the quick, brilliant footwork of classical ballet with the flexible back and shoulders of the moderns. He submitted that modern dance should be even more lifelike than it already was. He was convinced that movement was its own reason for being and that it needed neither plot nor musical structure to be compelling. Dancers didn't have to portray characters but could be interesting to watch as themselves. Among highly trained and specialized movements, Cunningham inserted nondance activities, such as riding a bicycle and doing a headstand. To structure his dances, he used chance methods such as the toss of a coin. His dances, like life, had no central focus. They were designed to be seen from any angle. The viewer could take in several images at once or would naturally be drawn to the most striking one. Cunningham collaborated with avant-garde musician John Cage, whose scores consisted mostly of electronic and vocal sounds or witty anecdotes read aloud. The dances and the music were created independently of each other and were brought together only in performance. The notion that dance movement should be strong enough to stand on its own was not a new one. Mary Wigman and Doris Humphrey worked from that premise when Cunningham was still a child, but he took it to its logical extreme. For years Merce Cunningham was ignored by the critics. Many people walked out of his concerts bewildered or infuriated. Yet his following grew steadily.

Cunningham taught dance composition at his studio in New York. His revolutionary concepts spawned another generation of modern dancers who gathered at the Judson Memorial Church in Greenwich Village in the 1960s. There a collective of experimental choreographers, musicians and artists presented a series of concerts that took Cunningham's ideas even further. They proposed alternative dance spaces, performing in lofts, on rooftops, in museums, parks and other outdoor locations. They worked with untrained dancers* and used—sometimes exclusively—nondance movement from every-day tasks, games and sports. The modern dance vocabulary burst wide open. The Judson Church group, which was comprised of such rugged individualists as Judith Dunn, Steve Paxton, Lucinda Childs, Tricia Brown and Yvonne

*This was not an entirely new idea either. In the 1920s and 30s Rudolf Laban, the German movement theoretician and forefather of European modern dance, had used masses of untrained dancers in his "movement choirs."

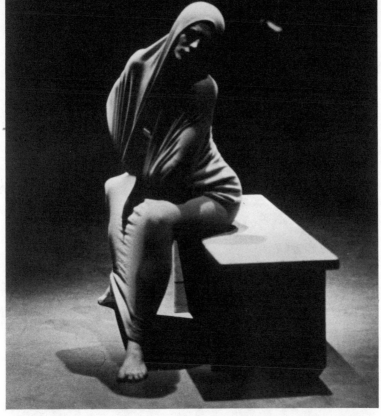

Janet Eilber in *Lamentation*, a solo choreographed by Martha Graham in 1930. *Martha Swope*

Rainer, was also the first to experiment with multimedia technology, including film and tape collages. Some even attached microphones to their bodies, accompanying themselves with the sound of their own muscles and bones moving. Not all their efforts were successful, but the post-modern dancers, as they are sometimes called, had a lasting impact on the choreography of the 1970s.

Because modern dance is predicated so heavily on personal expression, any slight shift in ideas, emphasis or way of moving can constitute a new style. And a new style may in turn become institutionalized as a new training system or technique, as did Hawkins' and Cunningham's. The numerous modern dance techniques and styles now prevalent, and the generations of choreographers begat by the second generation—Cunningham, Hawkins, Jose Limón, Alwin Nikolais, Paul Taylor, Alvin Ailey, Anna Halprin, James Waring and others—would take volumes to describe. Don McDonagh has done a good job in his two books, the *Complete Book of Modern Dance* and *The Rise and Fall and Rise of Modern Dance*.

Today we can see the work of five generations of American modern dancers, from reconstructions of Isadora Duncan's solos to the avant-garde dance-theater epics of Meredith Monk and the time-space explorations of Lucinda Childs.

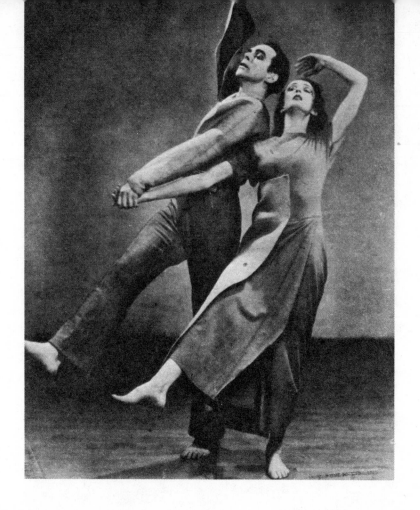

The modern dance class. Taking a ballet class is much the same anywhere in the world, but because of the great diversity in modern dance, classes vary enormously with regard to choreography, movement dynamics and teaching approach. Unlike ballet, which evolved at the leisurely pace of the sixteenth and seventeenth centuries, modern dance developed with the speed of twentieth-century future shock. Hundreds of modern styles are taught at present, some of which borrow liberally from ballet, jazz or ethnic dance. They are often so drastically different from each other that they require totally separate training. For instance, although Erick Hawkins' choreography grew out of Graham technique, a Hawkins dancer would have to train long and hard in the Graham method to be able to perform it properly.

The most widely practiced modern dance techniques are those of Martha Graham and Merce Cunningham. To some, an orthodox Graham or Cunningham class may seem as formal and codified as any ballet class, yet the two differ

Above: Charles Weidman and Doris Humphrey doing the suspended movement that was typical of their style. ***New York Public Library***

Right: Meg Harper and Merce Cunningham in Cunningham's *Rainforest,* with decor by Andy Warhol. ***James Klosty;*** Klosty's photos of the Cunningham company have been assembled in the extraordinary book *Merce Cunningham* (New York: E.P. Dutton, 1975).

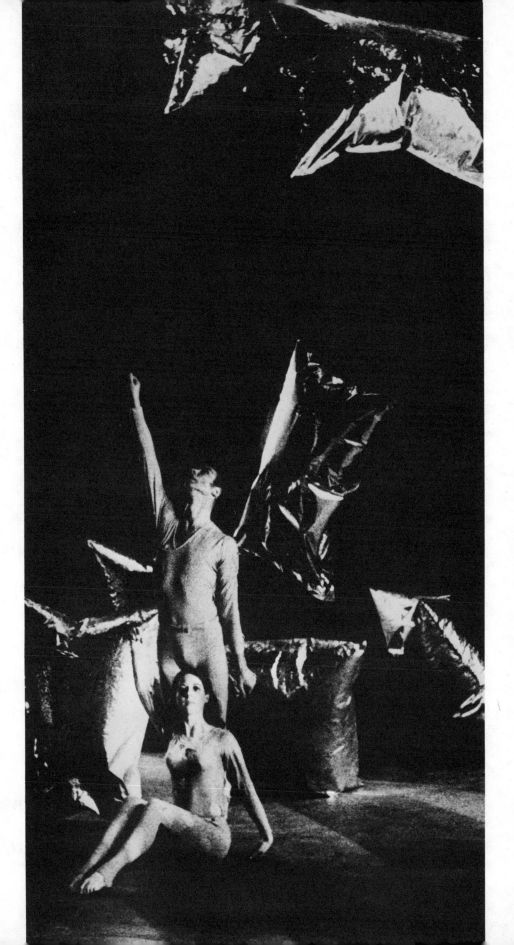

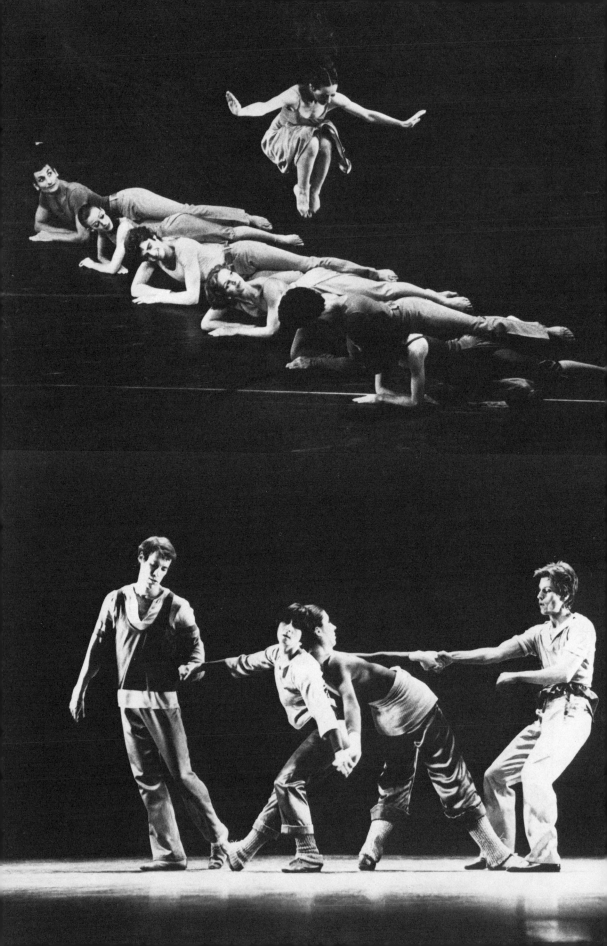

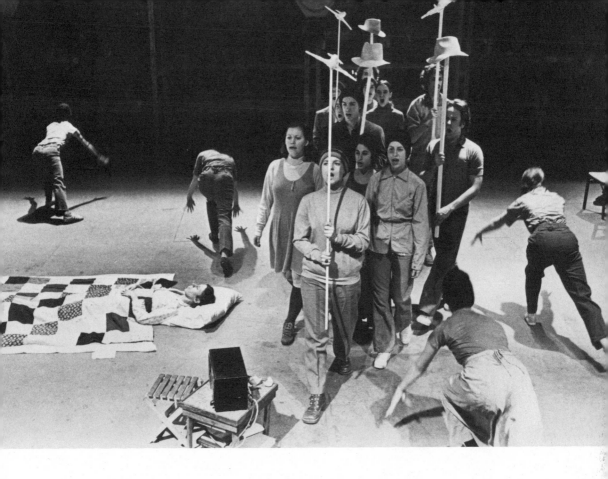

Above: A scene from Meredith Monk's *Quarry*. *courtesy of Meredith Monk/The House*

Top left: Lila York sails over members of the Paul Taylor Dance Company in *Esplanade*. *Jack Vartoogian, courtesy of the Paul Taylor Dance Company*

Bottom left: Sue's Leg, with original cast members Tom Rawe, Twyla Tharp, Rose Marie Wright and Kenneth Rinker, and choreography by Tharp. *Tom Berthiaume, courtesy of the Twyla Tharp Dance Foundation*

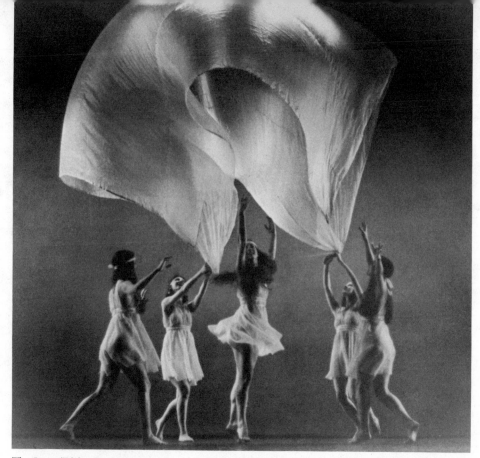

The Joyce Trisler Danscompany in a delicious moment from *Soaring*, choreographed by Ruth St. Denis and Doris Humphrey. Other historical modern dance works are being revived by the José Limón Dance Company, the Alvin Ailey American Dance Theatre, the Repertory Dance Theatre of Salt Lake City, the Isadora Duncan Commemorative Dance Company, and soloists Annabelle Gamson and Satoru Shimazaki.

as radically from ballet as they do from each other. Drama is choreographed right into Graham technique. The movement is the language of the inner conflicts of Graham's characters, and much of it comes from the pull of oppositional forces. Like its originator, Graham technique is forceful, sharp and intense. Classes begin seated on the floor with set exercises that start from a deep contraction of the pelvic muscles and develop into all sorts of twistings and coilings of the torso around the spine. Then pliés, brushes and battements are performed standing up in the center, to strengthen the lower body. Stretches of the sides of the torso, oppositional balances and turns, falls, jumps and leaps are added.

Cunningham classes also begin in the center of the floor, but standing. First there is a prescribed series of back stretches; next, pliés, and then a number of movement sequences combining back curves, tilts and twists with exercises to build strong and articulate legs and feet. In a Cunningham class dancers rarely get down on the floor. In fact, from the waist down many of the warm-up exercises resemble ballet barre practice done without the support of the barre. As in Cunningham's choreography, the movement is emotionally neutral; students

Right: A Graham floor exercise. *David Lindner*

learn to be agile mentally as well as physically and to think on their feet. Dance combinations are often repeated at double speed or slowed to half speed, and are reversed in space.

Other modern dance classes may begin with a ballet barre, with body swings and bounces, with some version of the Graham or Cunningham back exercises, with yoga stretches or with jogging around the room. Because the emphasis of this form has always been on choreography, many modern teachers are also experienced choreographers. Classes may end with a dance phrase freshly designed by the teacher, an excerpt from a famous concert piece, an exercise in composition or an improvisation.

The musical accompaniment for modern classes is equally diverse. It ranges from simple vocal sounds or percussion to a panoply of instruments. Modern dancers may move to contemporary, classical, jazz, folk, pop, lieder, baroque or romantic music; to experimental scores or even the word-music of poetry.

In spite of their differences, however, most modern dance classes adhere to certain underlying principles. In contrast to ballet's artificial positions, modern dance is founded on natural sources of movement. Isadora Duncan traced the center of all life and emotion to the solar plexus because it was the center of breathing. Since then, much modern dance movement has stemmed from a

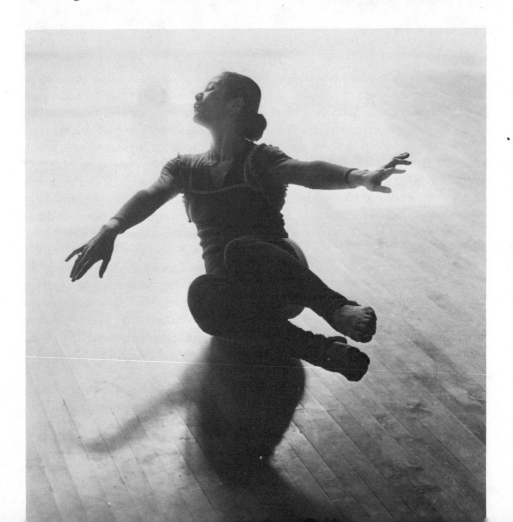

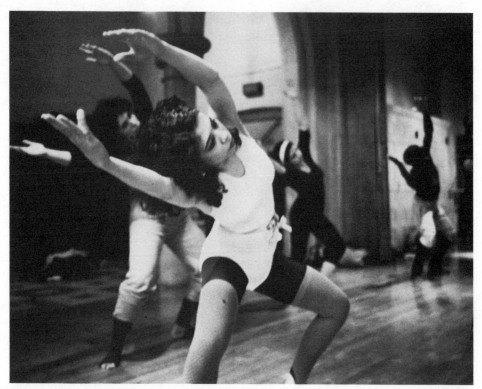

Warming up the torso in a Horton class. *Frank Gimpaya*

strong and supple torso. Natural, or parallel, as well as turned-out positions of
the hips are employed in modern dancing. Even when the legs are turned out, it
is to a comfortable degree. It is never an extreme stance. In many modern styles
the arms swing freely at the sides or respond spontaneously to body movement,
rather than maintaining fixed positions. One of the most obvious ways in which
modern dancing is natural is in the use of bare feet. The contact of bare foot
with bare floor immediately opens the dancer to new sensations and gives her
freedom to work the foot in different ways. Flexed and unformed positions of
the foot are practiced in modern dance along with pointed ones. Barefoot dancing also establishes a close connection with the ground, a feeling of being rooted to the earth.

    This brings us to another distinguishing feature of modern dancing: its
use of body weight. The ballet dancer defies gravity. Her body is lifted high, her
legs extend upward, and her arms float lightly above. She strives to maintain
the illusion of weightlessness against the forces of nature that pull her down.
The modern dancer, on the other hand, makes full use of her weight and the
downward thrust of gravity, both in choreography and to stretch and condition
the body in technique.

    The differences between ballet and modern dance become painfully ap-
parent when ballet dancers attempt to perform modern choreography without

adequate training. The movement never looks quite right; it often appears stiff and flat because of the contrary use of the torso and body weight in the two forms.

Since modern dance choreography is derived from the creative needs of the dancer rather than from a standard vocabulary of steps, there are endless possibilities for movement. A movement may start from the head or the shoulder or the hip as well as from the center of the body. It may be choreographed on the knees and on the floor as well as standing and in the air. An infinite variety of body lines and shapes—balletic and nonballetic, beautiful or grotesque—may be sought.

Modern dance companies are small. Unlike the hierarchical ranking system of ballet, each dancer performs as a soloist. Modern choreographers, therefore, like to work with dancers who have distinctive personalities and ways of moving. Similarly, in most modern classes, personal expression and creativity are encouraged. The first time I took a modern dance lesson I was surprised to hear the teacher correct a student by saying, ''Yes, that's nice, you can do it that way too, but for this class I want you to do it like this.'' For the first time it occurred to me that there was more than one way of dancing well. Recently another modern teacher told me, ''The more daring my students are about asserting their individuality, the more chances they take in that direction, the more interesting they are to me.''

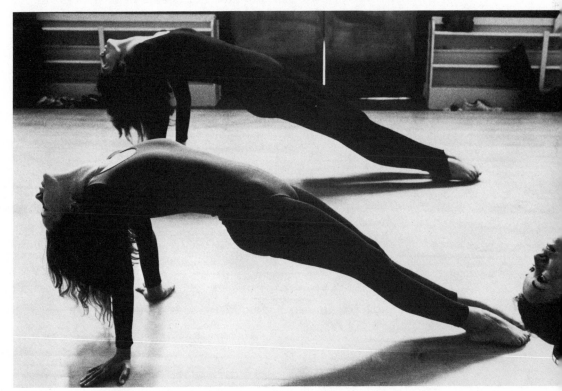

Sue Gaston Bridges, courtesy of the Room to Move Studio, Venice, California

Tap and Jazz: Pure Pleasure

These native American dance modes have traditionally appeared as popular entertainment rather than on the concert stage, though there have been a few notable exceptions. Tap and jazz have always been performed for the pure pleasure of movement and rhythm, the object being simply to have a good time and to give others a good time. That's what makes them so appealing—they are unpretentious, and their joyful spirit is truly infectious. Although it takes great skill to become an expert, almost anyone can master the basics of jazz and tap. Like modern dance, they are eclectic forms without any one standard technique. The personal style of the dancer or choreographer is the most visible and valued aspect of the performance.

The shared roots of tap and jazz. In essence, tap dancing concentrates on footwork and rhythm, while jazz focuses on body movement, but in many ways their origins are inseparable. They sprung from the same times and places, and often from the same performers. Both jazz and tap are derived from African dances brought to this country by black slaves. Both forms grew out of American vernacular, or popular, dancing. They have been developed, refined and transmitted over the past two hundred years by black and white entertainers in minstrel shows, vaudeville and nightclubs, and more recently in films and Broadway musicals.

For a long time jazz and tap were danced to the same music—jazz (and its progenitors, ragtime and minstrel music)—sharing with it highly sophisticated rhythms and the use of improvisation. During the golden era of the 1920s, 30s and 40s, tap and jazz were both called "jazz dance." Virtuoso dancers performed with the big jazz bands of Duke Ellington, Count Basie, Benny Goodman, Cab Calloway, Louis Armstrong, the Dorsey brothers and Paul Whiteman. As jazz archivist Ernie Smith says, in both ways of dancing "the most important thing was the rhythm, propulsive and compelling. You couldn't sit still and listen because this music was hard to ignore. It just *made* you dance." Tap dancers of this period combined the swivel-hipped, rubber-legged and acrobatic jazz movements with tap steps. They also incorporated current social dances such as the Charleston, the Shim Sham, the Lindy and Truckin'.* Jazz dancers, in turn, appropriated some of the agile tap footwork for their routines.

---

* Thanks to the efforts of old-time hoofers and their young protégés, this exciting form of tap dancing, known as jazz tap, is very much alive and well today.

138

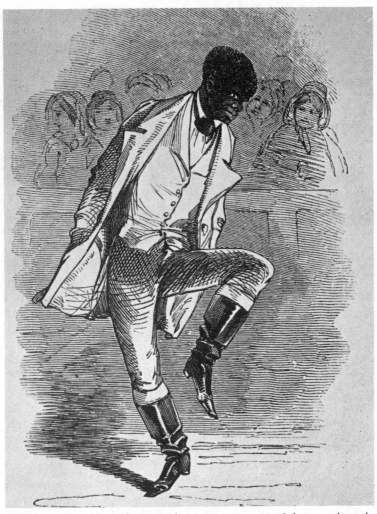

William Henry Lane, a freeman whose stage name was Juba, was the only black entertainer to get top billing in white minstrel shows. In 1848, when he appeared with Pells Ethiopian Serenaders at Vauxhall Gardens in London *(above)*, he received equal acclaim to that given ballerina Fanny Elssler. The first to combine European jig and reel steps with African rhythms, Juba is credited with having established tap dancing as a theatrical art form. It was Juba who instituted the practice of imitating other dancers' moves and inventing original variations. He and the great Irish jig dancer John Diamond popularized the custom of holding friendly tap competitions called challenge matches. Juba's frenetic body movements, which are described in Charles Dickens' *American Journals*, are also said to mark the beginning of American jazz dance. *New York Public Library*

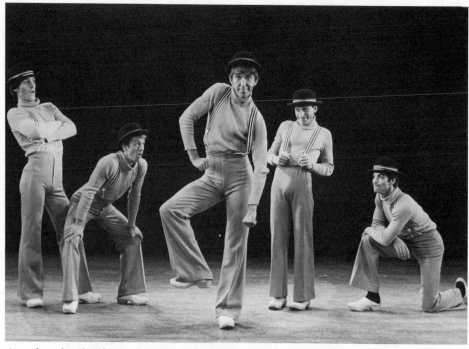

A modern-day clog dance created by Danny Daniels for the Broadway show *Walking Happy*. Here it is performed by the American Dance Machine, a New York-based group that preserves outstanding choreography from the American musical theater. *Martha Swope, courtesy of the American Dance Machine.*

Until recently, tap and jazz dancers had little formal instruction, since many of the best were banned from the "legitimate" theater because they were black. They learned their art on street corners, at carnivals and medicine shows, in saloons, brothels and dance halls, and in crowded ballrooms. The famous Hoofer's Club, where countless tap greats got their training, was the back room of a successful gambling establishment in Harlem. In their purest form, these dance modes still carry with them the high-pitched energy and hell-for-leather abandon of their birthplaces.

Also true to their ancestry, most tap and jazz classes don't place a great deal of emphasis on building the body or analyzing technique. But you'll probably see more good dancing in these classes than anywhere else because they really get students to loosen up and *move*. The advanced classes resemble musicians' jam sessions, where dancers pick up routines and embellish them in their own style.

Busby Berkeley choreographed lavish production numbers on land, sea and in the air for the 1933 film *Footlight Parade*. In this water ballet the girls still have their tap shoes on. *Museum of Modern Art.*

Tap dance

Tap dancing is a blend of the syncopated rhythms and tribal dances of the African slaves with step dances brought to America by the European settlers, such as the Irish jig, reel and hornpipe, and the English clog. It was made popular in the early nineteenth century by white minstrels in blackface parodying black people. Black men imitated whites imitating blacks. The Afro-Americans danced barefoot, but the English and the Irish wore wooden-soled shoes that made noise as they danced. By the early 1800s, copper pennies were screwed into the heels of the shoes to intensify the sound, and later these were replaced by metal tips known as taps.

For a variety of reasons, including the fact that segregation in the United States extended to the performing arts, an independent and quite tenacious black entertainment circuit flourished during the nineteenth and early twentieth centuries. It was called Theater Owners' Booking Association (TOBA), and tap dancing was one of its staples. But despite the separate black and white theater circuits, tap dancing was one forum where racial barriers broke down. At challenge matches and meeting places in New York and other cities across the nation, blacks and whites competed and traded the latest steps. They observed each other's performance styles, borrowed from each other's routines, taught and coached and inspired across racial lines.

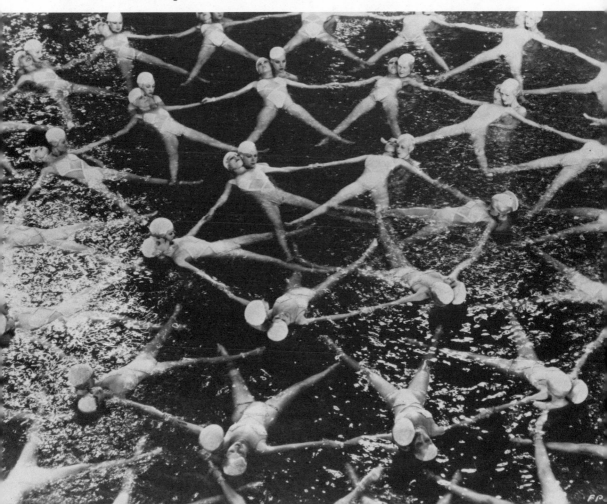

Tap was combined with ballet by such white stars as Fred Astaire, Eleanor Powell and Gene Kelly. Though they used more body movement than complex footwork, these dancers instituted an open, elegant carriage of the arms and upper body, and they added a spatial dimension to tap choreography by covering more ground. Paul Draper, who was trained at the School of American Ballet, invented a genre called ballet-tap. It was an amalgam of tap steps and balletic arm and leg movements, turns and jumps. Draper devised a tap barre and worked with ballet turn-out, and he danced in concert halls to the music of Handel, Vivaldi, Bach and Couperin.

Black hoofers primarily used their feet, but they were responsible for most of the major innovations in tap dancing and for bringing the form back to life in the 1960s, after a twenty-year decline. The late Marshall Stearns, founder of the Newport Jazz Festival, summarized their contributions in his book *Jazz Dance*, a complete and lively history of tap and jazz. King Rastus Brown started with flat-footed hoofing to a syncopated beat, Stearns noted. Then Bill "Bojangles" Robinson brought tap dancing up on the toes. Eddie Rector gave it traveling steps and graceful body movement, and John Bubbles added break-neck speed and rhythmic complexity, creating an idiom known as "rhythm tap." In the 1950s, even after Broadway and Hollywood had abandoned tap in favor of ballet, and many out-of-work hoofers had become messenger boys and factory workers, a hardy band of survivers was keeping the art alive. By coaching

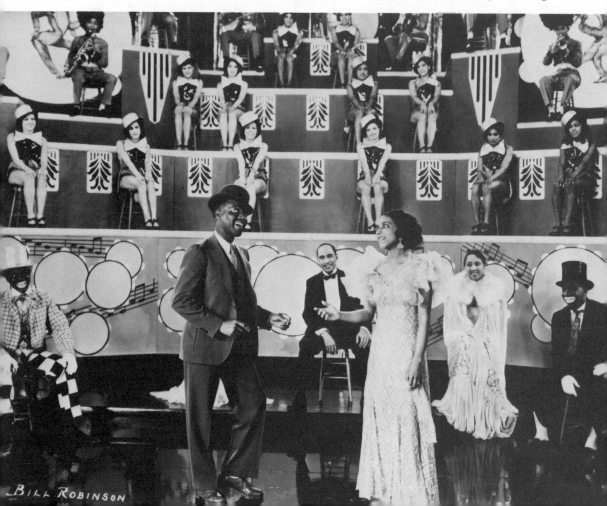

BILL ROBINSON

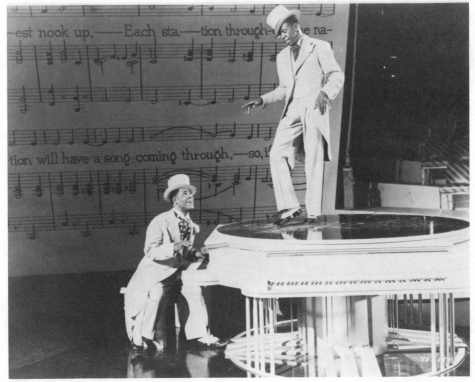

Above: Pianist Ford Lee "Buck" Washington and partner John Bubbles in the Warner Brothers musical *Varsity Show*. The smooth and elegant Bubbles, who invented rhythm tap, was a sensation in the Ziegfeld Follies of 1931. At the insistence of composer George Gershwin he played the part of Sportin' Life in the film version of *Porgy and Bess*. Bubbles taught Eleanor Powell how to tap dance, but because of the racial attitudes of the time he never received the widespread recognition that she did. *courtesy of the Ernie Smith Collection*

Left: The great Bill "Bojangles" Robinson in a number from the short subject *King for a Day*. The end men in blackface seated in the foreground are last vestiges of a minstrel tradition that survived into the twentieth century. *courtesy of the Ernie Smith Collection*

and choreographing for social dancers, television entertainers and rock 'n' roll groups, they passed their knowledge on to the next generation. They were still around to teach and perform when tap was revived during the nostalgia wave of the 1970s.

Stearns is credited with having started the recent tap revival by inviting seven virtuoso hoofers to perform at the Newport Jazz Festival in 1963: Cholly Atkins, Ernest Brown, Honi Coles, Charles Cook, Chuck Green, Pete Nugent and Baby Lawrence (Lawrence Jackson). Most of these men were members of the Copasetics, a Harlem-based fraternal organization of black showmen established in 1949 to commemorate the great Bill Robinson and preserve the old traditions. They brought the house down. Their success was followed by that of another critically-acclaimed revival group called the Hoofers, on Broadway. By 1971, when Busby Berkeley's tap classic *No, No Nanette* was resurrected with its

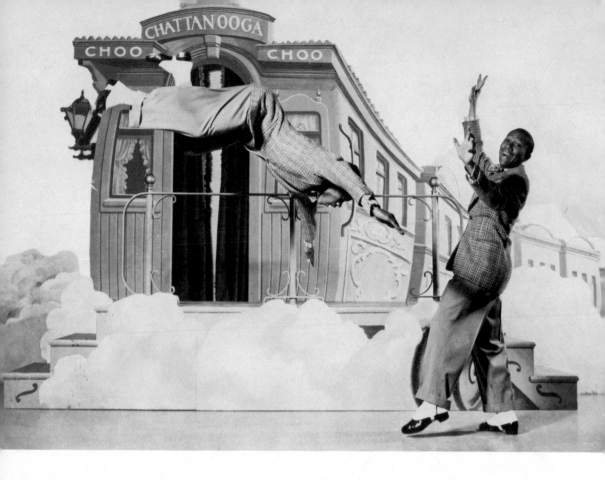

original star, Ruby Keeler, tap was well on its way to making a triumphant comeback. During the 1970s a generation of young dancers, who perform both in collaboration with the old-time tappers and on their own, arrived to insure the continuance of the tap renaissance. They include Jane Goldberg, Carol Hess, Gail Conrad and Andrea Levine in New York, and Los Angeles-based Lynn Dally.

The tap class. In tap the emphasis is, of course, on footwork and the expression of rhythm through sound. Tap is the only kind of dancing that is its own accompaniment. In that sense, tap dancers are the best musicians because they make their own "shoe music." When they worked with the jazz bands of the 1930s and 40s, tap dancers performed as percussionists. They took their solos with the rest of the band muted or playing stop time behind them. A variety of tap sounds and rhythms are possible. The more advanced the dancer, the more intricate the rhythmic patterns and the greater the range of sounds he can make. If tap dancers sometimes look introspective, it is because they are listening hard to the rhythms they are producing.

In order to make clear tap sounds and master the required weight shifts (which can be exquisitely subtle), the tap dancer must have a loose, relaxed stance and train for control and agility of the feet. The placement of the arms,

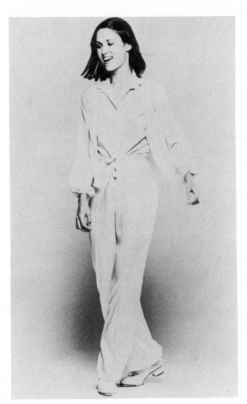

Right: New wave tap dancer Carol Hess. *courtesy of Carol Hess*

Left· The amazing Nicholas Brothers in an acrobatic tap sequence from the movie *Sun Valley Serenade. courtesy of the Ernie Smith Collection*

head and upper body are not prescribed in tap dancing; it is these elements that, according to their use by the individual performer, constitute personal style. Since the main concern of tap dancing is rhythmic expression—rather than the improvement of balance and line or the expression of emotions—most of the class time is spent practicing steps and learning routines. Most tap classes follow the ancient formula of the challenge match. Students learn the basic steps by watching and imitating their teacher, embroidering on these movements as they advance. (Now, as in the past, you aren't considered a good tap dancer unless you add something of your own style.)

A tap class usually begins with a brief warm-up, although this may be dispensed with in some advanced classes on the assumption that dancers will warm themselves up before class. The pliés, frappés, leg swings or grands battements at the barre or in the center of the room may recall ballet class, but here they are done with a relaxed knee and a fluid spine, the major purpose being to loosen the joints and muscles and to get the rhythms into the body. Students then practice the simplest components of the steps—toe-taps, steps, brushes, hops, slaps, shuffles, scuffs, ball changes, cramp-rolls, pull-backs and wings (the names are onomatopoetic). Soon students perform short combinations of steps; and finally everything is put together in a long dance sequence that is rehearsed several times to old show standards like ''Tea for Two,'' ''Singin' in the Rain'' or "Top Hat," tunes that were popular when tap was in its heyday. Tap dancing is customarily performed in an atmosphere of friendly competition and display, and this mood also permeates the classes as the teacher throws out steps and the students respond.

Though they are exciting when done in unison, tap routines can make a frightful noise when mistakes are amplified by many feet. So beware of over-crowded classes where it is hard to hear yourself and next to impossible for the teacher to hear you.

Master teacher Bob Audy in New York urges new tap students to be pa-tient. "Most beginners," says Audy, shaking his head, "want to learn routines right away. But if you don't understand the basics you still won't know what you're doing when you get to the routines. It's discouraging because you never really make progress. I have my beginners practice the basic steps and rhythms until they know them cold. Then they advance to a faster class where we work on routines.'' In his illuminating book *On Tap Dancing*, Paul Draper submits that "an instructor whose class consists of working on routines has no business teaching dancing at all. Not every student can learn to dance . . . whereas almost anybody can learn a routine, if it is simple enough. Those who can should have a chance to, and they never will if they learn only routines."

Audy, who has also written two instruction books on jazz and tap danc-ing, advises students to look for a teacher whose tap sounds are clear and whose rhythms are well defined when he demonstrates. "He or she should show a knowledge of several different styles and rhythms. Check your teacher's cre-dentials," Audy suggests. "Teachers who boast only a show-business back-ground tend to know only the repertory of the shows they were in and don't necessarily have a solid knowledge of other styles. On the other hand, those

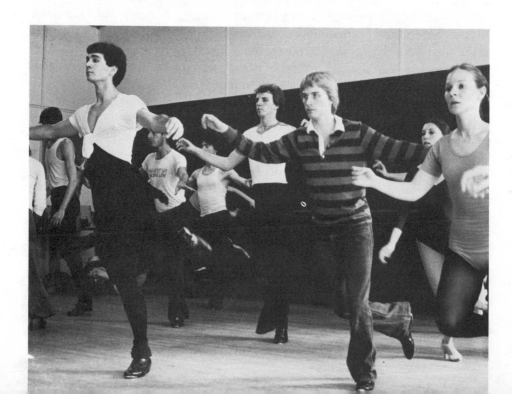

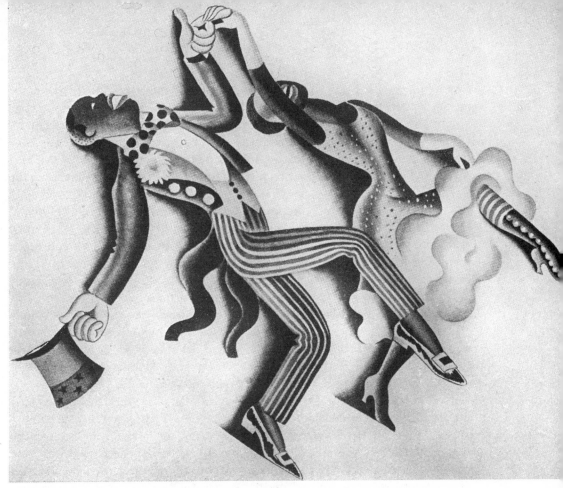

The Cakewalk, a high-stepping march popularized by ragtime music, was one of the first black jazz dances to sweep the country. *New York Public Library*

with only an academic knowledge of tap dancing don't necessarily make good teachers either. In general, a tap teacher with a broad background in ballet, modern dance or jazz will be more knowledgeable and complete as a teacher.''

Jazz Dance

Jazz is fundamentally popular dancing that has been stylized and polished to a theatrical brilliance. The original jazz dance was black social dancing done to jazz music. Based on folk forms of the rural South, it was performed by amateurs at parties and clubs and get-togethers. The term "jazz dance" was probably first used to describe choreography in 1917 when a song called "The Jazz Dance," composed by W. Benton Overstreet, came into prominence. As was the fashion in popular music then, the lyrics of the song instructed dancers in the appropriate steps to do—in this case the Texas Tommy, the Eagle Rock, the Buzz and the Shimmy.

In the 1920s and 30s—The Jazz Age—jazz became an international craze, the hallmark of an entire generation. Everyone was doing dances like the

Left: Tap students concentrate on a tricky routine. *Frank Gimpaya*

Charleston, which black showgirl Josephine Baker made fashionable with the French Follies Bergères; the Black Bottom, introduced by blues singer Alberta Hunter; and the Lindy, named after aviator Charles Lindbergh and later renamed the Jitterbug. Charleston dancers used body isolations for the first time in social dancing, swinging each part independently to different syncopated rhythms. Their torsos were pitched forward until they were nearly parallel to the floor.

In 1927 the Savoy Ballroom opened in Harlem. Dubbed the "Home of Happy Feet," it was the largest ballroom in the world—one square block to be exact. For thirty years the finest jazz dancers and swing musicians converged there, inspiring each other to heights of invention and virtuosity. The young crowd at the Savoy were the pace-setters, if not the originators, of the Lindy Hop. They danced lightning-fast, tossing their partners overhead in flying lifts and judo-like flips known as air steps. The Savoy's semiprofessional Lindy teams—who subsequently performed in vaudeville, nightclubs, and in Broadway and Hollywood musicals—were managed by an ex-bouncer with a flair for choreography called Herbert White. Whitey's Lindy Hoppers featured two of the greatest jazz dancers of all time, Al Minns and Leon James.

At places like the Cotton Club, Small's Paradise, the Savoy and Palladium ballrooms, and the Harvest Moon Ball in New York, new moves caught on as quickly as they were invented: the Shim Sham, the Suzy Q, the Bumps, the Mooch, the Grind, the Slow Drag, the Big Apple, the Snake Hips. Steps were named after dancers who created them and did them better than anyone else. Shorty Snowden made up the Shorty George, for example, and a shuffle step known as the Tack Annie was concocted by a pickpocket named Annie. "Nobody could do it like her, and it's all she could do, they said," reminisces choreographer Pepsi Bethel, who began his career as a Savoy Lindy Hopper and is currently reconstructing period dances for his Authentic Jazz Dance Theatre. "Anything else she couldn't do worth a nickel."*

Despite their phenomenal popularity, however, the original jazz dances, both as social and stage entertainment, went out with the 1940s. Modern jazz music, which replaced big-band jazz and swing, became too complex to dance to, and the phonograph made it possible for people to dance in their living rooms. One by one the fabulous ballrooms where vernacular jazz flourished closed down. But while the advent of mass media may have contributed to the demise of old-style jazz, it opened the way to new varieties of popular music and dancing that eventually gave rise to the jazz dance of the future.

In a truly American melting pot tradition, modern jazz dance is a highly stylized mix of the original jazz dances with steps from the subsequent dance crazes of the 1950s, 60s and 70s. It is a living history to which each generation has added and left its own trace. The jazz dance we see today retains the syncopated rhythms, body isolations, undulating torso and flat-footed steps of the

* From Mark Deitch, "Pepsi Bethel—Master of Jazz Dance," in *The New York Times*, August 6, 1978.

past, but it is no longer done exclusively to jazz music; it is performed to pop, rhythm and blues, rock and disco as well.

The new jazz dance cannot be neatly defined, for it is not any one thing; it is whatever is happening at the time in the popular culture. The essence of modern jazz dance is its very changeability, its ability to update itself by absorbing the music and dances that the general populace knows and enjoys. For this reason, it is always entertaining and always accessible.

Many of us have seen this blending of history take place in our own lifetimes. There is a two-way process: Some social dances are choreographed into

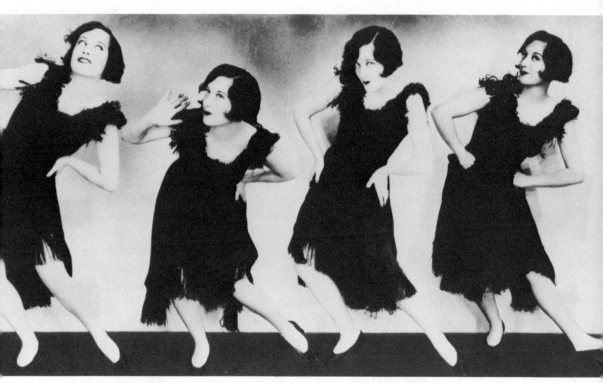

Joan Crawford doing the Black Bottom, 1927. *courtesy of the Ernie Smith Collection*

routines for television or stage after they have become popular and identifiable; others are invented by professionals and become popular because kids see them performed by television dancers and singing groups. In the 1950s and early 60s, old-time jazz dancers such as Cholly Atkins and Pete Nugent stayed around to coach and choreograph for such rock 'n' roll groups as the Cadillacs, the Cleftones, Frankie Lyman and the Teen-Agers, the Moonglows, the Five Satins and the Supremes. They taught them snatches of the Charleston, the Boogie Woogie, the Suzie Q, the Camel Walk, the Itch, the Chicken and other vernacular steps. And these reincarnated dances were imitated by teenagers who saw them on television variety shows and Dick Clark's *American Bandstand*. Thus, as Marshall Stearns has pointed out, the Camel Walk survived as the Stroll, the Jig Walk became the Slop, and the Slow Drag turned into the Fish. Jerome Robbins masterfully incorporated dances such as the Mambo and the Lindy in his choreography for *West Side Story*. And the steps we did in the 1960s—the Twist (really an old Negro folk step), the Bounce, the Boogaloo, the Frug (borrowed from the antiquated Shimmy), the Jerk, the Pony, the Watusi, the Mashed Potato (a latter-day version of the Charleston) and the Monkey—became more grist for the choreographer's mill. In the 1970s we saw sophisticated versions of disco dances added to the jazz lexicon.

Unlike the original jazz dance, which was performed by talented amateurs and self-styled entertainers, modern jazz is performed by professional dancers who are also trained in ballet, modern and ethnic dance. Not only do modern jazz dancers continually recombine old steps and create new ones in the same style, they blend jazz with other dance forms.

Back in 1936, George Balanchine merged jazz with ballet when he choreographed the "Slaughter on Tenth Avenue" number for the Broadway musical *On Your Toes*. Black choreographer Herbert Harper, who was Mr. Balanchine's assistant for the production, taught Ray Bolger to rhythm tap expressly for that scene. Two years later Balanchine worked with the incredible acrobatic jazz dancers Fayard and Harold Nicholas in his next Broadway show, *Babes in Arms*.

Since then several other ballet choreographers have lent a classical tint to jazz on Broadway, including Jerome Robbins, Michael Kidd, Peter Gennaro and Gower Champion. Another element that is integrated into modern jazz choreography is the African, West Indian and Latin ethnic dancing popularized by choreographers Katherine Dunham and Pearl Primus in the 1940s. Their influence can be clearly seen in the dances of Alvin Ailey, Walter Nicks and Talley Beatty, for example. Ailey, Jack Cole, Donald McKayle, Bob Fosse, Twyla Tharp and Eleo Pomare are among the choreographers who have successfully fused jazz with modern dance.

There is sadness in the assimilation of pure jazz with other dance modes, for some of the character and piquancy of the original dances has been lost in the process; but this fusion has also contributed to the survival of jazz dancing by broadening its expressive range and helping to establish it as a serious art form.

Jazz is the most widely viewed dance form in the United States because it is available through many channels in our culture—television, Broadway, nightclubs and the concert stage. Thanks to its marvelous adaptability, it continues to express the times we live in so well. Unlike most tap dancing, which is low-keyed and self-contained, jazz explodes through space with restless energy. Even after many transformations it is still a little raw and fast and naughty.

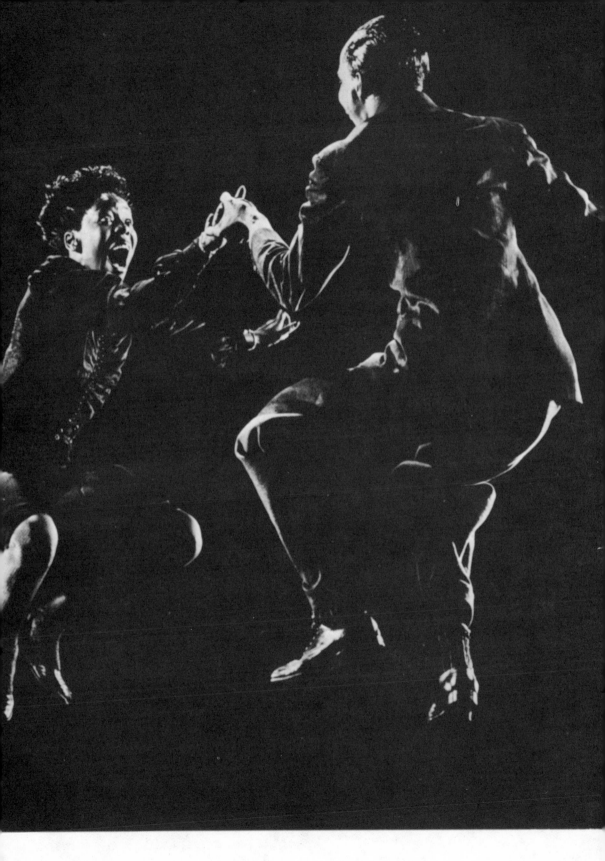

The Lindy Hop, 1943. *New York Public Library*

The jazz class. Jazz dancing as a system of training the body is a relatively recent development. Since jazz is a melting pot of dance styles that vary from choreographer to choreographer, there is no set way to teach a class. It is up to the teacher. Depending on her own background and training, she may combine jazz movement with other forms—by using ballet exercises or modern dance warm-up stretches, for instance.

Jazz warm-ups are normally about thirty minutes long. The standard plié makes its appearance as a limbering exercise; but in jazz class it is likely to be joined right away with relevés (rises on the balls of the feet), lunges and high, loose kicks. An ability to isolate body parts is central to jazz dancing. The pelvis, rib cage, shoulders, chest, arms and head must each be capable of a range of independent movements. Coordinating all of this can be tricky, with different parts of the body moving in different directions at the same time. So every jazz warm-up includes rhythmic work on various body isolations. Students then practice jazz walks and struts, and may also work on turns and adagio movements.

The remaining class time is devoted to learning routines. Sometimes individual steps are practiced separately first, follow-the-leader fashion, across the floor. The pacing of the jazz class reflects the choreography itself, which is high

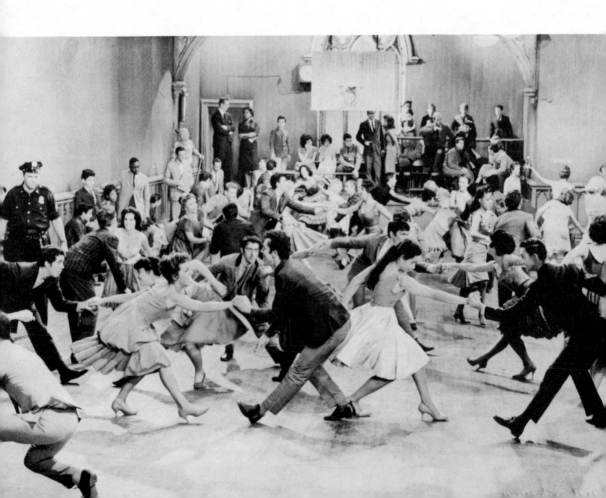

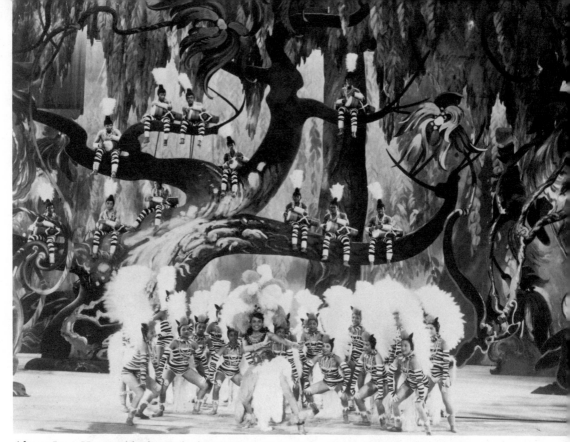

Above: Lena Horne with the Katherine Dunham Dancers in a scene from *Stormy Weather.* Dunham was the first choreographer to put authentic African and Afro-Caribbean ethnic dance on the concert stage and to establish a technique for its study. *courtesy of the Ernie Smith Collection*

Left: Jerome Robbins skillfully incorporated current social dances such as the Jitterbug and the Mambo into his choreography for *West Side Story.* *Museum of Modern Art*

in speed and energy. In advanced classes, the atmosphere often mirrors the orderly chaos of an audition. People leave the room and come back to take their turns. They change shoes or talk quietly. But once the music starts, they dance with a vengeance.

Jazz dancing is physically rigorous. It makes considerable demands on the body. Yet years ago jazz dancers didn't even warm up. Pepsi Bethel remarks of the old jazzers, ''You better not say warm-up, that's an insult to them.''*
Perhaps because of this carefree heritage some jazz teachers jump right into razzle-dazzle combinations in the center of the floor, without giving a proper warm-up. Unfortunately, this can lead to injuries. Dancers who are in good shape and have taken another class right before may be all right, but beginners should be especially wary. Look for a teacher who prepares you sufficiently for

* From Mark Deitch, ''Pepsi Bethel—Master of Jazz Dance,'' in *The New York Times*, August 6, 1978.

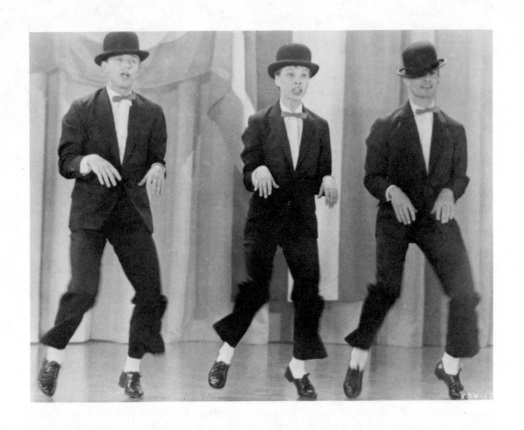

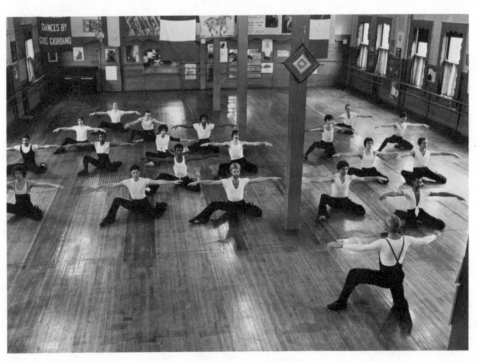

the workout. In jazz dancing the back and midsection need extra attention because they are used a great deal. A thorough warm-up should therefore include a full series of body isolations and stretches for the torso, as well as a complete progression of leg and foot exercises to warm and strengthen the lower body. Bob Audy adds that like all good teachers, jazz teachers should give a "consistent class in which the movement and principles presented in the warm-up are used later on in the dance combinations."

Nat Horne, the principal jazz instructor at the Alvin Ailey American Dance Center, agrees. "Because jazz dance by nature has no set form, it is particularly important for a teacher to stress body placement and conscientious application of technique," he says. "Just feeling the movement and having a good sense of rhythm aren't really enough to make a good jazz teacher; there must be a solid knowledge of technique along with the freedom of expression." Horne prefers live musical accompaniment for jazz classes because he feels the interaction between the dancers and musicians is vital. A teacher who handles records skillfully can be as effective, but this, Horne says, is rare.

Top left: Bob Fosse's "Steam Heat" number from *The Pajama Game* (1954) featured Buzz Miller, Carol Haney and Kenneth LeRoy. *Museum of Modern Art*

Bottom left: Gus Giordano leads a men's jazz class at his school in Evanston, Illinois.

Below: A jazz combination. *courtesy of the Suburban Cultural Arts Institute, Cleveland*

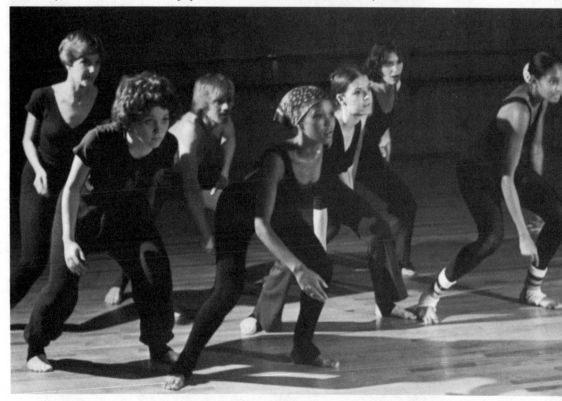

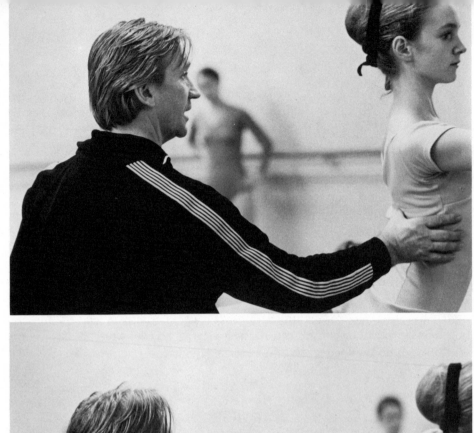

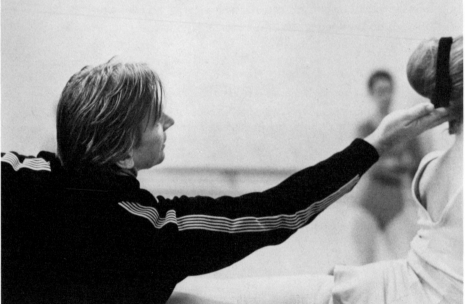

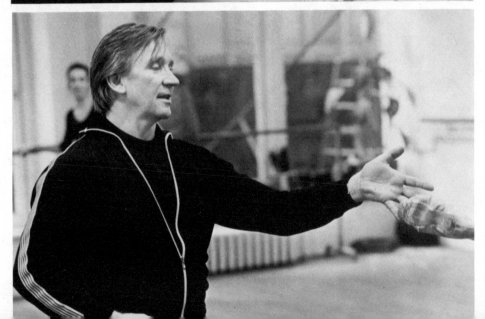

11

Teachers

*your teacher should
not only be good,
but good
for you*

Behind every successful dancer is a good teacher, yet how many times has a poor teacher stood in the way of a dancer's success? Your teacher is the single most important factor in learning to dance. He or she has the power to do both great good and great harm. These remarks from a respected performer really hit home to me:

> *One of the first good teachers I had taught folk dancing at a summer camp I went to as a teenager. She made a dance on us to a sea chantey, and I can still remember the words. She was extremely encouraging to me. Another teacher was wonderful because she had boundless energy that was contagious. And she was so well informed. But I had one teacher who said very destructive things that scarred me for life. I'm still trying to get over them. She knew her ballet all right, but she was very young, and I think more concerned with her own development as a dancer than with teaching. She told me that my legs were boring and straight and that I didn't have good feet and never would. My legs and feet have changed tremendously since then, but I still feel hounded by those words.*

Ballet teacher Don Farnworth fine-tunes a dancer's placement at his New York studio. *David Lindner*

Dance teachers can build bodies or twist them with bad training. They can build confidence or undermine it with a harsh word. Sometimes teachers who don't know how to help you put the blame on your lack of talent. More than the dance school you attend or even the type of dancing you do, your choice of instructor is a crucial one.

What makes a good teacher?

Though she needn't be a brilliant dancer, a good dance teacher demonstrates clearly and is able to make herself plainly understood. She instills a feeling for music in her classes and gives movement that is both strengthening and enjoyable to do. A sharp critical eye is indispensable, and knowing how and when to make corrections so they will be accepted is equally important. Able teachers structure their lessons so that each exercise leads logically to the next and students are properly warmed up. They utilize the entire body in a coordinated way—by this I mean that the back, hips, limbs and head move together rhythmically as a unit. Competent dance teachers work in an anatomically sound manner. They stress correct body alignment (see illustrations in chapter 18) and healthful working habits, such as getting the heels down on the floor in plié. They see to it that students use their muscles fully, with breath and flow, and without forcing or straining. A good teacher develops the body evenly. She avoids overworking any one muscle group by varying the exercises and alternating sides of the body. Strenuous movements are always counterbalanced with ones that stretch the muscles and release tension.

A well-constructed dance class is like a symphony in movement, satisfying and complete. Major themes are established, elaborated and restated as they are woven together to build to a rousing conclusion.

But the dance teacher's role extends far beyond simple instruction, past telling us which foot to place in front of the other and how. Undoubtedly one of the most valuable things she has to offer is her own enthusiasm. Time and again I have heard dancers say that their earliest teachers were found lacking in technique but they managed to transmit a sufficiently strong love of dancing for their pupils to grow and eventually seek out other instructors to develop themselves further. To inspire, to generate energy and excitement, is a vital part of the dance teacher's job. Day after day, she coaxes and cajoles the best efforts from her students, getting them to reach past their present abilities.

As opposed to merely teaching steps, a good instructor teaches you how to learn. She shows you how to look at movement and make it work on your own body. She is also part psychologist, sensing when to push an overcautious dancer or when to restrain an overambitious one. The good dance teacher opens doors, helping dancers to know themselves better and constantly revealing new avenues for growth.

In addition, she leaves you with a philosophy, a set of values to strive for that come from her own sense of what is interesting and important about dancing. Long after you have studied with her, you'll find that some part of her vision of dance is still with you, that you have taken it up and made it your own.

Finally, a good teacher is a good student who is herself continually learning. I once heard an Olympic diver pay tribute to her coach in very similar terms. "He is always thinking of new ways to attack our problems," she said. "If we keep making the same mistakes, he doesn't keep telling us the same thing; he tries different ways of explaining it until we've got it licked."

Good dance teachers, needless to say, are hard to find, but not impossible if you are persistent and go about it intelligently. The practical suggestions given in chapters 13 and 25 should help.

> *It sometimes seems to me that there are more bad teachers of dancing than of any other art. There is a great tendency to take advantage of people's ignorance, for it is impossible to make a judgment about a teacher unless you know something about dancing.*
>
> *I think the best thing to do in seeking a good teacher is to ask the advice of a well-known professional, an experienced dancer. If you admire a dancer, find out where she studied from* **The Dance Encyclopedia** *or write to her.* *
>
> *—GEORGE BALANCHINE*

What makes a teacher good for you?

For all that, having a good teacher isn't enough. What makes a particular dance teacher good for you is first and foremost her capacity to recognize your special qualities and cultivate you as a dancer. One way she'll show it is by giving you individual attention and encouragement, usually because she likes your way of moving and feels a rapport with you. Every dancer needs this kind of personal nurturing in order to thrive.

Even good teachers aren't always able to benefit all students because so much depends on how well you work together. Intangible barriers sometimes arise due to individual differences in personality and movement style. Even if

*From George Balanchine, "Ballet for Your Children," in *Dancemagazine*, June 1954.

she is excellent for others, her teaching methods may not mesh with your body type or the way you learn. You may have to experiment with several instructors before settling on the best one.

Until then you may have to choose from the opportunities available, set priorities and make some compromises. When you do find a teacher you like, stay with her, since only through regular contact will she be able to help you. As you grow and change you may eventually want to change dance teachers too. And at certain stages of your development you may wish to study with more than one instructor to satisfy all your wants and interests. There are few fixed rules as to teachers, but there are some general considerations which will help direct you to the right one for you.

Overall approach. There are at least two distinctly different types of dance teachers: those who instruct primarily by example, and those who analyze and explain. I call the former *action-oriented teachers* and the latter *analytic teachers*. Their methods correspond to the different basic ways we learn. Faced with learning a new language, for instance, some of us do best by plunging straight into conversation, while others need to study vocabulary and rules of grammar before attempting to speak. Just as some people have an ear for languages, some dancers have an eye for movement and can readily absorb unfamiliar motions. Others require a more thoughtful approach. It is unusual to find one teacher who is equally skilled in both the action-oriented and the analytic methods, although most good dance teachers adapt their approaches to the needs of their students by combining elements of both.

The action-oriented teacher. Often an impressive dancer himself, the action-oriented instructor teaches almost entirely by demonstration. His classes are packed with movement. He isn't given to long-winded explanations, nor does he dissect the steps; he presents them up to tempo, more or less as they are meant to be done onstage. Dance phrases are broken down into slower or simpler movements only for beginner classes, or when it becomes apparent that students are unable to follow.

This kind of teacher likes to keep his classes moving continuously. If he interrupts the flow of movement, it is only to give brief general directions or correct glaring errors. He seldom repeats exercises more than once. The fast pacing of an action-oriented class doesn't give you much time to think. You learn by watching and doing, by trial and error, by imitation and intuition. You must jump in and trust your body's instincts—which is the whole point.

You will find yourself dancing sooner, however imperfectly, in such a class. By throwing out lots of steps and combinations and expecting you to make them work, the action-oriented teacher gets you to balance, shift weight and travel through space as a matter of course. Because of the inherent continuity in this form of teaching, his class is something like a performance; you get caught up in the energy and spirit of the dancing around you. You learn *by* dancing, instead of merely learning *how to* dance. These lessons can be exhilarating and inspirational. They make you want to dance.

But sooner is not always better, and the action-oriented approach does have its shortcomings, especially for beginners. The success of this method depends very much on the teacher's ability to set a good example and on his students' ability to observe accurately and imitate what they see. If an action-oriented teacher is a poor model, beginners are likely to absorb his bad habits and personal mannerisms without learning any usable principles of technique. Even if the model is a good one, often the action-oriented approach doesn't leave dancers with enough conscious knowledge of what they are doing to yield consistent results. No matter how keen an eye you have, steady progress will not come from observation and unanalyzed experience alone, and for serious students, at least, this is ultimately very discouraging. Moreover, in a fast-moving class, there is little opportunity for dancers to deepen and refine their work.

The action-oriented teacher can therefore do the most good for students who already have a basic knowledge of technique and of themselves as dancers. His methods are particularly effective with those who have been working too tightly and need to break loose and dance. He is also good for dancers who are starting to perform because he develops their vocabulary and speed at picking up new movement. With an action-oriented instructor you can work on style and musical phrasing, gain stamina and learn to pace your energy simply by dancing a lot.

Such a teacher may also be best for recreational dancers who want to get moving rather than become bogged down in detailed technical analysis. The action-oriented approach produces a class which offers plenty of exercise and is generally more fun, provided there is enough explanation and individual supervision from the teacher to avoid injury.

The analytic teacher. In contrast to the intuitive, performance-like methods of action-oriented instructors, analytic teachers work slowly and carefully, stressing correct form and technique. Their classes begin with a long, thorough warm-up and progress systematically from there.

An analytic teacher gives precise instructions and works for precise results. She demonstrates the mechanics of the steps in detail, and she talks about the purpose of the exercises and the principles of movement behind them. She may, in addition, offer anatomical explanations, or suggest various mental images to help you get the right movement quality and dynamics (such as "imagine you are jumping over a fence on horseback," to get you to feel the lift and suspension of a leap). The nuts-and-bolts approach of the analytic teacher is aimed at giving students a clear understanding of movement so they can have consistent control and thus a reliable technique. Simple exercises are favored so that dancers can take the time to feel what is happening in their bodies and to work in a deliberate way. These are often practiced several times. Although the repetition may seem tedious, it fixes the movement in the mus-

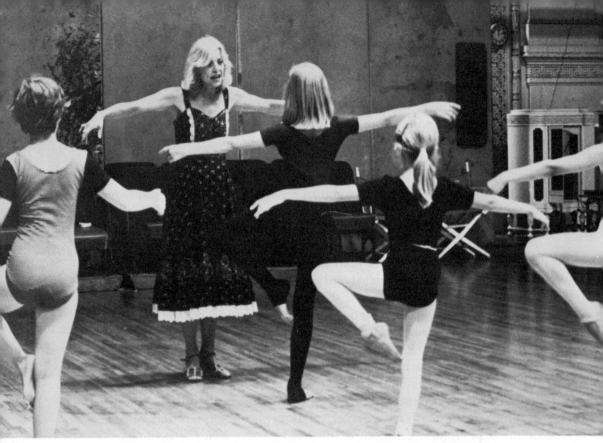

Loyce Houlton corrects youngsters at the Minnesota Dance Theatre and School.

cles and establishes strength as well as confidence.

Analysis is an intermediate step between seeing movement on someone else's body and making it work on your own. It gives you an explicit set of rules to go by, so you don't have to rely solely on your powers of observation or your teacher's execution. Eventually the students of analytic teachers are able to perceive for themselves when they are doing something wrong, and to correct their own mistakes. As ballerina Sally Wilson says of her teacher Margaret Craske: ''She teaches you to know what you're doing. You just don't copy, and do exercises. She gives you self-reliance. I know what she has taught me. I can teach it to someone else.''*

But the analytic approach, like the action-oriented one, has its pitfalls. Excessive analysis tends to paralyze movement rather than illuminate its art. A class with too much talk and repetition loses momentum, and if the wait between exercises is too long, the muscles cool off and cannot function efficiently. Students forced to stand around and listen may not get the workout they want and need. Dancing is above all a physical activity, and to be effective the analytic teacher must maintain a healthy balance between thought and action.

*From John Gruen, *The Private World of Ballet*.

On the whole, analytic teachers are best for beginning dancers because they are easy to follow, and they allow more practice time. There is less chance of developing bad habits or injuries with this kind of teacher, and the analytic method lays the most solid foundation for advanced study.

Analytic teachers are frequently dancers who have had to surmount physical difficulties themselves and as such they have a better understanding of how different bodies work. For this reason students with such problems as curvature of the spine, tight muscles and tendons or chronic tension are wise to study with them; so are dancers recovering from injuries or getting back into shape after a leave of absence.

Special interests / class emphasis. A dance teacher can teach you only what she knows. Thus the emphasis of the class will shift from teacher to teacher, according to their diverse backgrounds. Each will bring out different aspects of your dancing. Be aware that these are all choices—not inflexible answers—and try to find a teacher whose interests and objectives meet yours.

For example, some instructors get you very strong, others stress style and musical phrasing. Some train dancers to see and repeat movement accurately, others encourage individual interpretation. You may learn to dance with smoothness and control from one teacher, while another may urge you to take risks in order to push yourself further physically. One instructor may teach you to use your arms well; another may excel at teaching turns; another may give you a fine awareness of line. There are a few teachers, choreographers mainly, who have a genius for creating beautiful movement for class. Choreographer Lar Lubovitch has said of Antony Tudor, who was his ballet teacher at Juilliard:

> *Tudor choreographed phrases in his class which were so exquisite to dance that the whole sense of dancing them was, in itself, having mastered the technique. Just being in his class was a glorious dance.* *

Agnes de Mille used nearly the same words to praise Martha Graham's technique exercises:

> *The progressive workout is a collection of tiny dances, all lovely, all shaped and concluded, and all providing transition to the next group, so that even as he sits on the floor and starts the first contractions, the student is, whether he knows it or not, absorbing performance technique and, what is more subtle, dance form.* †

*Ibid.
†From Agnes de Mille, *To a Young Dancer.*

A Rogues' Gallery

"There is a kind of teacher who teaches class to her two prized students and ignores everyone else. There you are dancing your heart out, and you feel like the Invisible Man."

"I had a teacher who explained in repetitive detail the most elementary steps, which she had us practice over and over ad nauseam. Many days there wasn't even a pianist to break the boredom. All of a sudden, in the last twenty minutes of the class, she'd give us a combination from the last act of *Sleeping Beauty* or some other ballet, full of pirouettes and fast jumps and long balances which, of course, we weren't the least bit prepared to do. Her class went from the absurdly basic to the absurdly difficult."

"We would do a warm-up on the floor, which ended in a series of stretches. There was one in particular that was very uncomfortable to stay in for any length of time. The teacher would get us into this really excrutiating contortion and tell us to hold it—while he left the room for a quick smoke or chat with the secretary. By the time he came back we'd be practically blue in the face. It was sadistic."

"I was in an adult beginner ballet class taught by a Russian dancer from the Kirov Ballet. We certainly were a motley crew: There were young actors in their twenties, overweight housewives and silver-haired senior citizens with varicose veins popping through their tights. The class was supposed to make you feel good, but it was more like a concentration camp commanded by this teacher with dyed red hair plastered onto a purply rouged face—you know the kind, wearing heavy blue mascara and mauve lipstick. She must have expected a class full of lithe young swan queens, because she showed her contempt for us every chance she got. I guess there is no such thing as an adult beginner class in Russia. She would say to me, 'you don't have to do every step,' as though I was too hopeless to even try. I felt so ashamed of my unsvelte body and that I hadn't been studying ballet for ten years."

"One teacher spent the entire class admiring himself in the mirror. He was always taking deep breaths and expanding his chest and then staring at it. He'd give splits ten minutes after the class started, which was something his body could do easily. But I wasn't warm enough. I thought my legs were going to snap off."

Body type and movement preferences. Just as you have distinctive physical features, favorite ways of moving, and strengths and limitations as a dancer, so does your teacher. Consider her body build, the way she moves and the kind of movements she prefers in class.

A dance teacher composes the warm-up exercises and dance combinations, their timing and sequence, according to what works best on her body; but this may not necessarily work for you. An instructor who is loose-limbed and supple may start the warm-up with lots of stretching exercises because they are easy for her to do. You, on the other hand, may be a bit stiff. You may like the idea of loosening up with soft, spongy movement, but need to do it later in the class after you've had more time to warm up. Stretching when your muscles are not ready only creates more tightness and congestion and aggravates the tendency to grit your teeth and force your body.

Your teacher's way of putting steps together may or may not mesh with your own body logic; it may or may not click with your movement preferences. Maybe she always turns to the right when your body wants to turn to the left. Maybe she doesn't jump enough in class, or perhaps her tempo is too fast or slow. Some teachers like to challenge their students with intricate spatial patterns and tricky rhythms, while others give simple, straightforward movement with a natural musical flow, the kind you can let your body respond to instinctively. How do your movement choices compare with your teacher's? It is always more difficult to dance against the grain of your natural inclinations.

Other teaching variables

Pacing. Although in general action-oriented teachers give faster classes than do analytic ones, each dance teacher has her own characteristic pacing. Following it is like riding a wave in the ocean. If it comes at you too fast you are overwhelmed; if it is too slow you remain at a standstill. But if the wave catches you at just the right speed, its impetus will carry you much farther than you could go on your own powers. Some energetic instructors give hard-driving classes from start to finish; others begin slowly and gradually work up to a peak of intensity; and there are teachers who wind down with a quiet exercise at the end of the lesson. Of course, large dance classes and classes for beginners need to move slowly regardless of the teacher.

As you gain experience, you'll come to know the speed at which you work best. The pacing of a dance class should not be so slow that your muscles cool off between exercises, nor should it be so fast that you feel unprepared.

Counted or uncounted rhythm. There are two different ways of teaching dance rhythm: counting, or keeping time with vocal and other sounds. Some dancers find that counting the rhythm of a movement ("ONE-two-three, TWO-two-three") gives them a clear-cut framework within which to learn. (Incidentally, these are "dancer's counts," as opposed to musician's counts, because they are based on the timing and dynamics of the movement. They are an endless source of confusion to musicians.) Other students, who are bewildered by the numbers involved and have difficulty remembering them, prefer a teacher who keeps the pulse by singing ("DEE-da-da, DEE-da-da"), finger snapping, hand clapping or the like. This method lets the dancer feel the music and gets the rhythm directly into the body without the need for mental calculation.

Procedural differences. Some teachers work on certain steps or movements on certain days of the week (turns on Monday, balances on Tuesday, jumps on Wednesday, and so on). Others design classes that grow more difficult as the week progresses. Still others add more steps each day to the long dance combination at the end of class until, by Friday, their students have learned a full-length routine. All these stratagems assume daily class attendance, and may pose problems for dancers who study infrequently.

> *Good dance teachers are teachers by knowledge and conviction, not disappointed dancers, nor even practicing successful dancers who may be pulled away by the constant demands of a performing career. The performer who cannot teach can be as upsetting as the teacher who has no real knowledge of the subject. Not even all fine choreographers make good teachers, although they may be inspirational to those few advanced enough to profit by a master's advice.*
>
> —*AGNES DE MILLE,*
> **To a Young Dancer**

Chemistry. Never underestimate the effect your teacher's personality has on you. Make sure you feel comfortable with the person at the front of the room. In dance class as in life, some relationships take root and others don't. Try to find a teacher who speaks to you and whom you care about in return; someone, as my friend Ernie Pagnano says, whom "you not only respect as a teacher but trust as a person." One characteristic that always gets good results is a sense of humor. And you'll always want to do your best for a teacher who shows outright that she cares. Unless she is a full-blown messiah, there is no reason to put up with an instructor who is bored, insulting or temperamental.

Age is an aspect of teacher-student chemistry that is sometimes overlooked. Older teachers have had years of experience to develop and refine their methods. The good ones acquire an ease and clarity about teaching and can quickly see through to the heart of a problem. Teachers with their performing careers behind them are less apt to compete with students, and, what is terribly

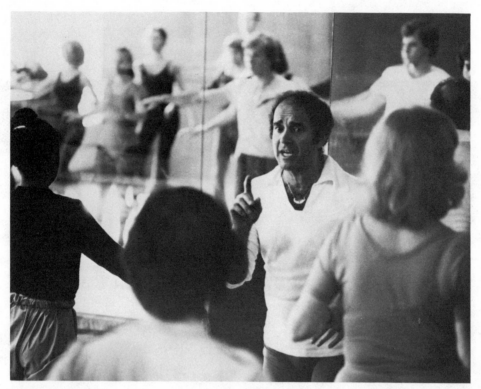

Bob Audy giving students a few pointers. *Frank Gimpaya*

important to young dancers, they serve as living links to past tradition. To hear, for example, octogenarian Vincenzo Celli talk about his teacher Enrico Cecchetti and his contemporaries Anna Pavlova and Vaslav Nijinsky is to inherit part of their legacy. A recent graduate of the School of American Ballet said of her teacher, former ballerina Alexandra Danilova: ''She knew the Balanchine ballets as they were originally danced, and she taught us about performing—the way she dressed, the broaches and scarves she wore, the way she even walked into a room. She taught us about soul.''

Young dance teachers have energy and physicality to offer. Their ability to demonstrate movement full out is both helpful and inspiring. Classes taught by younger instructors reflect today's tastes and technical advancements. If you are young yourself, you may be more at ease around a younger teacher with whom you feel you have more in common.

There are as many different kinds of dance teachers as there are people. You'll know instinctively when you find the right one. Go with your gut reactions.

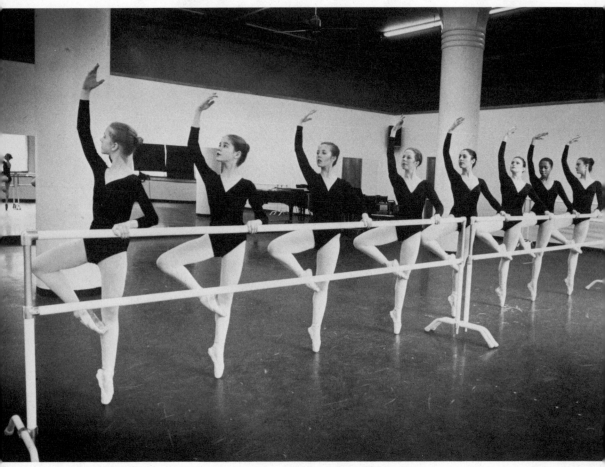

Michael Edwards, courtesy of the School of the Cleveland Ballet

12

Schools

*what to look for
in a dance school;
other places
to study dance*

Incredible as it seems, nearly half the dance studios operating in the United States were founded in the 1970s. Apparently overnight a bumper crop of schools has sprung up in such disparate locations as storefronts, suburban shopping centers, industrial lofts, churches and YMCAs. Today as you walk down the street, instead of seeing rows of pin-curled matrons sitting under beauty parlor hairdryers, you're likely to catch a glimpse of brightly clad dancers warming up at the barre.

But there are no government licensing requirements to regulate this unprecedented growth, and virtually anyone who can pay the rent can open up a dance school. Without any established standards to use as guidelines, how then should you go about choosing a place to study from the thriving but confusing variety available?

It's not always easy. Age and reputation are frequently used as indicators of a dance school's competence, yet the caliber of instruction varies so widely among the ones that survive that you cannot select a school on these grounds alone. While it is true that a school that has been in existence over ten years must be doing something right, and word-of-mouth reputation is often the most reliable kind, in dance training what is one dancer's meat can easily be another's poison. Besides, there are some excellent dance teachers who don't advertise and are scarcely known outside a small circle of devotees.

Through the years all dance schools undergo internal changes in administration, faculty and student enrollment which can profoundly affect their performance. Some of the older institutions rest too heavily on their reputations and, like elderly dowagers, become insular and set in their ways. New schools are often more eager to please and imaginative in programming classes. However, it takes about five years for a new dance school to prove itself, and during this time there may be a high turnover of teachers, with classes that are maddeningly uneven in quality. So although age and reputation can furnish some clues, in the end each school should be judged on its own merits and according to whether it meets your particular needs.

Not only are there more dance schools than ever before, but there is more diversity within the schools themselves. In recent years dance instruction, like choreography, has been moving toward eclecticism; and most schools now offer classes in more than one type of dance regardless of their individual specialties. The Marin Civic Ballet School in California, for example, provides jazz, modern dance and tap classes along with classical training. You can study jazz and ballet at Bill Evans' modern dance school in Seattle; and schools which specialize in musical-theater dance, such as the Gus Giordano Dance Center in Evanston, Illinois, and the American Dance Machine Training Facility in New York, round out their jazz and tap curricula with ballet instruction. Many schools offer classes in acrobatics, folk dancing or ethnic forms such as Afro-Caribbean and Spanish dance.

Keep in mind, though, that classes at a given dance school are not always uniform in quality. The jazz instruction may not be up to snuff with the ballet classes, or the tap may be better than the modern dance. It all depends on who is teaching what. Diversity can get out of hand, especially at a small school. One or two instructors teaching tap, toe, jazz and hula aren't likely to be experts at anything.

More and more dance schools are making expanded services available to students. Those in outlying areas, such as Ballet North in Fairbanks, Alaska, invite guest teachers and lecturers to conduct master classes and workshops. Many schools help find housing accommodations for visiting dancers, and some arrange for students to get academic credit at local secondary schools and colleges. The Fusion Dance School in Miami, the Nikolais-Louis Dance Theatre Lab in New York, and the Inner City Cultural Center in Los Angeles even publish their own newsletters.

Particularly in these times of rapid growth, one dance school can differ from another in surprisingly significant ways. This chapter examines some of the differences among schools and how they can affect you. Alternative places to study dance, such as dance academies, colleges, summer festivals and dance camps, are also discussed.

Size. Perhaps the most obvious way dance schools vary is in size. Big schools provide a broad selection of classes and instructors, and that is an enormous convenience if you wish to sample several at a time. Most sizable schools are associated with professional dance companies; they have the prestige and money to attract renowned teachers and to support scholarships. Such obvious enticements draw talented students. Hence, big schools can offer you the chance to study with dancers who are considered to be promising and, in the advanced classes, with ranking professionals.

Big dance schools serve as watering places for the dance community in their locales, where dancers, teachers and choreographers mingle and exchange news. Many of these schools are active information centers; their bulletin boards are crammed with notices of classes, concerts and other upcoming dance events, as well as job and apartment listings. If you want to know where to get a good massage, or which companies are coming to town on tour, or where the important auditions are being held, chances are that someone at a big school will be able to tell you.

There is a certain glamour and excitement to the well-oiled, fast-paced activity of a big school, yet due to the sheer size of the operation students may be treated impersonally. The biggest dance schools have upwards of a thousand pupils, and although enrollment may be limited, classes are apt to be large. You may not get the kind of individual supervision you need. In the extreme, such conditions can create a tense, competitive atmosphere.

Those who are looking for more relaxed and intimate surroundings may prefer a dance studio with a total student population of under four hundred. Most American dance schools fall into this category. Smaller does not necessarily mean inferior. On the contrary, there are certain benefits which only small schools can provide.

It is not unusual to see dogs, babies, plants and other homey touches around a small dance school. Its image may be less glamorous and its faculty less well known (though that is not always the case), but the small school invariably has a comfortable, informal feel to it. Since classes are not crowded, there is more personal attention to go around and less competition for scholarships. And payment terms are likely to be more flexible at small dance studios.

Entrance requirements. Because they are dependent on student fees to meet operating expenses, few American dance schools can afford to have stringent entrance requirements. These are usually reserved for scholarship programs. Several schools, however, have minimum age requirements, ranging from four years old for some ballet schools to high school age for schools that specialize in modern dance or jazz. Some dance schools may ask that you take a minimum number of lessons per week. Others, such as the School of Creative Arts in Salt Lake City and the Martha Graham School in New York, reserve the right to place students in appropriate classes. This saves time and trouble for all concerned and helps dancers progress faster. But mistakes are made occasionally, so if you feel you've been assigned to a class that is too fast or slow for you, talk it over with your teacher, and if necessary get a second opinion from another faculty member. You will generally find entrance regulations listed in the schedule of classes or the school brochure.

Facilities. Dance school facilities range from clean and spacious to dingy and cramped, with stopped toilets or only cold running water. These days just about all schools have dressing rooms and bathrooms, and many of the new ones are equipped with showers.

Practice studios also vary considerably. Some have adequate barres and mirrors and recently-tuned pianos, others don't. It goes without saying that dance classrooms should be well heated and ventilated, and their floors should be properly surfaced and have good rebound for jumping. But some floor coverings are sticky or slippery (both can cause injuries) or hard (if you jump on a hard floor long enough, you'll probably end up with shinsplints, knee trouble, or a sore back). Wood floors have been known to warp on occasion, leaving holes and bumps to stumble over, and heavily traveled Marley floors can stretch and buckle too.

It is possible to compensate for some minor floor deficiencies. If you are wearing ballet shoes, rosin or cleansing powder will give you traction on a slippery surface. If you are dancing without shoes, a dab of glycerin on the soles of the feet will reduce slippage, and a light dusting of talcum powder will help smooth your way across a sticky floor. But before using any foreign substance on a dance floor, get your teacher's okay. There is always the possibility that this may damage the surface or create problems for dancers working in the studio after you.

Now you may find a teacher who is so good that you are willing to put up with a few inconveniences for her sake. Often it is a matter of degree. Poor facilities can be merely irritating or downright hazardous—as in the case of a too small classroom. At best, overcrowding cramps your style, forcing you to spend the entire lesson holding back, watching out for other students and muttering to yourself. At worst, if the teacher is not alert, an overpopulated classroom can result in rather bad collisions.

Tuition. The average price of a single hour-and-a-half dance class is between $4.00 and $5.00. To this some schools add an annual or "one-time-only" registration charge of anywhere from $4.00 to $10.00. Special courses and workshops are normally priced separately, and different fees may be charged for different classes. For instance, ballet classes may cost more than jazz, and often children's dance classes are less expensive than adults' because they are shorter. Most dance schools give discounts to students who buy several classes at a time in a series card or semester package and, on a sliding scale, to students who take two or more classes per week (the more lessons you take, the less they cost). Lower rates are frequently offered to families with more than one child enrolled at the school, and to professionals—dance teachers and dancers who are union members. Professional discounts are also sometimes extended to advanced students who are training intensively for dance careers. Personal checks are almost always accepted at dance schools.

School policies vary, but by and large classes bought by the month or

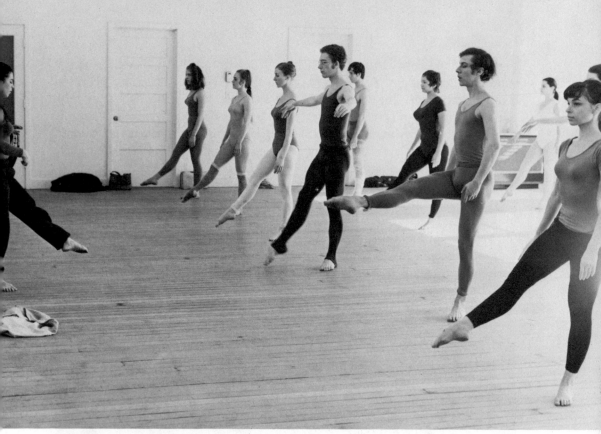

Modern dancers need good dance floors because they work barefoot. *Herman Arrow, courtesy of the Xoregos Dance Studio, San Francisco*

semester have to be made up or forfeited if missed. Students with series cards (five to ten classes purchased at a discount) are usually given a few months to use up the lessons before the card expires. This is the school's way of ensuring teachers that class attendance will not go up and down with the weather. Each dance school also dictates its own payment terms. You may be asked to pay the entire fee in advance or merely to make a deposit and pay the rest in installments. Tuition is nonrefundable, as a rule.

Scholarships. Scholarships offer much more than financial relief to an aspiring professional. Scholarship students are recruited from the best dancers in school. They are given special attention and encouragement in class, and special opportunities to develop. Most schools with extensive scholarship programs establish them to foster young talent for their affiliate dance companies, and a good many students on scholarship do eventually find jobs with these professional groups.

Most scholarship awards are decided by audition, although at small schools they may be based on the student's performance in classes over a period of time. Applicants are judged on talent, dedication and financial need. If the auditors are looking for future company dancers, a particular body type may be sought. By and large, ballet schools grant scholarships to intermediate and advanced students after their bodies have matured and their professional potential can be determined. The School of American Ballet, for instance, gives the bulk of its scholarships to fifteen-and sixteen-year-olds. Boys are accepted at slightly older ages since they mature later than girls. Schools that specialize in modern dance or tap and jazz may accept scholarship students through their early twenties. Scholarship auditions are publicized through notices on school bulletin boards or in the local newspaper; major schools may take out ads in *Dancemagazine* or in the trade papers *Backstage* and *Show Business* (see listings in chapter 20).

Scholarship students are usually expected to study exclusively at the sponsoring school and to follow its prescribed program of training. So accepting a scholarship entails making a strong commitment to dance in general and to the school, its policies and standards of excellence, in particular.

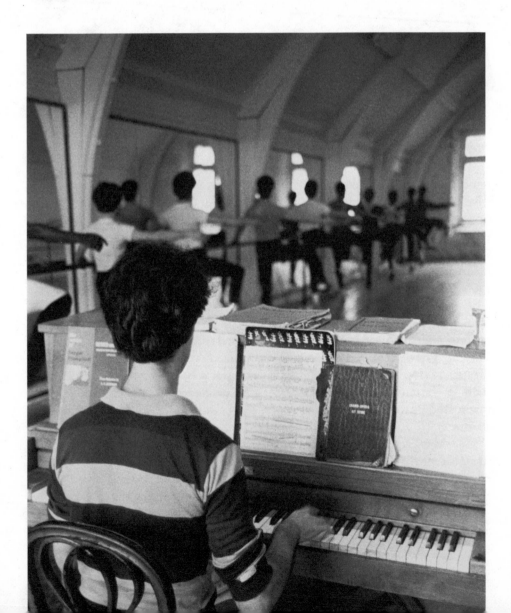

There are three kinds of scholarships. A *full scholarship* provides tuition-free study; a *partial scholarship* pays for part (normally half) of the tuition; and a *work scholarship* offers the student free classes in exchange for working at the school. A dancer on a work scholarship may be asked to man the front desk, answer phones, run errands, clean up the studio or assist at classes and performances. Some schools, such as the School of the Cleveland Ballet, and the School of American Ballet, the American Ballet Theatre School and the Joffrey School in New York, also grant short-term scholarships to students attending their summer intensive courses. Sometimes if the director of a school can't offer an official scholarship but feels you are deserving, she will try to find another way to help out—perhaps by giving you reduced tuition rates or allowing you to make deferred payments.

It is certainly no blot on your ability if you don't get a scholarship. Even for the most gifted dancer, a scholarship at a prestigious school can be discouragingly hard to win. Ballerina Cynthia Gregory was turned down three times before finally being granted one at the American Ballet Theatre School! Your best bet is to find a school where you are appreciated—and be persistent.

Musical accompaniment. As the great modern dance choreographer José Limón once remarked, we "hear music with the muscles and bones and blood and nerves." Music is the very heart of dance. It is what makes most people want to dance in the first place. It evokes moods, and helps the body remember movement by organizing it into rhythmic phrases.

Music is so important that most dance schools go to the trouble of providing live accompaniment for classes. It takes special skill to adapt a musical score to the needs of dancers. Music that is too slow or too fast, rhythmically awkward or otherwise inappropriate for the movement makes you feel as though you are running backward uphill. But the right kind of musician can discover untold riches in a routine combination of steps, as well as lend flavor and excitement to a dance class. Piano is the most commonly used accompaniment for ballet, modern dance and tap, while percussion is favored for jazz. Recorded music can be effective too, if skillfully handled.

Good music can literally transform your dancing. It can make you forget fatigue, sore muscles and the crowded bus ride to class. Violette Verdy, former ballerina with the New York City Ballet, has said, ". . . without the music I'm not that much of a virtuoso or of an athlete, I need it to give me the strength, the courage, the conviction, the desire, the pleasure, the emotion . . . to dance."* If you find a dance school that prides itself in furnishing first-rate music, you'll have a flying head start.

Class schedules and holiday closings. Classes fluctuate constantly at dance schools. New ones are always being dropped or added, meeting times change,

*From Cynthia Lyle, *Dancers on Dancing*.

teachers come and go. Most schools supply printed schedules which list current classes, teachers, fees and vacations, but these may change as often as twice a year. If you haven't been to class in a few months, it's wise to call first and confirm your information.

Most dance schools are open Monday through Saturday and closed on Sundays and legal holidays. Many follow the public school calendar, running from September to June with a shortened summer session; a few schools take breaks in winter and spring as well. But if you don't want to take a vacation, ask your teacher to recommend an alternative place to study in the interim.

Class observation. School policies vary with regard to class observation. There are convincing arguments for and against, and sometimes it is left to the discretion of the individual teacher in charge. Those who encourage visitors in the classroom claim it is good for students to get used to an audience and that this may improve their performance. Opponents believe spectators make students self-conscious—especially beginners, who should feel free to make mistakes and learn from them.

But even schools that don't normally allow visitors make some provision for parents to observe their children in class, usually by setting up special parent observation days during the year. At any rate, do check with the school before coming to watch a dance class.

Class offerings

Special instruction and graded classes. As the spectrum of dancers broadens, more dance schools are tailoring their classes to meet the diverse needs of their students and to provide them with comfortable and productive learning situations. For example, most schools today have evening adult beginner classes for dancers who are starting to train as adults. Children's classes are also widely available. Fewer dance schools offer classes for teenagers; and only a handful of major ballet schools, such as the San Francisco Ballet School, the Minnesota Dance Theatre and School in Minneapolis, and the School of American Ballet and the Joffrey School in New York, have ongoing men's classes.

Classes are more extensively graded at some dance schools than others. Several levels of beginner classes may be offered: introductory, fundamental, or basic beginner classes for students who have never been in a dance class before; beginner classes; and advanced beginner classes for more experienced dancers. There are advanced intermediate classes for students who have not quite reached the advanced level, and so on. Children's classes may be graded by age as well as technical ability. Be aware, however, that standards often differ from school to school. An advanced beginner class at one dance school may be an intermediate class at another, and occasionally one school's intermediate class may be the equivalent of an advanced class somewhere else.

A scholarship audition at the St. Thomas School of Dance in the Virgin Islands.

Non-technique classes. Besides the standard fare of technique classes, classes in related subjects such as dance therapy, history, and appreciation are available at some dance schools. Anatomy and kinesiology are taught at Raoul Gelabert's studio in New York and at the San Francisco Dancers' Workshop. Danny Daniels' Dance America School in Los Angeles offers instruction in voice and acting, as do the American Dance Machine Training Facility and the Nat Horne Musical Theatre School in New York. And classes at the New York-based Dance Theatre of Harlem include costume design.

Several dance schools sponsor teacher training courses, among them the Marin Civic Ballet School in San Rafael, California, the School of Fine Arts in Willoughby, Ohio, and the Farnworth and Hauer School of Dance in New York. The School of the Hartford Ballet has a two-year teacher certification program for high school graduates.

Although movement improvisation and dance composition courses are customarily held at modern dance schools, these studies are useful even if you are not a modern dancer. Improvisation requires no previous dance training; in fact, it seems to come more easily to those who haven't been molded by training and can respond freshly and unselfconsciously. Children are very good improvisors, but it's fun and illuminating for dancers of all ages to explore the ways in

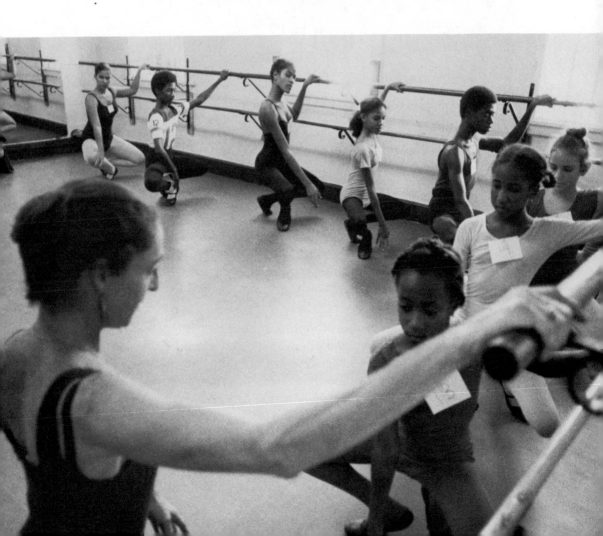

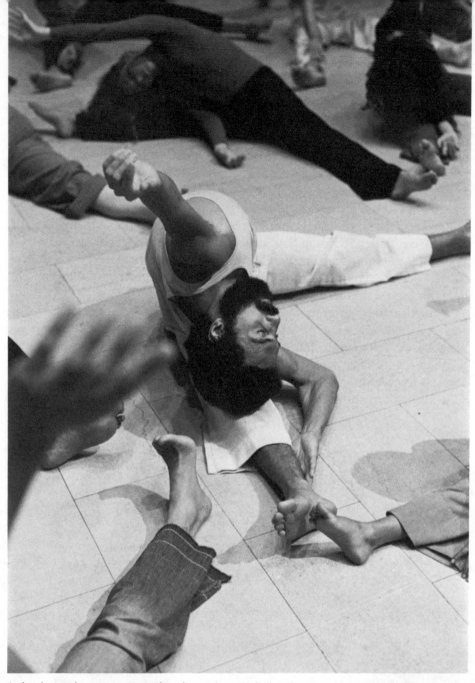

A class in creative movement exploration at Anna Halprin's San Francisco Dancer's Workshop.
Buck O'Kelly

which they move spontaneously. Improvisation classes also provide an opportunity for dancers to work together closely in much the same way as performers do onstage.

Choreography or composition classes carry the creative process into the formal craft of making complete dances. The Dance Theatre of Seattle and the Nikolais-Louis Dance Theatre Lab in New York, for instance, offer dance composition classes the year round; Merce Cunningham conducts a composition course twice a year at his New York studio; and students at the Louis Tupler Washington Dance Center in Washington, D.C. and Eleo Pomare's Vital Arts Center in New York get to show their finished works at studio performances.

Private classes and coaching. Not everyone can benefit from private dance instruction, and it should be restricted to those who can. Private classes best serve advanced students, professional dancers who need to develop audition material, and teachers. Coaching is for dancers who are preparing a role. Semiprivate lessons are sometimes available to small groups. The Academy of Dance in Wilmington, Delaware, for example, offers them to ice and roller skaters.

Beginners often ask whether they should study privately, thinking perhaps that they will progress faster with their teacher's undivided attention. In truth they have the least to gain, for the very reason that everything about dancing is new to them. They need other dancers around—to watch and ask questions of. By learning in a group, beginners get the help and moral support of several "teachers" at once.

Private dance instruction is expensive—between $10.00 and $25.00 a half hour—but fees may be negotiable depending on the individual teacher. For that matter, some teachers give free private classes to students in whom they take a special interest.

Intensive courses. These are short-term courses which enable dancers to study a technique or try out a school in a limited amount of time. Comprised of one- to six-week sessions of daily classes, they are held during school vacations so that teachers, out-of-town students and others who might not otherwise be able can

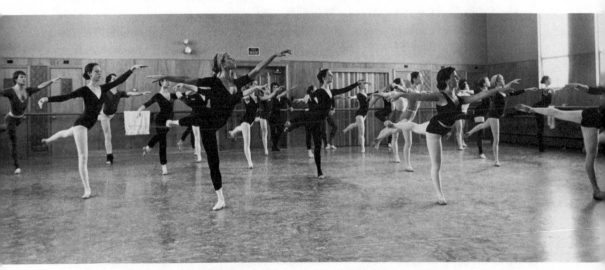

A summer master class at the Marin Civic Ballet School in California.

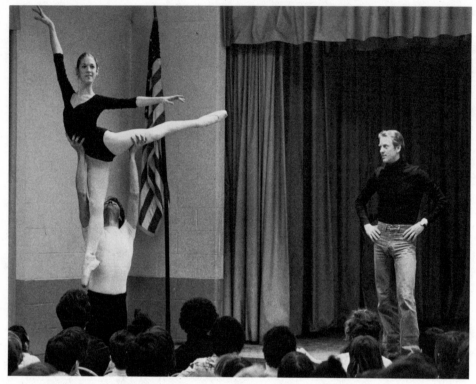

A public school lecture-demonstration conducted by the Boston Ballet's resident choreographer, Ron Cunningham. *courtesy of the Boston School of Ballet*

attend. Summer intensive courses, for instance, are given at the Connecticut Ballet School in New Haven, the Atlanta School of Ballet, the Dallas Ballet Academy, the School of the Cleveland Ballet, the Boston School of Ballet, and the School of Creative Arts in Salt Lake City. Dancers from all over the world come to New York to attend summer sessions at the American Ballet Theatre School, the Joffrey School, the School of American Ballet, the Martha Graham School and the Merce Cunningham Studio.*

Performing opportunities. Dance is, after all, a performing art, only part of which can be learned in the classroom. Realizing the importance of performing experience, a growing number of dance schools are establishing student dance companies and reviving the time-honored tradition of annual school recitals. Most of these programs are intended for young dancers, but occasionally adults participate too. Student productions not only give dancers the fun of performing and a chance to "get their stage legs," they bring dance to new audiences.

---

*For a complete listing of the intensive courses offered by New York City dance schools, see Ellen Jacob and Christopher Jonas' *Dance in New York: An Indispensable Companion to the Dance Capital of the World* (New York: Quick Fox, 1980).

Nowadays, almost every dance school provides one or more of the following performing outlets:

Annual student recitals. These range from elaborately staged concerts at local theaters to informal end-of-the-year studio showings of the students' accomplishments for family and friends. But even the workshop demonstrations are rehearsed and have the feeling of a performance.

Local dance companies. A great many dance schools are associated with student dance companies, or with semiprofessional and professional regional ballet companies (for more on regional ballet, see chapter 25). These groups perform at civic and social functions and at public schools and institutions in their communities. Some regional ballet companies engage internationally-known guest artists to dance the leading roles. The largest ones, such as the Atlanta Ballet, the Tulsa Ballet Theatre and the Dallas Civic Ballet, do limited touring.

Student apprentice programs. Many schools affiliated with professional dance companies train apprentices. Student trainees learn repertory and may do minor roles onstage. They are sometimes given a modest stipend to cover expenses. The American Ballet Theatre School, the Joffrey School and the Alvin Ailey American Dance Center maintain independent apprentice or "second" companies that are salaried, and that tour nationally.

Young students at company-affiliated ballet schools often perform when extended casts are needed for major productions such as *The Nutcracker* and *Coppélia*.

Professional company-affiliated schools. Company-affiliated schools are the official training grounds for professional dance companies. They tend to have a more serious atmosphere and more demanding teachers than other dance schools. They promise the career dancer greater access to job opportunities, and, through daily contact with company dancers who teach and rehearse at the school, a taste of what life with that company is like.

There are other advantages to attending a company-affiliated school. For one thing, classes are taught from a performer's point of view and they are charged with the excitement and energy of the stage. Technique is likely to be approached as a living process rather than a series of dry, academic exercises. As a matter of fact, you may see some dandy classroom performances from the teachers. Chances are the choreography will be better than average too, since it will probably be taken from the repertory pieces.

Especially at the advanced level, you may be able to study with the company's choreographer himself. Merce Cunningham and Erick Hawkins still teach at their schools in New York, as does Broadway choreographer Danny Daniels in Los Angeles. To see movement demonstrated and explained by its originator is a rare treat, a pure vision of his work to which ordinarily only his dancers are privy.

Other places to study dance

Although private dance schools are the primary source of dance instruction in this country, there are a number of alternative settings in which to study. You may wish to investigate these at one time or another.

Local colleges and universities. Apart from full-time degree programs in dance (see chapter 22), many colleges have schools of continuing education which hold a range of noncredit dance classes for adults. Some of them, such as the Cornish Institute of Allied Arts in Seattle, Washington, and the State University of New York at Purchase, also offer open classes for children and teenagers. Many college dance departments host summer study programs which feature guest teachers and choreographers and may be attended for credit or not. The Hanya Holm School of Dance Summer Session at Colorado College, the Green Mountain Dance Workshop at Johnson State College in Vermont, the Summerdance workshop at the University of Utah and the American University Fine Arts Festival in Washington, D.C. are fine examples. (For a complete listing of college summer programs, see the annual Summer Dance Calendar in the May issue of *Dancemagazine*.)

Dance academies. For serious dancers of precollege age, dance academies provide both academic study and intensive training in dance. Prior application and, in most instances, an audition are required for admission.

Alabama School of Fine Arts
Thor Sutowski, Chairman
Dance Department
820 North 18th Street
Birmingham, Alabama 35204
(grades 7-12; residential)

High School for Performing
and Visual Arts
Mary Martha Lappe, Dance
Coordinator
3517 Austin Street
Houston, Texas 77004
(public high school for city
residents, grades 10-12)

Interlochen Arts Academy
Suzanne Burns, Director of
Dance Department
Interlochen, Michigan 49643
(residential)

National Academy of Dance
Gwynne Ashton, Director

17 East University Avenue
Champaign, Illinois 61820
(grades 7-13; residential)

High School of Performing Arts
Lydia Joel, Director of Dance
Department
120 West 46th Street
New York, New York 10036
(public high school for city
residents, grades 9-12. Its
many successful graduates
include Eliot Feld, Rosemary
Dunlevy and Arthur Mitchell.)

North Carolina School
of the Arts
Martha Mahr, Director
P.O. Box 12189
Winston-Salem, North Carolina
27107
(grades 7 through college; state
school with low tuition for
residents)

Philadelphia College of the
Performing Arts
250 South Broad Street
Philadelphia, Pennsylvania
19102
(grades 1-12; state accredited
coed)

Walnut Hill School
Peggy Brightman and Sydelle
Gromberg, Chairpersons
80 Highland
Natick, Massachusetts 10760
(grades 7-12; residential)

The Wykeham Rise School
for Girls
Alicia Reisz, Director
Washington, Connecticut
06793
(grades 9-12; residential)

Summer festivals. These two long-standing modern dance festivals offer occasions to study with distinguished faculty and view performances by a variety of top-notch companies in an informal environment. Both promise close contact between teachers and students and maintain student dance companies which give public performances.

American Dance Festival
Charles Reinhart, Director
Duke University
P.O. Box 6097
College Station
Durham, North Carolina 27708
(919) 684-6402
Open June and July; established in 1934 and formerly located at Connecticut College. Previous performers have included the Alwin Nikolais Dance Theatre, the Erick Hawkins Dance Company, Kei Takei's Moving Earth, the Paul Taylor Dance Company, the Twyla Tharp Dance Foundation and the Pilobolus Dance Theatre. Classes are conducted in modern dance, ballet, and ethnic and jazz dance, as well as in related subjects such as choreography, acting, massage, injury prevention, dance history, dance therapy and education. In addition, the American Dance Festival sponsors a Critics' Conference for professional journalists.

Jacob's Pillow Dance Festival
Liz Thompson, Artistic Director
P.O. Box 287
Lee, Massachusetts 01238
(413) 637-1322
Open July and August. Situated on a picturesque farm in the Becket township of the Massachusetts Berkshires, Jacob's Pillow has remained essentially unchanged since Ted Shawn founded it in 1932, save for the modernization of plumbing and electrical equipment. Shawn's eclectic formula for dance education has also been faithfully preserved. There are classes and performances in modern dance, ballet, jazz and ethnic dance, and the Jacob's Pillow theater presents both foreign and American companies. Studies include dance composition and music.

Summer dance camps. These combine dance training with outdoor sports. Although most dance camps are for youngsters, the Green Mountain Academy of Dance listed below has an adult extension session at the end of summer. This is only a partial listing; for further suggestions, consult your dance teacher and check the advertisements in the spring issues of *Dancemagazine*.

Beaupré-Dance
Mrs. Stanley T. North, Director
Stockbridge, Massachusetts 01262
(413) 298-3235
(girls 9-16)

Briansky Saratoga Ballet Center
Skidmore College
Saratoga Springs, New York
(coed, ages 9-20)
Inquiries should be sent to:
220 West 93rd Street
New York, New York 10025
(212) 799-0341

Green Mountain Academy
of Dance
P.O. Box 223

Londonderry, Vermont 05148
(802) 824-5948
(girls 8-16, June 27-August 8;
adult extension, August 8-22)

Rabovsky Ballet Summer Camp
Ferndale, New York
(girls 6-17)
Inquiries should be sent to:
11-20 154th Street
Beechhurst, New York 11357
(212)767-8998

Stephens College School of
Dance and Creative Arts Camp
Steamboat Springs, Colorado
(junior high school through
college-aged women; offers
college credit)

Inquiries should be sent to:
Admissions Office
Stephens College
Columbia, Missouri 65201

Summerdance at West Virginia
University
Fine Arts Music Camp
Susan Abbey, Director of Dance
288 Coliseum
West Virginia University
Morgantown, West Virginia
26506 (grades 9-12)

Svetlova Dance Center
P.O. Box 206D
Dorset, Vermont 05251
(802) 867-5596
(girls only)

I am grateful to the following dance schools and their directors for supplying data for this chapter:

Alabama
Alfonso Figueroa
Birmingham Ballet School
1830 South 29th Avenue
Birmingham 35209
(205) 879-1047

Alaska
Joan R. Welsh
Ballet North
P.O. Box 81067
Fairbanks 99708
(907) 452-3963

California
Christopher Beck
Centerspace
2840 Mariposa Street
San Francisco 94110
(415) 861-9759

Barbara Crockett and Al Gallo
Crockett Dance Studio
3839 II Street
Sacramento 95816
(916) 452-1436

Dance/L.A. School
2504 West 7th Street, #5
Los Angeles 90057
(213) 382-2426

Karen Goodman
and Florence Tsu Sinay
Danceworks
7315 Melrose Avenue
Los Angeles 90046
(213) 933-7069

Bernice Giagni
Danny Daniels Dance
America School
310 Wilshire Boulevard
Santa Monica 90402
(213) 395-7331

Roland Dupree
Dupree Dance Academy
8115 West 3rd Street
Los Angeles 90048
(213) 655-0336

Stanley Holden
Stanley Holden Dance Center
10521 West Pico Boulevard
Los Angeles 90064
(213) 475-1725

C. Bernard Jackson
Inner City Institute
for the Performing
and Visual Arts
1308 New Hampshire Avenue
Los Angeles 90006
(213) 387-1161

Claudia Chapline
Institute for Dance
and Experimental Art
522 Santa Monica Boulevard
Santa Monica 90401
(213) 395-0456

Vera Lynn
Vera Lynn School of the Dance
469 West Fourth Street
San Bernardino 92401
(714) 888-5440

Maria Vegh
Marin Civic Ballet School
100 Elm Street
San Rafael 94901
(415) 453-6705

Steven Peck
Steven Peck Dance Studios
2855 South Robertson
Los Angeles 90034
(213) 837-3775

also at:
516 North Harbor Boulevard
Fullerton 92632
(714) 427-4725

Julie McDonald and Nina Lilly
Room to Move
312 Venice Way
Venice 90297
(213) 822-3032

Carlos Carvajal
San Francisco Dance Spectrum
3221 22nd Street
San Francisco 94110
(415) 824-5044

Anna Halprin
San Francisco Dancers'
Workshop
321 Divisadero Street
San Francisco 94117
(415) 626-0414

Virginia Storie-Crawford
Storie-Crawford Dance Theater
1329B Fifth Street
Santa Monica 90401
(213) 393-3962

Joe Tremaine
Joe Tremaine Dance Center
10960 Venture Boulevard
North Hollywood 91604
(213) 980-3336

Shela Xoregos
Xoregos Dance Studio
70 Union Street
San Francisco 94111
(415) 989-3167

Colorado
Gwen Bowen
Gwen Bowen School
of Dance Arts
714 South Pearl
Denver 80209
(313) 722-1206

Connecticut
Joseph Albano
Albano Performing Arts Center
15 Gerard Avenue
Hartford 06105
(203) 232-8898

Robert Vickrey and Robin
Welch
Connecticut Ballet School
1044 Chapel Street, 1st Floor
P.O. Box 1081
New Haven 06504
(203) 865-4936

Alice Martin DeMund
Institute for Movement
Exploration
15 Lewis Street
Hartford 06103
(203) 549-5527

Enid Lynn
School of the Hartford Ballet
308 Farmington Avenue
Hartford 06105
(203) 525-9396

Delaware
James Jamieson
Academy of the Dance
209 West 14th Street
Wilmington 19801
(302) 656-8969

Florida
William Lord and Mary Luft
Fusion Dance Company
4542 SW 75th Avenue
Miami 33155
(305) 264-0661

Georgia
Merrilee Smith
Atlanta School of Ballet
3215 Cains Hill Place NW
Atlanta 30305
(404) 237-7872

Idaho
Jeannette Allyn
Ballet Folk School
Ridenbaugh Hall
University of Idaho
Moscow 83843
(208) 882-7554

Illinois
Gus Giordano
Gus Giordano Dance Center
614 Davis Street
Evanston 60201
(312) AL 1-4434

Craig Pollock
Jack Benny Center for the Arts
1917 North Sheridan Road
Waukegan 60085
(312) 244-1660

Kansas
Judy Gillespie
Kansas City School of Dance
Ranch Mart, 95th and Mission
Overland Park 66206
(913) 642-6688

Louisiana
Harvey Hysell
Ballet Hysell
3110 St. Charles Avenue
New Orleans 70115
(504) 895-3113

Maine
Andrea Stark
Ram Island Dance Center
103 Exchange Street
Portland 04111
(207) 773-2562

Maryland
Ethel Butler
Ethel Butler Studio
5204B River Road
Bethesda 20016
(301) 652-5178

D. Foster and Carol Vaughn
Feet First Jazz and Tap
Dancing Studio
7244 Wisconsin Avenue
Bethesda 20014
(301) 656-9076

Charles Dickson
Metropolitan Academy of Ballet
4836 Rugby Avenue
Bethesda 20014
(301) 654-2233

Massachusetts
Carol Jordan
and Gerald Schneider
Cambridge School of Ballet
15 J. R. Sellers Street
Cambridge 02139
(617) 854-1557

Trish Midei
Dancers' World
268 Bridge Street
Springfield 01103
(413) 739-5318

Sandy Hagen
Sandy Hagen's Jazz
Dance Centre
295 Huntington Avenue
Room 206
Boston 02115
(617) 843-6185

Ken Estridge and Jill Greenberg
The Joy of Movement Center
536 Massachusetts Avenue
Cambridge 02139
(617) 492-4680

Michigan
Rose-Marie Gregor
Birmingham Community
House
280 South Bates
Birmingham 48009
(313) 644-5832

Carol Kimmel McKush
Carol Kimmel Dance Studio
518 East 4th Street
Royal Oak 48067
(313) 548-5060

Sylvia Hamer
Sylvia Studio of Dance
525 East Liberty
Ann Arbor 48108
(313) 688-8066

Kay Wise
Kay Wise Ecole de Ballet
1009 Maryland Avenue
Grosse Point 48230
(313) 822-2310

Minnesota
Marcia Chapman
and Hank Bourman
Minnesota Dance Theater
and School
528 Hennepin Avenue
Minneapolis 55403
(612) 339-9150

Mississippi
Thalia Mara
School of the Jackson Ballet
P.O. Box 1787
Jackson 39205
(601) 948-5768

Missouri
Stanley Herbert
Stanley Herbert Ballet
Arts Academy
7620 Wydown Boulevard
St. Louis 63105
(314) 727-1705

Nathalie Levine
and Gary Hubler
Nathalie Levine Academy
of Ballet
11607 Olive Boulevard
Creve Coeur 63141
(314) 872-7165

New Hampshire
Jean Davidson Graney
Pine Brook Studio of Ballet
37 Proctor Hill Road
Hollis 03049
(603) 465-7733

New Jersey
Yvette Cohen
The Yvette Dance Studios
118 Walnut Avenue
Cranford 07016
(201) 276-3539

New York
Alvin Ailey and Pearl Lang
Alvin Ailey American Dance
Center
1515 Broadway
New York 10036
(212) 997-1980

Edith D'Addario
American Ballet Center
(Joffrey School)
434 Avenue of the Americas
New York 10011
(212) 254-8520

Patricia Wilde
American Ballet Theatre School
3 West 61st Street
New York 10023
(212) JU6-3355

Louise Roberts
Clark Center for the Performing
Arts
939 Eighth Avenue
New York 10019
(212) 246-4818

Michael Bloom
Merce Cunningham Dance
Studio
463 West Street
New York 10014
(212) 691-9751

Dance Center
92nd Street YMHA
1395 Lexington Avenue
New York 10028
(212) 427-6000, Ext. 721

Arthur Mitchell
and Karel Shook
Dance Theatre of Harlem
466 West 152nd Street
New York 10031
(212) 690-2800

Don Farnworth, Robert Hauer,
and Charles Kelley
Farnworth and Hauer
School of Dance
1697 Broadway
New York 10019
(212) 581-0135

Raoul Gelabert
Gelabert Studios
255 West 86th Street
New York 10024
(212) TR4-7188

Linda Hodes
The Martha Graham School
316 East 63rd Street
New York 10021
(212) TE8-5886

Erick Hawkins
Erick Hawkins School of Dance
78 Fifth Avenue
New York 10011
(212) 255-6698

Finis Jhung
Finis Jhung Ballet
2182 Broadway
New York 10023
(212) 877-4740

Henry Le Tang
Henry Le Tang School of Dance
1717 Broadway
New York 10019
(212) 245-9213

May O'Donnell
May O'Donnell Modern
Dance Center
439 Lafayette Street
New York 10003
(212) 777-0744

Hope Moss
New Dance Group Studio
254 West 47th Street
New York 10036
(212) 245-9327

Julio Tores
Puerto Rican Dance Theatre
215 West 76th Street
New York 10024
(212) 724-1195

Nathalie Gleboff
School of American Ballet
144 West 66th Street
New York 10023
(212) 877-0600

Ohio
Jefferson James
Contemporary Dance Theatre
School
P.O. Box 1355
Cincinnati 45201
(513) 721-1919

Ian Horvath and Dennis Nahat
School of Cleveland Ballet
1375 Euclid Avenue
1 Playhouse Square Building
Suite 110
Cleveland 44115
(216) 621-3633

Janice and Raymond Smith
Dance Department
School of Fine Arts
38660 Mentor Avenue
Willoughby 44094
(216) 951-7500

Michael Falotico
Youngstown Academy of Ballet
260 Federal Plaza West
Youngstown 44503
(216) 746-1400

Oregon
Catherine Cassarno
Catherine Cassarno Ballet
Studio
696 McVey Avenue
Lake Oswego 97034
(503) 636-5529

Jeanne Maddox Fastabend
Maddox Dance Studio
224 Astor Building
Astoria 97103
(503) 325-3961

Tennessee
Wanda Rehfeldt
Wanda Lenk School of Ballet
5407 Harding Road
Nashville 37205
(615) 383-7541

Texas
Jerry Bywaters Cochran
Jerry Bywaters Cochran School
of Modern Dance
3541 Villanova
Dallas 75225
(214) 361-5360

George Skibine
Dallas Ballet Academy
3601 Rawlins
Dallas 75219
(214) 526-1492

Pat George Mitchell
Studio of Creative Arts
1116 North 3rd Street
Longview 75601
(214) 758-3882

Utah
Mikal Cichy Casalino
School of Creative Arts
1597 South 1100 East
Salt Lake City 84105
(801) 466-4633

Virgin Islands
Katherine Atcheson
St. Thomas School of Dance
P.O. Box 1741
St. Thomas 00801
(809) 774-4712

Washington
Bill Evans
Bill Evans Dance Company
School
Dance Theatre Seattle
704 19th Avenue East
Seattle 98112
(206) 322-3733

Martha Nishitani
Martha Nishitani Modern
Dance School
4205 University Way NE
Box 5264
Seattle 98105
(206) 633-2456

Washington D.C.
Louis Tupler and Terry Parresol
Louis Tupler Washington
Dance Center
4321 Wisconsin Avenue NW
Washington, D.C. 20016
(202) 686-9847

Wisconsin
Nikolai and Juanita Makaroff
Makaroff School of Ballet
109 East College Avenue
Appleton 54911
(414) 734-7073

Jean Paul Comelin
Milwaukee Ballet School
536 West Wisconsin Avenue
Milwaukee 53203
(414) 276-2566

13

Adding It All Up:
An Evaluation Checklist

how to quickly
size up a dance class;
how to tell whether you're
making enough progress
and what to do
if you're not

Most of us find dance classes the way we do everything else—through experimentation, happenstance or perhaps a recommendation (for suggestions on how to track down first-rate dance training in your locale, see chapter 25). Some mistakes are inevitable, but usually no harm is done unless you stay with a poor choice too long. Whenever possible, therefore, it is best to test the waters by evaluating a trial class or two before committing yourself to a series of lessons. Most dance schools will let you take a single class, and many allow you to observe classes free of charge if you arrange it ahead of time. Once you have found a class you think you can stick with, though, it is important to give it enough time to do you some good. Otherwise you will never really know what it has to offer.

Dance styles, teachers and schools are not as separate as they may seem from the analysis in the preceding chapters. The experience of the dance class is a combination of these elements and the sum total of their effect. Hence much of this chapter serves as a quick review of key points raised in chapters 10 through 12, as they arise in a real-life classroom situation. Since the perspective of time plays a crucial role in any meaningful appraisal of dance classes, the evaluation checklist has two parts. The first is a guide for choosing classes; the second, a follow-up questionnaire for use after several weeks of study.

The first day

There are two ways to evaluate a trial dance class: by taking it yourself or watching from the sidelines. When you take the lesson you feel the movement on your body and you are treated as a member of the class group. When you observe a lesson, you get a broader view and tend to notice things that a participant might not—for instance, how the students are responding to the teacher and the overall caliber of the dancing in the class. If you are a beginner who, besides being unfamiliar with this particular teacher and movement style, is unaccustomed to taking dance classes, you will probably get more out of watching the first lesson. But whichever method you choose, don't let premature judgment cloud your vision. While you're in class, try to be open and receptive. Draw conclusions after all the evidence is in.

Don't worry if your initial reactions are vague or mixed. My first lesson with a teacher who turned out to be one of the best I've known was crowded and tedious, I thought, and I didn't especially like the movement she gave. Yet despite these misgivings, something about the woman compelled me to go back day after day, until I could understand what she was trying to do—did do—for her students. In all likelihood you too will come away from a new class with an intuitive conviction that it is worth pursuing or not.

- Are the school's facilities adequate for your needs?
- Do you feel comfortable with the teacher's personality?
- Is her attitude toward the class positive and encouraging? Does she take a genuine interest in her students' progress?
- Does she seem to enjoy teaching? dancing? Does she make you want to dance?
- Does the teacher demonstrate both the form and the rhythm of the exercises clearly, so that the class seems to understand? Do you understand what is demonstrated?
- Does she use her body smoothly and fully when she dances? Does she practice correct postural alignment (see illustrations in chapter 18)? Are her movements free and unstrained?
- Is the lesson intelligently planned, with each exercise setting you up mentally and physically for the next?

- Do you feel warm after the warm-up? Do you feel that certain parts of your body are overworked, while other areas are neglected?

- Are you getting enough explanation to know what you are doing? Are the exercises repeated often enough to give you a chance to improve?

- Do you like the movement? Does it click with your body logic?

- Is the teacher's pacing right for you? too fast? too slow? erratic? Does she keep the energy of the class high?

- Does she make corrections clearly, repeating them if necessary until students show improvement? Does the teacher give enough individual correction?

- Does the music enhance the class?

- Do you feel comfortable with the size of the class and the mixture of students?

- Are the other dancers inspiring to watch? Do they move in a free and unmannered way? Do they look alive? coordinated? Are they dancing on the music? Are they breathing normally when they dance?

- For the most part, do the students' bodies look evenly developed, without any obvious muscular imbalances such as bulging thighs, swayback or flaccid arms? Are there an inordinate number of bandaged knees and ankles?

- Once accustomed to the class routine, do you think you could keep up with most of the students? Would you find it not challenging enough?

A good class has a thorough warm-up with adequate time to establish alignment and placement. The teacher should be constructive and inspiring, and should push you beyond your limits physically by increasing your range of movement and strength; and mentally, by breaking through barriers of fear. Avoid an inhibiting atmosphere in which too much discipline prevents you from making mistakes and learning from them; a frustrated, negative teacher; overcrowded classes, and rushed classes, especially the warm-up. Also stay away from classes that are so slow and intellectual that the body has no chance to incorporate what is learned into its muscle memory. Dancing is nonverbal. Words can help, but eventually you have to understand in your body.

—SARA MAULE
American Ballet Theatre

If, after answering these questions, you are still undecided about the class, talk to the other dancers. Ask whether this was a typical class. Ask why they like the teacher. Ask about other good classes and teachers at this school or elsewhere. If possible, catch the teacher after class. If you took the lesson, ask whether it was the appropriate level for you. Ask whether this was a typical class, and about any specific problems you had.

After a while

There are no fixed formulas to determine how much time you'll need to properly judge whether a dance class is working for you. It may take anywhere from a week to six months, depending on how rapidly you adjust to new situations, how often you study and how experienced you are as a dancer.

Regardless of how long it takes, the ideal time to evaluate a dance class is after you've learned the exercises and understand at least some of the basic principles of technique that the teacher is trying to convey. You should be used to the teacher and feel comfortable in the class group. Until then you cannot get the full benefit of training, much as an actor cannot do justice to a role before he has mastered his lines. Beginners and those tackling a new dance style should allow themselves a minimum of ten to sixteen lessons before making a final decision. This interval is needed just to learn the mechanics of the movement and acquire the physical stamina to get through the class tolerably well. Besides, many dance teachers leave newcomers alone to get acclimated and don't correct them for several lessons.

Of course you have to use some common sense. If the class is overtaxing your body, or the teacher is endangering your safety through negligence or incompetence, don't wait for disaster to strike. There are always a few teachers, for example, who yank their students' bodies into impossible positions or demand that they do difficult movements without adequate preparation. I'm reminded of choreographer Marcus Schulkind's little quip: "If a teacher told you to jump off a bridge in fifth position, would you do it?"

- Is the teacher sensitive to your individual needs as a student? Does he time corrections well, so that you are not overwhelmed or discouraged, yet keep growing and progressing? Does he know when to give you personal attention and when not to put you on the spot?

- Does he give you an appreciation of your special strengths and weaknesses (such as "You've got a lot of energy but you move with too much tension")? Does he know how to work with your body type?

- Do you continue to find his classes stimulating and enjoyable? Are they still hard on your body? If so, you are probably working incorrectly or you need to be in a slower class.

- Does the movement feel good to do? Is it expressive for you?

> *Look for good basic principles of movement, plus the individu-*
> *al freedom to explore. A good teacher provides a total learning*
> *atmosphere where there can be physical, emotional and intel-*
> *lectual growth. Avoid superficial, undefined, personality-*
> *oriented techniques, with too much imitation and not enough*
> *learning about how your own body works.*
>
> *—DON REDLICH*
> *choreographer*

Signs of progress. The best way to measure progress in dancing is not by comparing yourself to other dancers, but rather by the improvement of your own insight and ability over what they were in the past. There will always be students
in class who are more advanced and less advanced than you; what is important
to remember is that everyone has their own learning style and speed and these
cannot be compared (see chapter 15 on learning how you learn). Look for the
following signs of progress:

*You are enjoying yourself, and can do things with your body you couldn't do
before.* You are stronger and more supple. Dancing is easier, and there is less
strain. The movement feels more natural. You don't have to think so much and
can relax and feel the flow of the movement. You are able to put more of yourself—physically and emotionally—into dancing.

You are feeling new things in your body. This heightened awareness allows you
to work more deeply.

You look better. Your body proportion and muscle tone are improving. You see
longer, better defined muscles. You may even appear taller, due to improved
posture.

You can pick up the steps faster. You see more in the teacher's demonstrations
and hear more in the music.

Your dancing has consistency. You are able to get the same results over and over
again. This is the acid test for true understanding and control.

You have more confidence and a stronger sense of yourself as a dancer. This
comes both from sound technique and reliable feedback from your teacher.

Progress in dancing is as much qualitative as it is quantitative. Two
clean, well-balanced turns, for instance, are far superior to four jerky ones, hopping and bobbing around with your lips pursed and your arms frozen in space
like broken wings. Dancing an entire movement phrase with continuity and
with the right feeling and musical phrasing is infinitely more valuable than going for a single spectacular trick at the expense of the transition steps leading up
to it. Often the simplest actions are the hardest to perform successfully because

they are so revealing: plain walks and runs; clear, open arm gestures; or just standing beautifully still in space. Most dancers feel strangely exposed when they can't hide behind showy movement, but learning to be simple and direct is perhaps the greatest achievement of all.

Moving on. If after two months' study you feel you are not improving, don't stay where you are and get discouraged. Talk to your teacher after class. He may not even be aware that you are having problems and may be able to help in some way. If you think he knows you well enough, ask for a progress report. He may recommend a slower or faster dance class, or even another teacher.

Learn from your mistakes as well as your triumphs. Before going off in search of greener pastures, stop a minute and take stock of your complaints. What went wrong? Did something put you off about the school? Was it the movement that didn't agree with you? You may, for example, do better in a tap class than in ballet because you are interested in working more rhythmically or because ballet is too hard on your body; or you may want to continue with ballet but find a less competitive school or a more responsive teacher. If the teacher wasn't satisfactory, try to pinpoint the reasons why and keep these in mind as you experiment with other teachers. The clearer you are about what you don't want, the better your chances of finding what you do want the next time.

Even if you are happy where you are, what works for you at one stage in your development may work against you at another. Eventually you may outgrow your teacher or need the stimulation and fresh challenge of a new class. Remember, too, that your teacher's corrections are only one type of input. Working on your own, observing other dancers in class and onstage, seeing how people move in sports or everyday life, studying other art forms such as music, painting and sculpture—all these and more are valid sources for learning about how you want to dance.

Part IV

A leg up: Making the most of dance classes

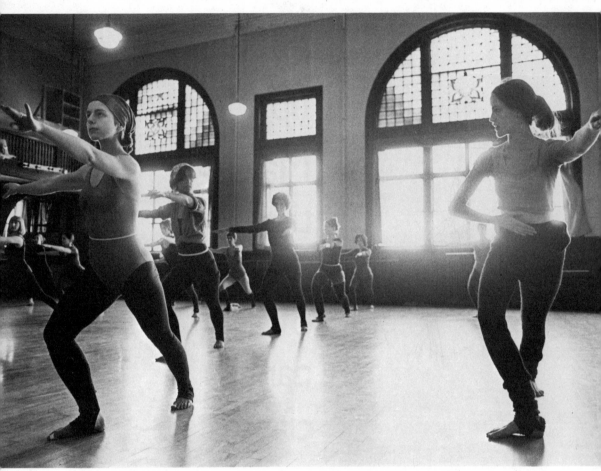

George Simian, courtesy of the Joy of Movement Center, Cambridge, Massachusetts

14

If You're Just Beginning

what to expect,
classroom protocol,
learning from
corrections

There is no one who has cooked but has discovered that each
particular dish depends for its rightness upon some little point
which he is never told.

—HILAIRE BELLOC

What to expect

Often our expectations about dancing are based on what we see on-stage—highly polished, seemingly effortless performances that are made to look even more so by the illusion of lights, costumes and makeup. But the dancers we admire are in reality the end product of many years of good training and experience. They work months in intensive rehearsals to prepare their roles, frequently under inspired direction and expert coaching. What we don't see on-stage is the rutty process of learning and creating—the imperfection out of which grow those few glittering moments of perfection. Most people never see all the bad dancing that goes on at the first rehearsals of a new piece, or the daily battles that even great artists wage to stay in shape and keep growing.

Some years ago, on assignment for *Dancemagazine*, I had occasion to observe an advanced class at the School of American Ballet. Lined up at the barre were several members of the New York City Ballet corps and, to my delight, a well-known principal dancer from the company. I expected a great show. But of course they weren't there to impress me. The same man who had given a bravura performance in *The Prodigal Son* the night before was now just another student in class. Watching him struggle to get through the preliminary exercises with a painfully stiff body, I actually felt sorry for the guy. Many times since then I've wished that I could have witnessed that scene when I first started to study dance. It would have saved me considerable worry and self-doubt.

Right off the bat, beginners can do themselves a big favor by coming to class as free as possible of expectations. Besides being unfamiliar with the movement and the teacher, you don't yet know the ropes of the very process of learning dance. It takes time, cultivation and a sense of humor to dance. Try to adopt an attitude of curiosity and self-discovery, rather than one of judgment—which can only be premature at this stage of the game. Don't expect to pick up everything at once, but be ready and willing to try new ways of moving and being with people.

Ideally, you should begin your studies in a *fundamentals, basic* or *introductory class* (the terminology varies from school to school), and many dance schools will require that you do so. Such classes will start you out slowly so you can build a firm foundation for your technique, while also getting you accustomed to classroom procedures. If there are no prebeginner classes available, a beginner class is fine—but you may have a little catching up to do and should be that much more patient with yourself.

In the beginning it is natural to feel awkward and strange. You may feel as though you are trapped inside a suit of rusty armor, or you may find your legs wobbling and unsure of where they are going. You may think you are hopelessly uncoordinated, that the rhythm of the music is eluding you, or you may simply wonder how your body is ever going to accomplish what you have planned for it in your head. You may be shy about floundering across the floor while your classmates watch.

Relax. There isn't a dancer alive who hasn't had these misgivings. When you know your classmates better, you'll discover that almost all of them feel as self-conscious as you do and are too preoccupied with their own troubles to take much notice of yours. Give yourself permission to experience and then transcend these difficulties. In dance, the way you get over shyness or stage fright or the unknown is to do the difficult things and to keep on practicing. Sometimes beginners just have to tough it out and trust they'll do better the next time. Try to move smoothly without pushing or jerking or tensing-up. Get in the habit of finishing each exercise on the music, even if you don't yet know what you are doing. The only way you will learn to dance is by getting the movement and the rhythm into the kinesthetic memory banks of your muscles. This is what dancers call "muscle memory." No matter how shaky you feel, with each attempt you develop strength and coordination. You gain confidence and you feel the music a little better. The effects of dance training are rarely immediate: They are cumulative.

In ballet, to begin to learn to dance is to be born again, know-ing nothing. The body is suddenly a stranger, deaf, uncontrolla-ble, incapable . . .

It looks simple. The teacher does it easily, simply. Plié in fifth, tendu to the side with—which foot? Not that foot? Every-body else is going in the other direction? The foot isn't point-ed? The supporting leg is wobbling at the knee, heel and toes scrabbling for purchase, and now it isn't in plié anymore, the arms are flailing, the supporting leg hopping crazily, shoulders swiveling and swaying, torso breaking, everything totally off balance, out of control, what? Staggering? Falling? What's go-ing on?

"All right, let's try it again. Fifth position, right foot in front. Plié—"

And the body won't obey, it doesn't understand. The eyes see, the ears hear, the mind thinks it understands and tells the body what to do. But the body doesn't do it, because the body doesn't understand. The body must learn. Through the help of the mind's analysis, through imitation, through trial and error. . . .

Try it again. Again. Again. Again. Feeling for it. Groping. Finding a little part of it. Losing it. Groping for it again. The body must learn. It must be taught until it knows within itself, without the mind's intervention. . . . Something happens, there is some kind of click, and for the first time, look, they dance.

They dance!

—FRANKLIN STEVENS,
Dance as Life

Let your teacher help you. That's what she's there for. Feel free to ask questions if you don't understand. Watch the good dancers in your class; you can learn a great deal from them. Ask your teacher or an advanced student to help you after the lesson. If you tire before the end of class, sit out and observe. When your legs are trembling and buckling under you it's time to stop. A grad-ual regimen is best for those who are out of shape. You might start by taking only the warm-up or the first hour of class and, as your stamina improves, work your way up to the entirety. But while you are dancing don't sit in between exer-cises. The muscles cool off and it's hard to regain your concentration once you've removed yourself to the sidelines.

If like many new dancers your muscles are tight, don't get discouraged. Remember that it is possible to increase muscle length up to one and a half times with regular stretching. In your very first dance class you will probably experience the "stretch reflex," that unpleasant recoiling of the muscles when you try to stretch them beyond their customary resting length. This is nature's way of protecting them from overstretching. The shorter your muscles, the sooner you will feel them tug back. But if you stretch a little after every class—when you are warm—eventually the muscles will lengthen and you will be able to go much further before you feel resistance from the stretch reflex.

Stretching is also much easier if you think of letting go in the muscles and allowing the energy to flow through them, rather than forcing or holding them in a rigid position. Deep breathing helps too; in fact, some teachers will have you do breathing exercises while stretching. If your muscles are very tight, try alternating *ballistic* stretching (controlled bouncing in and out of the stretch position) with *static* stretching (maintaining the stretch position for thirty seconds to one minute before releasing; this method entails ignoring the discomfort of the stretch reflex, but it has less tendency to cause muscle soreness and tearing). Suppleness is so essential to good dancing that many dance schools offer special *stretch classes*, where there is concentrated work on limbering the body.

Classroom protocol

A dance class is a cooperative venture that depends on certain ground rules for its success. As a beginner, one of the first things you have to learn is the conventions of the classroom. Arising out of practicality, tradition and performance requirements, they hold true everywhere, whether you study in Omaha, New York or Paris.

When you walk into the dance studio you may notice a pile of dance bags deposited under the piano or some such out-of-the-way place. To avoid petty thievery—which sometimes occurs in even the best schools—take your valuables into the studio with you and park them where you see the others. Especially in crowded classes, some dancers arrive early to reserve a favorite place at the barre or on the floor by leaving a towel, ballet slipper or other article of clothing as a marker. You may wish to do the same.

Once the lesson begins, the basic protocol is that you come to class on time, alert, properly dressed and ready to dance. These simple requirements are not mere etiquette but are vital to getting the full benefit of the class. If you miss part of the warm-up, for example, you won't be physically or mentally prepared and you may risk injuring yourself later. It's only fair—particularly if you are in a class with more advanced students—that you pay attention to the teacher. Stay alert, so that others' time isn't wasted by needless repetition of instructions. Excessive talking, letting your mind wander, hanging back and hold-

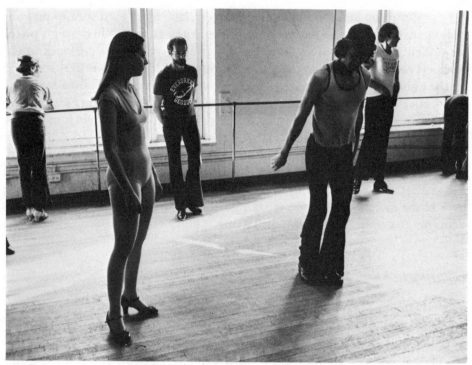

Frank Gimpaya

ing up a line are all drains on precious class time. If you are unclear about the movement, go to the end of the line or stand near the back of the room where you won't be in anyone's way; then take your turn wholeheartedly, mistakes and all.

Most especially, be aware of your neighbors as you move. It's an important part of dancing. Crowding and bumping are not only distracting and annoying, they can be hazardous in a studio full of moving bodies. Before each exercise begins make certain that you have enough room to stretch and extend your arms and legs in all directions or to travel where necessary. If the dancer in front of you is drifting into your space it is perfectly all right to ask him or her to move up. When dancing in a line across the floor, keep moving or the person behind you won't have anywhere to go. If you blank out or get lost, whatever you do, don't stop. Keep the pace of the dancer in front of you, even if you have to wing it. When changing from barre work to center floor, or from the center to lining up to move across the floor, get there quickly and be ready to go in turn.

In most dance classes the more advanced students stand in the front line during center work and go first across the floor. They serve as models for students who are less sure of the combinations. Use them as examples, but with a grain of salt. They are students too, and they can make mistakes. If you get overdependent on following others, you'll never know how to do anything yourself. And you'll be in trouble when you are moved to the front line.

Once you feel comfortable in a dance class, it's a good idea to periodically change your spot at the barre or in the center. Some teachers assign places for students to stand; but if placement is left up to you, don't get stuck in the back left corner of the room every day. During one class each week try standing on the right side, or in the center. You don't want to learn the routines from one perspective only, or to be hidden most of the time from the teacher's correcting eye. If you always rush to the front, other dancers won't get their turn for the teacher's attention.

Be sensitive to the codes of behavior in your class. Classroom protocol varies slightly with each teacher. For example, in some classes students applaud the teacher at the end. Some teachers don't mind if students practice in the back of the room while others are taking their turn in the center; others ask students not to because they find it distracting.

Learning from corrections

Most beginners make the mistake of being afraid to make mistakes. There will be times when you are so unsure of yourself that you will be tempted to hide behind a classmate, fudge an exercise or sit it out entirely. But you cannot be noncommital about dancing. Either you do it or you don't. If you don't make visible blunders that come from an all-out effort, you won't get corrected and you won't improve. There is nothing to be embarrassed or apologetic about. Nobody expects you to get it right the first time. Only when you make clear mistakes can your teacher see where you need help; and a correction is an indication of her belief in your ability to progress. If you are not certain of a step, do what you think it is. Then you'll have a definite starting point.

Much of the learning process in dance has to do with applying corrections. A teacher may correct students by giving verbal instructions, by demonstrating the mistake and the right way, or by physically manipulating the student's body into the proper position. You can learn from corrections, whether they are directed to you, to the whole class or to another student. Sometimes it's easier to relax and absorb criticism when class attention isn't focused on you. When the teacher corrects someone else, take that time to apply the same criticism to yourself. Are you making the same mistake? Are you making the opposite mistake? Watch the correction as it is made on your classmate; transfer it to your own body. Can you *feel* what you have just *seen*? Learn to observe other students when you are not dancing yourself; notice their errors, see what they are doing right, how and why, and eventually you will become your own teacher.

Be open and receptive to the instructor's criticism of your work. Even if you think you are doing the exercise the way it was demonstrated, there is often a gap between what you feel in the body and what the teacher sees. Sometimes a correction doesn't take hold right away—that is, you may not understand it immediately or be able to make the change physically at the time. But if you work steadily, keeping it in mind, eventually you will find that you are able to accomplish the task. In Mary Clark and Clement Crisp's book *Understanding Ballet* ballerina Natalia Makarova talks about long-term results:

> . . . I know that even if I put all my concentration and effort into something I want to achieve the result is never immediate. You work on something so that some day there will be a result—but it is a long-term result. When I was a younger dancer I was impatient and looked for immediate results; and I never got them. Then suddenly, after a year, there came the result of what I had done a year before.

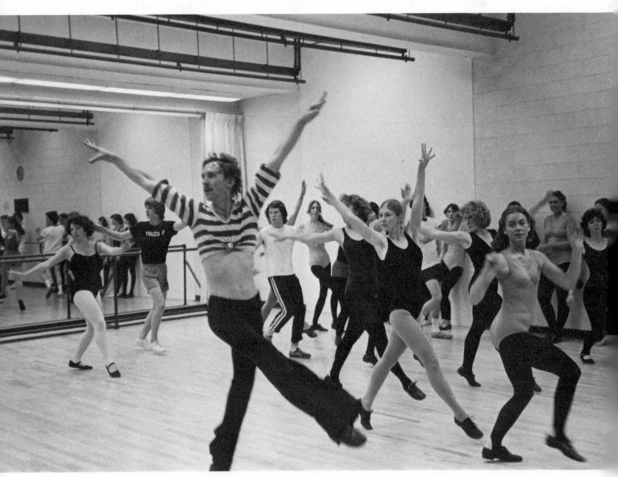

Everyone has their own way and rate of learning to dance. *courtesy of the Joe Tremaine Dance Center, Hollywood, California*

15

Treating Yourself as an Individual in Class

learning how you learn,
dealing with limitations,
warming up and cooling down,
day-to-day variability

Learning how you learn

When learning new material, musicians play from a written score and actors read their lines from a script, but a dancer has to memorize every move she makes. You cannot dance well unless you have a clear idea of the steps. Learning to accurately see and repeat movement is therefore a critical part of dancing.

There is no right or wrong way to do this. You'll get all sorts of suggestions from teachers and other dancers. Try them out, but realize that they may or may not work for you. Eventually everyone finds his or her own learning tricks. Some people need words and analysis in order to absorb new movement, while others seem to soak it up like a sponge, without any conscious reference points. Some dancers get the general shape, direction and feeling of the movement first and fill in the details later; many find rhythm the key. Some start by learning the beginning and end of a phrase, others concentrate on the transitions, or joining steps. One dancer with a near-photographic memory for movement told me that she had a total gestalt approach to learning. ''I try to place myself inside the choreographer's body and feel what it would be like to be him doing that movement—with his body, weight, facial features and voice," she said. "I try to feel what that person is feeling when they dance."

Learning movement involves all the senses. It is not strictly visual, not purely rhythmic; it is also kinesthetic and intuitive. It doesn't really matter where you begin. The secret is to begin with a receptive mind and to go with whatever works for you. Open up your intuitive antennae and trust that learning goes on at many levels. Don't worry if you don't always know intellectually what your body is doing. Often the body understands before the mind does. Sometimes you need a different learning approach for different kinds of movement. Kinesthetic or intuitive learning (feeling and doing rather than thinking) work best with natural movement that has an organic flow. Tricky movement takes conscious analysis of detail to master, and dancing that is rhythmically complex demands that, above all else, you pay close attention to the rhythm and music.

Dancers have different learning speeds, too. Unless you feel grossly out of place in your class, don't get flustered if you learn at a slower or faster rate than other students. Ultimately this has nothing to do with talent or ability, and there are advantages and disadvantages to both. Facile learners are a godsend to teachers, and they frequently become the unofficial demonstrators for the class. But their very speed may rob them of the opportunity to digest all they take in, and they have a tendency to be superficial. As a slow learner, I have found that although—or maybe because—it is a struggle, once I learn a step it becomes a part of me, as if I had choreographed it myself. Never throw yourself into movement you don't understand just to keep up with the rest of the class. A quick snap of the head or a hastily planted foot can easily give way to injury. Instead walk through the combination, slowly if you have to, in the back of the room where you'll be out of the way.

Naturally, the more familiar you are with your teacher's way of moving, the easier it is to pick up her steps. Mental attitude is also important. From time to time all dancers have to be reminded that they are not in class to look good. Don't berate yourself for making mistakes. You'll only create mental blocks and make it harder to try again. Don't forget that the dance class is a laboratory, a place to work and to try new things. You are there not to hide your mistakes but to learn from them. Not worrying about how you look frees you to get fully involved in what you are doing. And the more actively you take class, the more you'll get out of it. Teachers respond well to students who ask questions, try hard and contribute as full human beings. Learning is a partnership, after all.

Another thing to keep in mind when learning new movement is that no two dancers look or move alike, due to individual differences in physique, timing and movement quality. Long, lean people look different doing small, quick movement than short, compactly built people, though they may be equally skillful. A lyrical adagio doesn't have the same impact on a stocky, muscular type as it does on a willowy body. Sometimes it is hard to resist wanting to look like someone else, particularly because one learns to dance chiefly by imitating others. But expect some movements to register very differently on you than on your teacher or classmates, and remember that this is what makes you unique as a dancer.

Limitations

Many physical limitations can be overcome with good dance training, which usually entails both remolding the body through daily conditioning and expanding the dancer's notion of what he or she can do (see chapter 2).

Say, for example, that you are having trouble with pliés. Every time you do a plié you think about how tight your muscles are and how your joints refuse to bend. In keeping with that mental image of yourself fighting to do a plié, you brace yourself by holding your body rigidly and, with grim determination, you try to force the muscles to stretch. They, of course, only jam up more and reinforce your image of yourself with a short, tight plié. In addition, faulty posture may be causing you to grab and tense your muscles just to stand up on your feet. A good teacher will correct your stance so that each body part is carrying the proper workload and the muscles are free to stretch fully (see illustrations in chapter 18). She'll give you feedback on how far your body can go ("You have much more plié than that, if only you would start the movement from your hips and relax your feet and ankles.") She'll also give you a clear picture of what you should be aiming for by demonstrating the plié with the right muscular feeling and rhythm. Eventually the tone and performance of your muscles will change in response to working them differently, and your physical range will grow along with your mental understanding of the movement. Once they are working well, most dancers discover that they have greater physical capabilities than they thought possible. But it takes time to learn to work with your body and you should give yourself the time to explore.

Slumps often lead us to make mistaken assumptions about our limitations. Nobody knows exactly what causes these temporary setbacks, but they affect all athletes. During a slump progress levels off. There may be no noticeable improvement in your dancing for several weeks, and you may even backslide into old problems. This is sometimes due to an information overload: You may need more time to assimilate new concepts and experiences. Sometimes the body isn't ready for change and needs to make connections or develop strength; or your dancing becomes stale because you need a change of pace. In the latter case, taking a short break from classes is often the best tonic. Try sports, or folk, ethnic or ballroom dancing. The best thing about slumps is that after they've blown over you'll usually find that something new has jelled for you.

But the day will come when you'll know that your leg simply won't go up any higher, your hips won't turn out any further, your back will bend only so far, and your plié will stop at such-and-such a point; to defy these structural limits is to invite injury. So at the same time that you are forging ahead, be realistic. Understand not only what you are capable of but what you really need in order to accomplish your goals. Your enjoyment of dancing and quality as a performer are by no means determined by the height of your extensions or the quantity of turns you do. In chapter 1, I noted several outstanding artists who have founded careers on their so-called limitations. Too many dancers—especially beginners—think that the most interesting thing about dancing is technical skill. They don't realize that the most interesting thing to watch is themselves and that technique is only exciting when it is given meaning and expression by a complete person.

Warming up and cooling down

If you find yourself in a class where you don't feel warm after the warm-up, do your own before the next lesson. Even if the warm-up is adequate for your body, it is still a good idea to take a few minutes beforehand to center yourself and shift gears for dancing. A preliminary workout needn't be long, and it can consist of almost anything that feels good. Massaging the feet, easy bounces and back stretches, head circles, arm circles, body swings, pliés, foot brushes, yoga exercises, jogging, sit-ups and push-ups are some of the things that dancers do to get the circulation moving and gently limber the muscles. You may want to do the warm-up exercises you've learned in class, ask your teacher for suggestions or devise your own routine. On cold days or days when you feel stiff, allow yourself extra warm-up time.

After a strenuous workout it's best for your heart and helps prevent muscle soreness if you wind down gradually with stretches, easy pliés or just walking around the room for a few minutes. If you are going out into freezing weather after class, be sure you are fully dry and dressed warmly. Otherwise your muscles will contract sharply when they hit the cold. Since hot temperatures make added demands on your body during exercise, you should give yourself a cooling-off period in the summer too.

Allowing for day-to-day variability

Every person varies from day to day in terms of concentration, energy level, mood, weight, stretch, balance, timing and so many other factors. If you fell asleep last night in a twisted position, for example, you'll have some kinks to get out of your back today. You'll need to concentrate on those muscles more than usual and perhaps to do some additional stretching and warming-up before class. Having a fight with your roommate, fatigue, muscle soreness, wearing new dance shoes—all take their toll on dancing. The challenge is to learn to work in a manner that achieves consistency despite day-to-day variability. To do this you have to be sensitive to how your body is functioning each day and to be aware of those areas that want more attention on a particular day.

If you are having lapses in concentration or trouble with your turns, or all of a sudden you can't seem to hold a balance, don't let it throw you. Take the ups and downs in stride and try to work with whatever is happening. You may learn something new about yourself. Choreographer Viola Farber once told me that her best performance in class occurred on a day when she wasn't in the mood to dance and couldn't care less about how well she did.

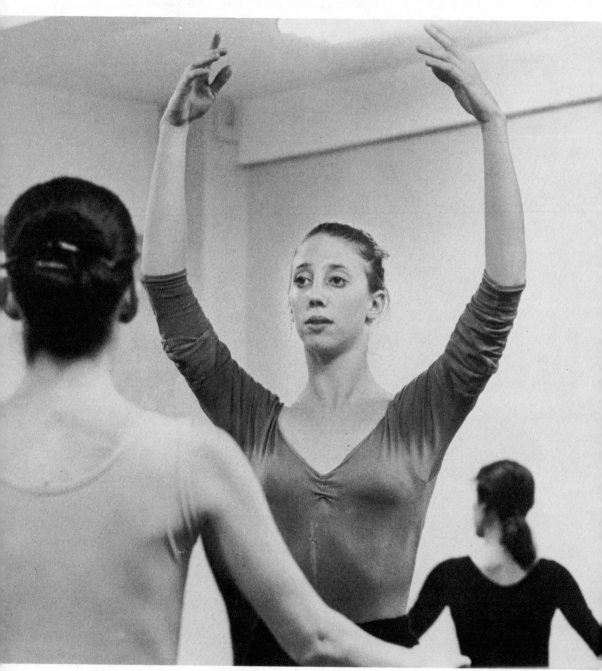

David Lindner

16

Uncommon Sense

tools of the trade,
how to tell
if you're trying too hard,
taking time out,
practicing on your own,
and other matters

Tools of the trade

Concentration. Sometimes in dance class it is hard to concentrate; then, when you make the effort, you overdo it and tense the muscles. You lean against the barre while the other students are going across the floor, and your energy drops. You work so hard at turning out from the hip that without noticing you've let your hands become spastic-looking claws. Dancing entails a different kind of concentration than most people are accustomed to. It takes relaxed effort with focus. Classes are most fruitful when you are able to clear your mind of everything else and simply concentrate on what is happening inside the classroom. If you daydream or let your thoughts drift while an exercise is being demonstrated, it requires twice the effort to get started again or to pick up the combination on your own.

At the same time a dancer's concentration must be flexible. Although your mind is focused inwardly on what you are doing, you have to be aware of what is going on around you—the teacher, the other dancers, the music. You need *both* freedom and control. Like a Zen archer, the dancer often finds that the way to improve skill is by letting go rather than pushing so hard; by directing the body without forcing, by concentrating steadily, yet going with the flow of feelings and sensations and retaining the freedom to respond to spontaneous events. Once you have learned to concentrate like a dancer, you have learned a great deal.

As you gain experience, it grows easier. You find that you can be aware of what several parts of the body are doing at once, instead of feeling that one leg is enough of a problem. You can control your arms in space as you accomplish the footwork. You learn to see more details in a demonstration and take in the music at the same time. You are able to handle more corrections at once. Finishing each exercise with the music will come as naturally as collapsing once did.

Discipline. It is normal to get sidetracked sometimes by momentary doubts. From time to time everyone is plagued by fretful inner voices that interfere with dancing. "I'm such a clutz," they say, "I'll never be able to do that. What if I make a fool of myself?" But if you want to progress, you have to keep on going in spite of your misgivings. It's important to do the plié you thought would leave you stuck on the floor, to do the tap routine one more time before you despair of getting a particular rhythm, or to go up on half-toe when you fear you may fall over on your nose. It is likely to be that final go at it that sets the new skill firmly into your body. That's where discipline comes in. The only way to improve is to make yourself keep the rhythm of the music, even if it's a struggle, and to finish each exercise no matter how badly you think you've done. Dancer's discipline means coming back and trying again—*especially* when you feel discouraged.

Discipline isn't beating yourself with a strap; it's keeping yourself moving on the right track. To have feelings of inertia or resistance or fear is the nature of the human animal. But part of becoming a better dancer is learning how to cope with these distracting inner voices. Trying to silence them completely or viewing them as the enemy will only leave you tense and driving yourself harder and harder. A sense of acceptance of these common beasties, on the other hand, will usually allow you to deflect them with a sense of humor.

Breathing. The ultimate skill that every dancer strives for is to work with concentration and calm control of the body, but without tension. To achieve this, the breath is instrumental. Yogis have known for thousands of years that breathing is the key to the concentration and discipline that enables them to perform many extraordinary feats. The human breath cycle was the impulse for the modern dance styles of Isadora Duncan, Martha Graham and Doris Humphrey. Ballet dancing, which seems to mask ordinary human function, achieves its characteristic lightness and elegance with the use of breath. The inhaled breath can literally lift you in the air as you jump or are raised by a partner; the exhaled breath can pull you over into a fall or contraction. All movement must have breath and flow; otherwise it looks flat and lifeless.

Breath supplies your bloodstream with oxygen and gives you the energy to continue dancing. Deep, steady breathing makes strenuous movements much easier to do. It is curious that we tend to hold our breath at critical moments, when we need it most, and that dancers have to be constantly reminded to breathe, of all things. Breathing, moreover, is a great tension-breaker. Most of us carry around a burden of excess tension which worsens when we are under emotional stress or are making a special effort. We try to get hold of ourselves by tightening the muscles of the throat and neck, the jaw, hands, stomach—wherever we are trying to assert control. Once you tense up you are fighting yourself because the muscles can't respond freely. Dancing isn't very enjoyable in this condition, and it looks terrible. If you feel you are holding your muscles anywhere, breathe deeply and let the movement of air through your body flush out the tension. It also helps to shake yourself out between exercises, like a dog shedding water from its coat.

How to tell if you're trying too hard: distinguishing among pain, strain and healthy effort

How many times have you heard it said that good dancers make dancing *look* easy? Behind that innocuous-sounding cliché lurks a rather harmful misconception. Effortless dancing is not at all an illusion. Dancing *is* easy when you are working correctly and are in good shape. Contrary to popular belief, it isn't supposed to be labored or painful. Because many dancers expect dancing to be uncomfortable, it is often difficult for them to tell when they are courting danger by pushing their bodies too far. Dancing demands the paradox of trying not to try so hard.

Pain is a warning. Heeded in time, it can prevent injury. Pain means you are placing unsupportable stress on a body part, probably due to improper technique or insufficient strength. Here is a case in point: During a series of intensive rehearsals for a new piece, a colleague of mine repeatedly complained of foot pain but continued to work because the discomfort wasn't unbearable. Within a week she had broken two metatarsal bones, one so badly that it required surgical repair. Needless to say, she was sidelined for several months. The knee, back and ankle are the most commonly injured parts of the body in dancing, so even mild pain in any of these areas should be taken seriously. Stop dancing if you suspect trouble, tell your teacher and try to determine the cause as soon as possible. When I get careless about turning out my legs from the hips, I feel a twinge of pain in my knees. After suffering a disabling knee injury a few years ago, I have learned to stop and think about my leg alignment before taking another step (see illustrations in chapter 18).

"Grabbing," "clutching," "tensing," "gripping," "forcing" and "locking" are terms that dance teachers use to identify *strain* (not to be confused with a tearing of the muscle tissue, which is also called a strain). Steady strain on a body part can lead to injury too. I know a dancer who actually broke a rib by forcing the muscles in her torso over several years. Strain is frequently caused by improper body placement or muscular effort. Many people in our achievement-oriented society believe that if they don't work violently hard they are not accomplishing anything of value. But for a dancer this is nothing short of self-sabotage.

Make a fist, then clench it—hard. You'll see the cords popping out of your forearm. That's what strain looks and feels like. It blocks circulation and energy flow, and it tightens the muscles, making movement difficult. Try bending your wrist when it is held in a tight fist; relax and see how much more easily it flexes. Choreographer Erick Hawkins tells his students that tight muscles cannot feel or love. Strain does indeed have a deadening effect on the body. The dancer who is straining cannot feel what he or she is doing and thus loses both expression and control. However, since it is more easily tolerated than pain, strain frequently goes unnoticed for years. Watch out for chronic tightness or soreness in the back, ankles, hips, shoulders and knees. If you are gripping in the neck, grabbing in the buttocks or bracing the back by squeezing your shoulder blades together, or if your muscles are trembling, you are straining. Strain often shows on the face. You may catch sight of yourself in the mirror pursing your lips, knitting your eyebrows or clenching your jaw. Your teacher should help you to recognize when you are straining and continue to remind you until you are able to feel it for yourself.

As opposed to the tight, stiff body movement that characterizes straining, wholesome movement has energy, strength and elasticity. *Healthy physical effort* is a full, free-flowing and vigorous use of the muscles. It has breath and release and it is efficient, involving only the muscles needed to do the job. If you are not used to all-out physical work you may tire, feel shaky or breathe heavily as you dance, but it won't hurt or feel stressful. The worst result may be a charley horse the next day.

Taking time out

There are many reasons why dancers may interrupt training temporarily —vacation, illness or injury, work, lack of funds. Respites aren't necessarily detrimental. They can give you a needed perspective on dancing. If you have over-developed your muscles through strain or misuse, some time off will rest and relax them, and you may find yourself surprisingly more supple than when you were "in shape." Returning to dance class is a chance for a fresh start and, with a little patience, dancing can be better than ever for you.

But no matter how good you feel, your muscle tone, timing and coordination won't be what they should for a while, and your concentration may be a bit scattered. As a rule it takes about as long to get back into condition as it did to get out of it. If you are working daily the retraining period may be somewhat

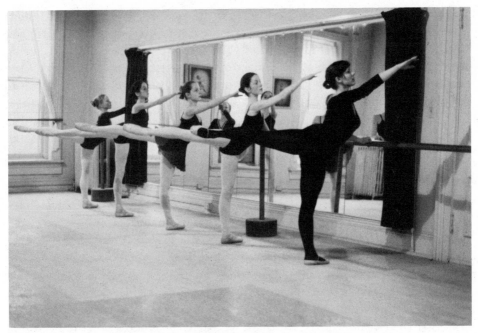

Tony Flannery, courtesy of the Makaroff School of Ballet, Appleton, Wisconsin

shorter. Take your time getting back. Work carefully and in a slower class than usual. Pick up stamina and strength gradually, don't overdo. You might take only part of the class at first and work up to a full class by degrees. Strenuous jumping should not be attempted for several weeks. If you've been weakened by illness or injury, make sure you have a teacher who will watch you closely. Use the knowledge you've retained from the past, but remain open to new ideas and sensations. If you train regularly, before long you'll be back to your former level of skill or beyond it. Keep that light in view as you work your way gently through the tunnel.

Practicing on your own

"Practice makes permanence," says Jon Devlin of Dancercise. It does make perfect if you're practicing correctly, but you don't always know if you are (tap dancers have an advantage here because they can listen for errors). For this reason, if you're a beginner you should first find out what your teacher's feelings on the subject are. She may be so wary of possible bad habits forming as a result of unsupervised practice that she advises against it until you have gained a basic understanding of the technique.

For more advanced dancers, practicing alone can be an excellent tool if used in conjunction with—not as a substitute for—classes. You have the opportunity to experiment on your own and do the exercises as slowly and as many times as you need to do them. Home practice can reinforce your class work and lead to a better understanding of how your body works. Yet even if you are an experienced dancer, there is the danger of merely reinforcing bad habits when working by yourself. Without the support of a teacher and class it is difficult to keep your energy high or to maintain a uniformly high quality of movement. It is tempting to allow the rhythm to slacken, to favor one side of the body over the other and to do what is easiest when no one is watching. Considering all these stumbling blocks, practicing alone is not generally a good idea unless you are certain that you can work productively.

Uses and misuses of the mirror

At times we all like—and need—to look at ourselves in the mirror. But the story of Narcissus and his reflection is a good one for dancers to remember when using the mirror. Undoubtedly the mirror is a valuable teaching aide. Mistakes such as incorrect body positions and postural distortions can be quickly corrected by checking in the mirror. Glancing at your reflection allows you to dance and watch others at the same time, so you can follow the class more easily. Yet the mirror can also draw you into yourself like quicksand. People who spend a lot of time "dancing in the mirror" develop a dull stare which cuts off their movement and makes them look like zombies. Every dance studio has a "fat" and a "thin" mirror—the thin mirror is the one in front of which most of the class is crowded—and some dancers use these to obsess about their weight. Probably the worst hazard of all is the tendency to become overdependent on the mirror and not be able to work without it. Dancers must know what their bodies are doing and where they are located in space by feeling rather than looking. The mirror doesn't even give you a true picture. Besides the slight distortion of the actual image, it is often necessary to alter your body position, direction and speed in order to gaze at your reflection.

17

What to Eat, What to Wear

what you put into your body
and what you put on it
can make a big difference
in your dancing

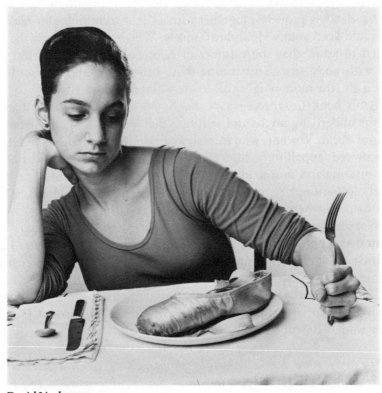

David Lindner

Dancers can obsess endlessly about diet and dress, but the basic requirements for both can be summed up in a few words: Eat the right kind of food at the right time; and dress warmly, comfortably and in such a way that your teacher can see how your body is working.

Nutrition

Like any other physical exercise, dancing demands a well-nourished body. Sound nutrition helps reduce the risk of injury by bolstering your resistance against fatigue and helping the body cells to repair themselves. You should follow a steady, well-balanced diet on the days you're dancing as well as on those you don't. In fact, you may feel the need to eat slightly more on dancing days because your body needs the extra calories. Everyone has an optimum dancing weight, at which they look and feel their best. You should be thin enough to move efficiently for your particular frame and build, but not so thin that you feel listless and look like a bag of bones.

Dancers are always trying to lose weight, but depriving your body of essential nutrients is the most damaging way to shed pounds. The dance grapevine abounds with horror stories of bones and muscles impaired by mineral and vitamin deficiencies due to fad diets. In the art of dance your body is your instrument, and its care and feeding are vitally important. The vigorous exercise that dancing provides, together with a slight trimming of overall caloric intake, should keep your weight down nicely. Weight-watchers may be further encouraged to know that the number of calories burned in physical activity increases with body size. This means that, barring metabolic disorders, the heavier you are, the more weight you'll lose while dancing.

In his book *Competing with the Sylph* Dr. L. M. Vincent explodes many of the underlying myths and attitudes that lead to rampant dietary abuse in the dance world. Vincent, who interviewed hundreds of dancers in New York City, uncovered appallingly high incidences of voluntary starvation, self-induced vomiting and misuse of laxatives and diuretics. Such cases, he says, are particularly commonplace among young female ballet students at major company schools, where competition and preoccupation with thinness are the keenest. Not only is poor nutrition counterproductive to good dancing, Vincent warns, but over a period of time undernourishment and chronic water loss may cause dehydration and kidney problems, as well as difficulty with menstruation and other sexual functions.

Chief among the self-deceptive and potentially harmful dietary pitfalls into which dancers often tumble is the "feast or famine" syndrome. Here's how one young woman described it:

> *The only time I had a weight problem was when I started*
> *skipping meals. I had just begun to dance professionally and I*

used to starve myself to look thin before rehearsals and per-
formances. It was a vicious cycle: When I was dancing I'd feel
light-headed all the time, and afterward I would spend the
night raiding the refrigerator. The next day I would wake up
bloated and feeling guilty; I'd pump myself up with vitamins
and coffee and repeat the same process. I managed to gain
twenty pounds that way. This went on for nearly a year, until for
some reason — probably because I was feeling more secure in
my roles — I went back to eating three square meals a day. I was
down to my normal weight in a few weeks, and amazed at all
the energy I had.

Even if you are not on a diet, somewhere along the line you're bound to hear that you shouldn't eat for hours before a class or performance. I think it depends on the individual. You can best determine when and how much you need to eat. If you come to class or performance so hungry that you are weak or dizzy, it will be a foggy experience. If you dance on a full stomach, you'll probably feel sluggish. In general, eating a well-balanced meal one or two hours before dancing, or a judiciously chosen snack right before, will boost your mental alertness and energy level. If you have a nervous stomach, eat two or three hours before dancing. All dancers should have a diet rich in vitamins and minerals and drink plenty of fluids to replenish those lost in perspiration. On hot days it's a good idea to add extra salt to your food to combat the effects of heat stress (see chapter 18 on keeping fit).

Another common misconception is that eating a candy bar right before dancing will give you a slug of energy. That's true in a way, but misleading, since the energy provided by sugar-rich foods will soon dissipate, depleting your blood sugar, dehydrating your system and ultimately leaving you feeling hungrier than ever. A far better snack would be fruit, fruit juice, milk or the dancer's favorite, yogurt. Both yogurt and milk supply carbohydrates for immediate spurts of energy, and calcium and protein for long-range muscle fuel. They are convenient and low in calories. Yogurt has the added advantage of being readily digestible because of its friendly bacterial cultures.

I couldn't attempt here to cover the entire subject of nutrition, but there are several good books on the subject, including Dr. L.M. Vincent's *Competing with the Sylph: Dancers and the Pursuit of the Ideal Body Form* (Kansas City: Andrews and McMeel, Inc., 1979) and *The Dancer's Book of Health* (Kansas City: Sheed, Andrews and McMeel, 1978); the excellent textbook *Nutrition and Physical Fitness,* 9th edition, by J. Bogert, G.M. Briggs and D.H. Calloway (Philadelphia: W.B. Saunders Company, 1973); Dr. Nathan Smith's *Food for Sport* (Palo Alto, California: Bull Publishing Company, 1976); and the Adelle Davis classic *Let's Eat Right to Keep Fit* (New York: New American Library, 1970).

Dress

Dance clothes are worn almost as much outside the classroom as in. Leotards, tights, leg warmers, ballet slippers, jazz oxfords and tap shoes (without the taps, of course) can bee seen at home, office and night spots. Dancer's garb seems made to order for our active modern lives; it's versatile, comfortable, easy to care for and fun to wear.

Only a decade ago dancewear was limited to a few basic designs and dreary colors. But thanks to the rising popularity of dance and the appropriation of dance apparel for fashion, today there is a riot of styles, materials and tantalizing colors to choose from. There are costumes to flatter every figure and fill every dancing need. Given the variety available, your dance clothes should express you. They should make you feel good and make you feel like dancing.

You can spend as much or as little on dance clothes as you like. The prices of a plain nylon and lycra-spandex scoop neck leotard ($9.00), a tank top leotard ($7.50), a tee-shirt (about $2.00) and tights ($6.00) are well within the average budget; while a wool leotard may cost up to $24.50 and a sleek lycra and nylon unitard (leotard and tights combined) sells for $32.00. There are numerous ways to economize, and dancers are quite resourceful about putting together practice "rags" from shreads of old clothing. Snug-fitting sweat pants and a sweater wrapped around the waist, or thermal underwear, for example, make frugal substitutes for knitted leg warmers and body suits that normally run from $10.00 to $28.00. Low-cost women's camisole tops and tube-style leg warmers manufactured by sock and hosiery companies are widely sold at department stores. Some dancers wear inexpensive plastic exercise pants (cut off at the knee or hip) instead of leg warmers, but I don't recommend these because they don't allow the skin to breathe. They crackle noisily whenever you move and get cold and clammy as soon as you stop.

Sometimes dance schools and teachers sell or give away marked-down remainders from bulk purchases of dancewear, so be sure to inquire. Bargain hunters should also keep an eye out for end-of-season sales at local stores (these are usually held in late summer and winter). Many dancewear shops sell seconds or irregulars at reduced rates and offer student discounts.

One place you definitely shouldn't skimp, though, is in buying dance shoes. Anything you put on your feet must fit well and allow full mobility. Otherwise your feet and your dancing will suffer. And who needs to be discouraged by a pair of shoes?

Some dance schools have dress regulations governing the style and color of clothes and shoes that may be worn in classes. In some dance classes, too, there is a tacit dress code, and often you will feel more comfortable if you fit in. If you are a beginner, check with your teacher before investing in new equipment. He or she will be able to recommend the best brands and local suppliers and help you with fitting problems. Never buy anything without trying it on first. Twist, bend, kick and stretch in the clothes and move around in the

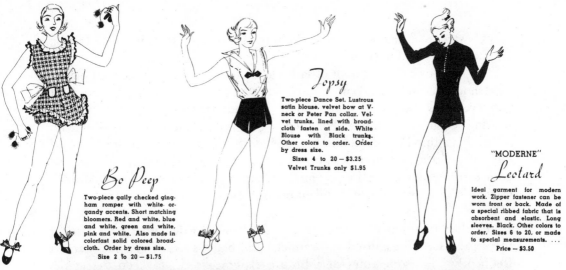

Bo Peep

Two-piece gaily checked ging-
ham romper with white or-
gandy accents. Short matching
bloomers. Red and white, blue
and white, green and white,
pink and white. Also made in
colorfast solid colored broad-
cloth. Order by dress size.
Size 2 to 20 — $1.75

Topsy

Two-piece Dance Set. Lustrous
satin blouse, velvet bow at V-
neck or Peter Pan collar. Velvet trunks, lined with broad-
cloth fasten at side. White
Blouse with Black trunks.
Other colors to order. Order
by dress size.
Sizes 4 to 20 — $3.25
Velvet Trunks only $1.95

"MODERNE" Leotard

Ideal garment for modern
work. Zipper fastener can be
worn front or back. Made of
a special ribbed fabric that is
absorbent and elastic. Long
sleeves. Black. Other colors to
order. Sizes 6 to 20, or made
to special measurements. ...
Price — $3.50

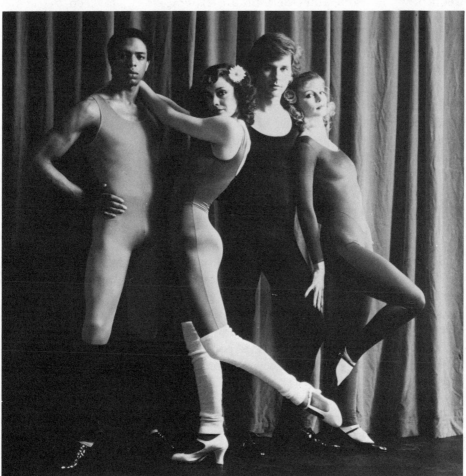

Top: What the well-dressed dancer wore in 1937, from an old Capezio mail-order catalog.

Bottom: Capezio's slick new lycra and nylon unitards with sculptured torso and leg that can be worn at the ankle or pulled over the foot. **courtesy of Capezio Ballet Makers**

219

shoes—walk, plié, relevé, jump, and point and flex your feet. If you're buying tap shoes, try out a few steps.

Although there is a lot of latitude for personal taste, in general dance-wear should feel warm and comfortable; it should let you move freely, look neat and reveal how your body is functioning. The standard way to achieve this is by wearing leotards and tights. For men, tights are pulled over a tee-shirt and rolled over a thin belt or held up by suspenders. A dance belt, which is a special kind of athletic supporter designed for dancing, is worn underneath. In this basic costume you would be prepared to take any kind of dance class, though each form adds its own details and embellishments.

Ballet. The traditional practice clothes for ballet are leotards (tee-shirts for men), tights and/or knitted leg warmers, and ballet shoes. Over this, dancers frequently add—sometimes to a bizarre extreme—socks to keep the ankles warm, sweaters, shirts, skirts and other layers which may be removed as the muscles warm up. Be careful, though, that these extras don't hide bad habits, such as locking or neglecting to stretch the knee. I am sorry to say that I wasted months of perfectly good ballet training just because I wore baggy sweat pants to class. While I had them on I never straightened my knees, nor did I get corrected for this. When I stopped wearing them I found that I got better corrections from the teacher and I became much more aware of what my knees were doing. Many ballet teachers encourage, or require, students to wear light-colored tights or body warmers so that the use of the leg muscles will be totally visible.

Ballet shoes cost about $13.00 a pair and come in a range of makes and styles. A shoe that is well chosen enhances the shape and use of the foot; a poor choice impairs both looks and function. For these reasons, you should try on several different brands before deciding on one. Since ballet shoes are hand-made, even pairs of the same size and style can vary considerably in softness of the leather, cut, fit and color. Shoes are so critical to the ballet dancer's per-formance that when Soviet danseur Leonid Koslov defected to the United States late in 1979, the only thing he took with him was a pair of favorite ballet slippers, which he had mailed to a friend in Los Angeles a few days before.

Soft shoes offer more freedom and enable you to feel the floor, while stiffer shoes last longer and give you support (this is important for dancers with very flexible feet and men who do a lot of jumping, but unless you fall into these categories it is better to get soft shoes). The size of the vamp (the forepart of the ballet shoe covering the toes) also makes a difference in the way your feet look and work. A high vamp gives more support to flexible feet and a low-cut vamp makes a stiff foot look better by allowing the forefoot to come out of the shoe and bend more easily. Canvas ballet slippers are less expensive ($10.00) and more durable than leather, but not as flexible.

Most manufacturers recommend that you buy ballet shoes a size and a half smaller than your street shoes, and on the snug side because they stretch with wear; canvas shoes can be slightly larger because they don't give as much. Ballet slippers should not be fitted loosely for children to grow into because this may cause accidents and conceal the functioning of the foot from the teacher's view. The shoes should fit like a second skin, but your toes should not be cramped together or curled up when you stand. You may want to experiment with sizes. I've even worn men's shoes on occasion.

Although they are much softer than pointe shoes, ballet shoes require breaking in, too. Stiff new shoes can put a strain on your feet and throw your balance off. It takes a few classes for the leather to soften and mold to the shape of your foot. Before you wear them in class, try wearing your new slippers around the house for a couple of hours; then use them for only part of a lesson, with a comfortable old pair nearby ready to slip into.

Some dancers dislike wearing new ballet shoes so much that they put off buying them until their old pair literally falls apart. You can prolong the life of your shoes by repairing the holes with masking tape (try to find a matching color), and you can take up the slack in overstretched shoes by wearing heavy socks.

The first pointe shoes were nothing more than soft ballet slippers stiffened with glue or starch and reinforced with stitched ribbons. Early toe dancers could stand on their pointes only for short periods of time, and often with a great deal of pain. But modern-day toe shoes come in a variety of styles and weights for support. Since they have a complex construction and are handmade, toe shoes are expensive—about $21.00 a pair—particularly so because they wear out quickly with moderate use. Students taking three to five toe classes a week may go through two pairs of shoes a month (the stronger the foot and the lighter the dancer, the less wear and tear there is on the shoe). Custom-made shoes are available for hard-to-fit feet, but they are expensive. To squeeze a few more weeks of use out of their pointe shoes, some dancers coat the inner lining (including the toe box) with Future, an acrylic floor wax which hardens when dry.

Pointe shoes differ in all the ways that ballet slippers do, as well as in the weight and size of the supporting toe box, and the shape and size of the pointe or tip. Beginning pointe students usually start out with heavier shoes and graduate to lighter, more flexible ones as they gain strength. Square pointes are generally favored over round ones because they afford more room for the toes and a larger surface on which to balance.*If possible, bring your teacher or an experienced dancer along when you buy your first pair of shoes. Mistakes can be costly in more ways than one. Toe dancing is difficult enough without the sheer torture of working in a pair of ill-fitting shoes.

Breaking in a pair of brand-new pointe shoes is a project in itself. The strong leather inner sole, called the shank, and the stiff toe box need to be

*Square-tipped toe shoes are a relatively recent design innovation. In the old days, ballerinas used to darn a square platform at the tips of their pointes.

softened before use. There are a number of time-honored ways to do this. Some dancers take the shoe in hand and bang the tip vigorously against the floor, then bend the sole back and forth; others slam the shoe in a door. Shoes that are too tight can be stretched by moistening them with water before wearing. Work the foot into the shoe by doing some simple exercises, such as relevés, échappés and foot stretching.

Those who are using ballet slippers or pointe shoes for the first time should ask their teachers how to sew on elastics and ribbons so the shoes are securely and neatly fastened to the feet.* Ribbons should be knotted and the excess snipped; drawstrings should be pulled tightly and knotted, and the excess tucked under the vamp or cut off. You'll look more professional that way and won't risk tripping.

Modern dance. Modern dance attire is the simplest and least expensive because you work barefoot. Leotards and tights or leg warmers are all you need. Heavy socks with the heels and toes cut out can also be added to keep the ankles warm. Special footless tights are sold for modern dance, but many dancers prefer to cut the heels and toes off their ballet tights or to slit the foot seams so the same pair of tights can be used with or without shoes (thin white ankle socks can be worn with footless tights for classes that require shoes). If you bruise easily, you may want to buy a pair of knee pads to protect your knees during floor work (see chapter 18 on keeping fit). These should not be too tight and can be purchased at any sporting-goods store.

Jazz. Jazz clothes should provide maximum mobility. Normally a leotard or tee-shirt and tights or knitted "jazz pants" (about $20.00) are worn in class. For safety, the pants should not be too long, and the dancer's feet should be fully visible. Blue jeans are not recommended because they are restricting. Jazz dancers sometimes add colorful adornments, such as bright scarves to hold back the hair, halter tops, sweat pants or socks.

Although some teachers conduct the warm-up barefoot, jazz dance is meant to be done in shoes. You can buy specially made jazz shoes for about $28.00 to $45.00. The leather should be buttery soft and the soles made of nonskid rubber or suede. Your teacher may prefer a particular style, so check with him or her before investing in a pair. Sneakers should be used for jazz only if nothing else is available, since they make it difficult to point the foot properly. If you are only taking a trial class, you can wear ballet slippers or dance in bare feet temporarily.

Tap. Besides tights or socks under their tap shoes, tap dancers wear leotards, skirts or loose street pants; men wear tee-shirts and jazz pants or loose street

---

*A free pamphlet on toe-shoe care is available from Capezio Ballet Makers, 1860 Broadway, New York, New York 10023.

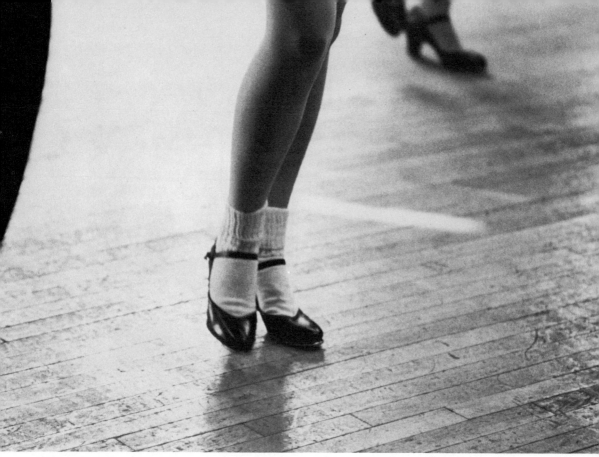

Frank Gimpaya

pants. Don't be surprised· if you see some wild deviations, though; in some informal tap classes students may be dressed in shorts or even baggy overalls.

You can buy tap shoes at dancewear stores (for women, pumps ranging from a low to a two-inch heel; for men, flat shoes), or use a pair of street shoes with taps added. Ready-made tap shoes cost from $18.00 to $60.00, and a customized pair can run up to $150.00. The shoes should fit tightly when new, since they tend to stretch quite a bit with wear. Taps, which cost about $7.00, come in different pitches and sizes (the size determines the volume). Solid aluminum, glass or metal taps are best. They should be fastened by screws rather than nails. Most teachers disapprove of "jingle" taps, which make extra noise but are in fact a cheat device. Here is tap virtuoso Paul Draper's advice on selecting taps:

> *The first requisite of a good tap is that it be firmly fixed to your shoe. Any looseness, jingle or rattle, whether on the front tap or the heel tap, is a great detriment to the production of clear tap sounds. The second requisite is that it be as small and as light as possible in order to produce clean, audible sounds. There are taps which cover half of the front of the shoe and all of the heel. Shun them as you would the plague. They serve no useful*

223

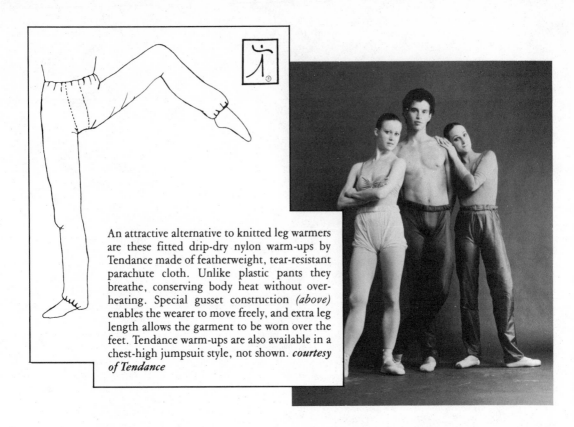

An attractive alternative to knitted leg warmers are these fitted drip-dry nylon warm-ups by Tendance made of featherweight, tear-resistant parachute cloth. Unlike plastic pants they breathe, conserving body heat without overheating. Special gusset construction *(above)* enables the wearer to move freely, and extra leg length allows the garment to be worn over the feet. Tendance warm-ups are also available in a chest-high jumpsuit style, not shown. *courtesy of Tendance*

purpose whatsoever. The taps should not protrude beyond the sole at any point, and any sharp edges should be rounded off with a file. *

Hair and jewelry. Women who don't like its severity will be glad to know that the tight ballerina-bun is no longer the regulation hairstyle for dancing, though admittedly it is the simplest way to keep long hair in place. Hair should be worn neatly, out of the eyes and off the neck, so that the neck, shoulders and upper back are exposed and the head is free for turning and spotting; but this can be accomplished with a scarf, headband or some well-fastened barrettes and hairpins. Remove your jewelry, including pierced earrings—an earring that flies off during a turn can be a dangerous weapon.

Care of dance clothing. Hand in hand with dancing goes a lot of laundry. To save time, a friend of mine showers with his dance clothes on; but however you prefer to do it, practice clothes other than knitted warmers or pants should be washed in a mild detergent after each use. Follow the laundering instructions on the garment and, if possible, avoid electric dryers because they are hard on the clothes and cause them to shrink. Most dancewear today is made of nylon and lycra-spandex, which dries in a few hours anyway.

*From Paul Draper, *On Tap Dancing.*

If you lose an article of clothing at a dance school, report it to the person at the front desk and look through the lost-and-found box—every school has one. Keep trying. Things have a way of mysteriously reappearing a few days later.

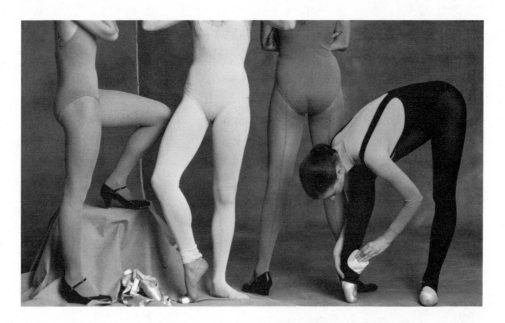

Above: Because of their flattering effect, mesh tights *(left)* are preferred for performances. They allow the skin to show through, creating shadows which slim thick legs and contour underdeveloped muscles. Full-fashion tights *(right center)* have seams, with the shape knit into them. They are heavier, warmer and more durable than mesh, but may be restricting to delicately built dancers. **Gordon Munro, courtesy of Danskin**

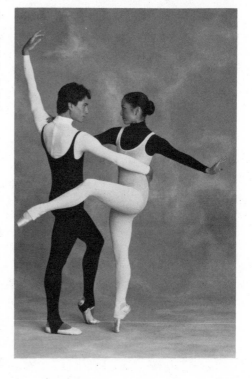

Right: Advanced technology in the use of synthetic fibers has produced highly practical dancewear. These Danskin body warmers, made of top-quality acrylic specially processed to retain heat and pass off moisture, are washable. The acrylic yarn has similar properties to cashmere but moves better, is sturdier and far less expensive. The seamless design offers lots of stretch and doesn't add bulk. **Gordon Munro, courtesy of Danskin**

Dancewear suppliers. The following companies are manufacturers of their own product line and/or distributors of a variety of dance apparel produced by others. They will sell directly to you by mail order, or refer you to the nearest retail shop that stocks their line. Dancewear catalogs are often sent free to teachers and other professionals who request them in writing on business stationery, and at a nominal charge (50¢ to $3.00) to the general public.

Albert's Hosiery Shops
591-595 Eleventh Avenue
New York, New York 10036
One hundred locations

Apollo Dance and Gymnastics
157 Franklin Turnpike
Waldwick, New Jersey 07463

Bal-Toggery
48 East 21st Street
New York, New York 10010

Baum's, Inc.
106-114 11th Street
Philadelphia, Pennsylvania
19107

Johnny Brown Theatrical
7300 Hutchison
Montreal, Quebec H3N1Z1
Canada

Capezio Ballet Makers
1860 Broadway
New York, New York 10023
Fifty dance-theater shops

Chacott Company
1-20-8 Jinnan, sbibuya-ka
Tokyo 150, Japan

Costume Gallery
1150 East Orthodox Street
Philadelphia, Pennsylvania
19124

Curtain Call Costumes
16 West Maple Street
East Prospect, Pennsylvania
17317

Dancetown, U.S.A.
P.O. Box 30692
Santa Barbara, California
93105

Dans-ez International
35 Sloan Gardens
London SW1, England

Danskin, Inc.
1114 Avenue of the Americas
New York, New York 10036

Flexatards
1544 20th Street
Santa Monica, California
90404

Footlights
126 Post Street
San Francisco, California
94108

Frederick Freed Ltd.
108 West 57th Street
New York, New York 10019
Also has stores in Boston
and Houston

Gamba, Ltd.
5 Northfield Park Estates
Beresford Avenue Wembley
Middlesex HAO 1GW, England

Gym-Kins, Inc.
749 Commerce Street
Sinking Spring, Pennsylvania
19608

Herbet Dancewear
902 Broadway
New York 10010

Hollywood Dancewear
6512 Van Nuys Boulevard
Van Nuys, California 91401

Kling's Theatrical Dancewear
218 South Wabash Avenue
Chicago, Illinois 60604

La Mendola
1795 Express Drive North
Smithtown, New York 11787

Lady Oris Dancewear
358 Fifth Avenue
New York, New York 10001
Stores in the East.

Lebo's, Inc.
4118 East Independence
Boulevard
Charlotte, North Carolina
28205

Leo's Advance Theatrical
2451 North Sacramento
Chicago, Illinois 60647

Loshin's Dancewear
215 East 8th Street
Cincinnati, Ohio 45402

Maurice Danswear
P.O. Box 874
119 South Main Street
Royal Oak, Michigan 48067

Mondor
785 Mercier
Iberville, Quebec Canada

Protogs, Inc.
P.O. Box 678
Syosset, New York 11791

Selva
47-25 34th Street
Long Island City, New York
11101

Star-Styled of Miami
465 Northwest 42nd Avenue
Miami, Florida 33126

Stein Imports
Box 468
Arlington, Virginia 22201

Les Steinhardt, Inc.
15841 Stagg Street
Van Nuys, California 91406

Art Stone Dance
and Gymnastic Supply
1795 Express Drive North
Smithtown, New York 11787
Other retail outlets in
Atlanta, Houston, Minneapolis,
St. Louis; Fairfax, Virginia;
and Metairie, Louisiana.

Taffy's
701 Beta Drive
Cleveland, Ohio 44143
Other stores in Atlanta,
Boston, Cleveland, Dallas,
Fort Worth and Seattle.

Tendance/Warm-Ups
66 East 7th Street
New York, New York 10003

Tunics, Ltd.
343A Finchley Road
London NW3 6ET, England

Wendy's Knits
1206 Maple Avenue, Suite 350
Los Angeles, California 90015

Weissman's Theatrical
801 North Skinket
St. Louis, Missouri 63130

Wolff-Fording and Company
1302 McTavish Street
Richmond, Virginia 23230

18

Keeping Fit

*preventing injury
and getting the best results
from your body design;
coping with minor aches
and pains*

A dancer's instrument is her body; she can only go as far as it will carry her. A little preventive maintenance will go a long way toward reducing the risk of injury and helping you get the best possible performance out of your body design. Although a good teacher will work carefully in order to avoid mishaps in class, most dance schools disclaim any liability for injuries sustained on their premises. So in the end the wise dancer must take full responsibility for her own well-being. Learn how to keep fit. Take care of your instrument, it's the only one you've got.

Practice good body alignment

Body alignment is quite simply posture, or the way we stand. Good alignment is the positioning of various parts of the body in relation to a central axis, so that each part works efficiently and the whole structure functions harmoniously. It serves both to center the body and to balance it mechanically—legs over feet, pelvis over legs, spine over pelvis and head over spine. Poor alignment occurs when parts of the body stray from the central axis, resulting in such distortions as a forward-thrusting head or a pelvis tilted behind the legs. Because it throws you off balance and places extra strain on the body, poor posture is often to blame for anything from chronic tension to really serious injuries. What's worse, there is a domino effect. When one body part is out of line, it usually pulls others out to compensate for the imbalance.

In the same way that the wheel alignment of your car should be periodically checked if you don't want your tires to wear out prematurely, you should maintain good body alignment in order to keep your human machine in good working order. This will let you dance years longer by building strength in the right places and putting a minimum of stress on each body part. When you are standing correctly, it's amazing how much freer and easier your movements become. Breathing is deeper and there is less wasted effort.

Good alignment is also the foundation of a strong technique. Balancing is not, as the word suggests, a precarious circus trick, but really a matter of stack-

Standing Up Straight
Some Common Mistakes and How to Correct Them

The rules of good body alignment are essentially the same for all styles of dancing, though occasionally they are waved to achieve a desired choreographic effect. Even then, it's important for dancers to know when they are distorting their bodies and to try to work correctly most of the time.

The back and pelvis

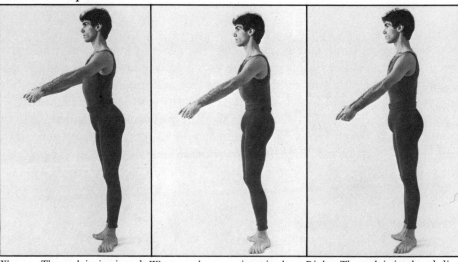

Wrong. The pelvis is tipped behind the spine, resulting in a swaybacked posture. The dancer has pulled his weight off his legs and is rocking backward on his heels. In this stance the spine is weak and the legs can't turn out from the hips. This mistake is the primary cause of back strain and grabbing in the legs and feet.

Wrong—the opposite mistake. The pelvis is tucked under, flattening the lower spine and making it very difficult to straighten the knees without straining.

Right. The pelvis is placed directly over the legs and the weight is carried on the whole foot. The back is long, but with a normal curve in the lower spine. The groin and inner thigh muscles are working to turn out the legs.

ing the bones correctly. A well-placed dancer is secure on her feet. She has control over her movements and she can change direction or shift weight at will. A body that functions efficiently is well proportioned and always produces good line.

Standing up straight ought to be one of the most natural things in the world to do, but in fact it's among the hardest. Habit, social custom and psychological pressures all affect the way we hold ourselves. By the time we reach adulthood most of us have an assortment of postural problems to correct, and one of the most immediate tasks of a dance teacher is to help students establish good body alignment. Although the basic principles remain the same, every body is different. Each dancer needs a slightly different approach to help her feel the right stance for her particular body build, as well as personal supervision to keep her from backsliding into old habits.

Since the way you stand is very much a part of who you are, changing your posture is bound to feel strange or uncomfortable at first. Postural patterns are deeply ingrained in the musculature, and it may be necessary to stretch or strengthen certain muscle groups before you are able to stand up correctly. But after you've been working in the new alignment for a while, it will become second nature and you'll feel better even when you are not dancing.

The legs

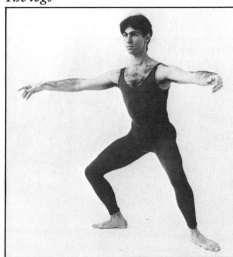 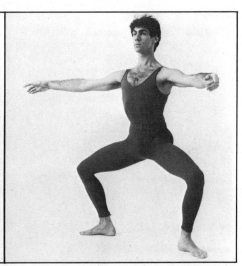

Wrong. The legs are turned in from the hips, the knees are twisted and the feet are rolling over on the arches. This misalignment is especially dangerous when landing from jumps because it puts enormous stress on the knee and ankle joints. Ultimately it can result in a sprained ankle or torn knee cartilage.

Right. The legs are rotated from the hips and the knees are positioned directly over the feet, so that an imaginary line can be drawn through the center of the hip socket, the knee joint and the foot. The dancer's weight is evenly distributed between both legs and he is standing on all his toes. His spine and pelvis are straight and right up on his legs.

Position of the hips in tendu

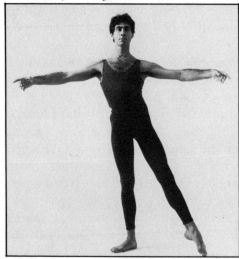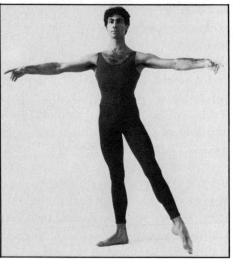

Wrong. The working hip is lifted and turned in, and both hips are twisted to the dancer's left, throwing his balance off center and straining his lower back. This happens quite often in a ronde de jambe action.

Right. The hips are level and squared off to the front. The working hip is down and turned out evenly with the standing hip, and the dancer's spine is long.

Position of the hips in leg extensions

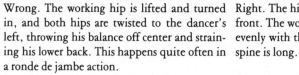

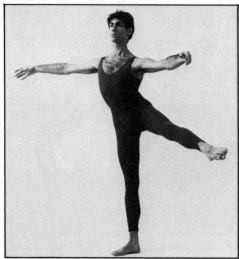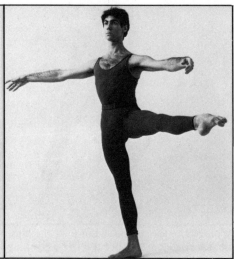

Wrong—the same mistake as above. The working hip is lifted and twisted, with the leg turned in and the spine distorted. This posture forces the dancer to grab the muscles of his working leg. It's hard to lift his leg because he is lifting his much heavier hip as well, and almost impossible to balance securely because his spine is not centered.

Right. Both hips are even and facing front. The spine is long and straight. The working leg is free and isolated from the hip and is thus much lighter and easier to turn out.

The shoulders

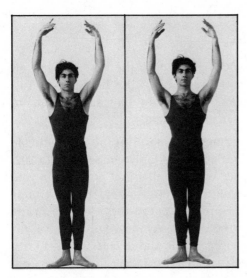

Left: Wrong. The dancer is trying to raise his arms by lifting his shoulders along with them. This mistake is particularly tempting if the joints are tight, but it shortens the neck, produces shoulder strain and looks terrible.

Right: Right. The shoulders are down. The arms are moving freely from the spine and they are isolated from the shoulders. The head, neck and upper body have an open, elegant look.

The feet in relevé

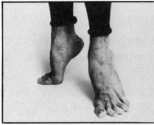
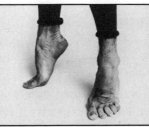

Wrong. The dancer is rolling badly on his arches, with most of his weight being borne by his big toes. This is a frequent cause of painful bunions.

Wrong—the opposite mistake. The dancer is rolling on the outer portion of his feet, with his weight teetering on his little toes.

Right. The weight is evenly distributed over the center of the feet. This is the strongest and healthiest position in relevé.

The head

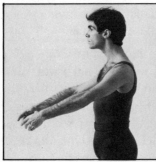
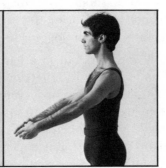

Wrong. The dancer is jutting his chin forward in an attempt to stretch his neck. He is actually shortening it.

Right. The head is directly in line with the spine and the neck is long.

dancer: Earnest Pagnano
photos: Frank Gimpaya

231

Dress warm, get warm, stay warm

Given a choice, most dancers would gladly skip the warm-up and get straight to the fun of dancing, but a good warm-up is the closest thing to a miracle I know. It takes a tired, stiff or reluctant body and transforms it into one that is supple, energetic and free—a dancer's instrument.

Warming up your body is very much like warming up a car in cold weather. It circulates the blood and raises the internal body temperature to 102-103 degrees Fahrenheit, which in turn speeds up the chemical processes in your body. When you are warmed up, nerve impulses travel faster, so your timing and coordination are better. The warm-up also paves the way for greater exertion by preparing the heart and lungs for action. As you begin to move, the muscles soften and lengthen, becoming more supple and thus less likely to tear under stress. At the same time, warming up helps the dancer to focus her concentration and tune the mind to the body. By the end of a proper warm-up—which ought to be at least a half hour long—you should have worked up a respectable sweat. The kinks should be out and you should feel warm, loose, up in energy and ready to dance.

Sometimes you don't miss a good warm-up until you've experienced one and can see how much more deeply and freely it enables you to work. As you gain experience you will come to know your own requirements. Some dancers need more time to warm up than others and some parts of your body may want more work than the rest. Generally, if you are tight in the joints and muscles, have special problems or injuries, or are over thirty, you should do a slow, thorough warm-up every time you dance. Look for a teacher who gives the best one for your body. Unfortunately, some teachers who are imaginative choreographers and wonderful dancers give inadequate warm-ups. To a certain extent you can make up for this lack by doing your own warm-up before class—provided, of course, that the class is otherwise worthwhile.

To be effective a warm-up should immediately precede full physical activity. If there are any long breaks in dancing (for explanations, changing shoes, etc.), you should briefly rewarm yourself. Jogging in place is often enough.

If you dress warmly and work out in a warm room, your temperature will rise faster and your body heat will be retained longer. That's why most dancers don't like air conditioning and refuse it even in the hottest weather. Occasionally performers and management get into squabbles over the thermostat setting in the theater: Should it be cool enough for the audience's comfort or warm enough for the dancers' safety? But superficial heat alone, however helpful it may be, is not enough to prepare your body for dancing (this includes hot soaks, saunas, massage and sunbathing). Although it's fun to dream about instant warm-ups, the only way to raise the temperature *inside* the muscles is to work the body itself.

Go to class regularly

Unlike most other students, dancers never graduate from their classes because, strange as it sounds, dancing by itself isn't enough to keep you in shape for dancing. A dancer is also an athlete who must stay in training. He goes to class not only to dance but to improve his technique and keep his body fit. Good technique is no mere academic nicety, it gives the dancer a sure and efficient way of moving and it spares his body unnecessary wear and tear by eliminating extraneous actions. The methodical conditioning exercises performed in dance classes build strength and firm, resilient muscles that are able to react quickly and smoothly and to offer the joints protection from stress. Strength must be developed evenly throughout the body: You cannot have a strong back without having strong stomach muscles. And muscle development must be the same on both sides of the body as well as in the opposing sets of muscles (flexors and extensors) in a limb. Dance classes also improve muscle stretch—for long, lithe muscles that produce free and supple movement—along with timing, coordination and heart-lung endurance.

Dancing is more fun when you go to class regularly because your body is up to it. Moreover, dance classes are intended for people who are in shape. If your attendance is erratic, you won't stay in the optimal condition needed to do the work. Then you are more likely to push yourself into an injury in an effort to keep up.

Conditioning requirements vary for each individual. The amount of physical exertion that is beneficial for one dancer may be too much or too little for another. That's why it is important to experiment with different teachers and classes, and to be sensitive to your body's responses. The class you take should be on a par with your present exercise tolerance level. If it is too easy you won't progress, and if it's too demanding it may overtax your body and cause harm. In order to better your performance it is often necessary to push yourself a little beyond what is comfortable—to pull a stretch further and hold it longer than you are accustomed, to move a little faster or to repeat an exercise more times than you'd prefer—but never to the point of faintness or pain. After a desirable level of fitness is attained, it may be maintained with less effort so long as there are a minimum of two or three workouts per week.

Most dancers know only too well how rapidly fitness declines once training is broken. Muscle strength is lost at a rate of about ten percent a week; cardiovascular endurance diminishes a bit more slowly, and motor skills eventually deteriorate too, though never entirely. Whenever they are not being actively worked, the muscles shorten and their stretch has to be renewed daily.

Rest up

The dancer's body needs rest as much as it needs to work, and muscles can get as stiff from too much dancing as from too little. A certain amount of fatigue is all right, even pleasant. It helps you sleep. In fact, you may require more sleep than usual when you are dancing, especially while you are getting into shape. Rest restores overcharged muscles by allowing them to relax, shorten and get rid of accumulated wastes called metabolites.

If, however, a good night's sleep doesn't relieve your fatigue, you are overtired. Extreme fatigue produces stiff, painful movement. It is a primary cause of injury, because tired muscles frequently respond too quickly, too slowly or in a jerky fashion. When you are exhausted the best thing to do is give your body the extra rest and sleep it craves. Massage also relieves weary muscles by improving circulation, relaxing the body and helping it to eliminate metabolites. Try to avoid dancing when you are very tired, but if you absolutely must, conserve energy by pacing yourself and proceed cautiously. Missing a class once in a while or taking only part of it won't hurt either.

Correct physical conditions

When I started dancing I was terribly swaybacked. For two frustrating years my teachers corrected and corrected me, but as hard as I tried I just couldn't straighten out my spine. I was urged to drop my lower back and pull up my stomach muscles. Nothing happened. I was told to tuck my buttocks under; this only caused tremendous strain and gave me a formidable derrière. One day, purely by chance, a substitute teacher noticed that tight muscles were preventing me from improving my posture. She gave me two simple stretching exercises to do every day, one for the lower back and one for the front of the thighs and the hip joints. Within a few months I stopped thinking that I had the wrong body for dancing because I could stand up straight without straining.

Many people have a swaybacked condition or a curvature of the spine, an asymmetrical spinal column that creates an uneven arm hang or one shoulder and hip that are higher than the other. Most dancers have some degree of bow-leg, knock-knee, or hyperextended knee (when loose ligaments in the back of the knee, combined with weak hamstring muscles, pull the kneecaps backward beyond the normal alignment of the leg). Tibial torsion, or inward-rolling kneecaps caused by a twisting of the lower leg bones, is fairly common too.

Mild physical conditions can be improved by correcting one's body alignment and studying under the supervision of a competent teacher. Severe structural deviations, however, call for a special way of working plus remedial exercises* to stretch or strengthen the involved muscle groups. The more dancing you do and the more rigorous the style, the more troublesome these

*Raoul Gelabert's two-volume book *Anatomy for the Dancer* (New York: 1964, Danad Publishing Company) prescribes corrective exercises for many common physical conditions. It is available at libraries or from *Dance-magazine* (at $17.50, including a $1.00 postage and handling charge), 1180 Avenue of the Americas, New York, New York 10036.

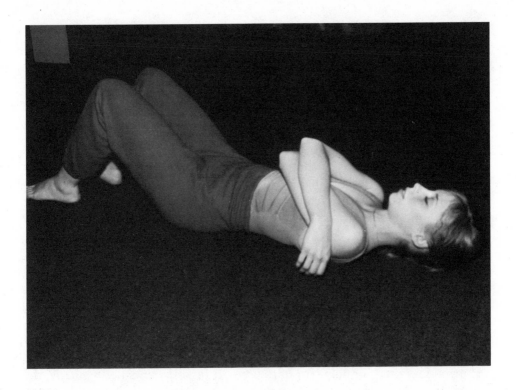

Lying in the Constructive Rest Position (CRP) is the best way to relax when not sleeping because no muscle effort is required to maintain it. Developed by Dr. Lulu Sweigard, the CRP relieves muscle strain by using the weight of the body to loosen and open the muscles. It is very effective in easing backache. For best results, lie on a rug, mat or folded blanket placed over a level floor. Bend your legs, with your knees pointing toward the ceiling. Place your feet a comfortable distance away from your torso and several inches apart, so they are in line with your hip sockets. If your legs tend to flop open, move your feet slightly further apart. Hang your arms loosely across your chest with your elbows almost overlapping, but not so much that your shoulders hunch. This crossed-arm position releases tension in your shoulder girdle by allowing your arms to fall back in their sockets and by stretching the muscles across the width of your back. Close your eyes. Feel that your body is very heavy and let it be completely supported by the floor. Feel the length of your spine on the floor, but do not deliberately flatten your lower back by pressing it down. Try conjuring up a restful image of yourself soaking in a warm tub or sinking into a field of soft spring grass; or imagine that your body is a large hollow cavity which each inhaled breath expands with air and each exhaled breath empties of wastes and tension. *dancer: Conni Brunner; photo: John Wisdom*

problems become. Acute conditions demand the attention of an analytic teacher (see chapter 11), because they can affect other parts of the body and lead to injury.

Coping with minor aches and pains

You are far more likely to encounter some of the garden-variety aches and pains associated with dancing than the serious injuries discussed in the next chapter. These are generally harmless, of short duration and easily alleviated by simple home remedies. Everyone gets them, and they are certainly no cause for alarm. If trouble persists, ask your teacher's advice, since this may indicate that you are working incorrectly.

Soreness and stiffness. Soreness comes from tiny muscle spasms or muscle tears which cause mild inflammation and pain. The result of a sudden overexertion, it can occur in just about any place you are not used to moving. Some charley horse is inevitable if you are taking a new dance class or intensifying your training. It can also arise from gripping the muscles or working with tension. You'll get less sore if you ease into the unaccustomed activity gradually, perhaps by taking a slower class or only part of the class at first. If you dance regularly, the discomfort will soon go away. Stiffness, on the other hand, is usually due to metabolites that have collected in the muscle tissue as a result of overwork or fatigue. It signals the need for more rest.

Wearing warm dance clothes, massage, soaking in a warm tub and applying a heat rub (such as Ben-Gay or Absorbine Jr.*) will relieve both soreness and stiffness. So will a slow, thorough warm-up. Gentle stretching at the end of class helps decrease muscle spasms.

Shinsplints. Caused by inflamed muscles and tendons along the tibia, or shinbone, shinsplints are often experienced as a dull ache which intensifies as the muscles cool off. Like charley horse, shinsplints occur with unaccustomed activity. Even if you are not out of condition you can get them from jumping on a hard floor or dancing when cold. Rest, massage, warm baths, heat rubs and aspirin help. Dress warmly, and if you're out of shape resume dancing gradually. If the shin pain lasts over ten days or occurs when you are in good shape, consult a doctor to make sure you don't have a stress fracture (see chapter 19).

Muscle cramps or spasms. These are involuntary muscle contractions that can be painful. They normally come from overworking the muscles with insufficient

*Heating balms work by irritating the skin and causing a dilation of the small blood vessels, which brings a flood of blood and warmth to the area. They'll burn if you put too much on or use them with strong heat from lamps or electric heating pads. Be careful, too, not to rub your eyes absentmindedly while the medication is still on your hands.

relaxation between exercises. Cramps of the instep and toes are common in beginners, who aren't used to pointing their feet. Some dancers get thigh or back spasms. If you get a cramp, stop moving. Grasp the area firmly, applying constant pressure until the contractions subside; then massage it to break up the spasm. Keep warm. When the cramp has melted away, the muscles can be gently stretched and, if necessary, a heat rub or other superficial heat applied. Wearing warm practice clothes and working slowly with the body relaxed will help prevent cramps from recurring.

Sore feet. *Blisters* and other foot maladies are, alas, one of the occupational hazzards of toe dancing, though they diminish as the dancer acquires strength and protective foot calluses. Properly fitting toe shoes and tights help minimize the friction that produces blisters; so does a light dusting of talcum powder between the toes. Toenails should be well trimmed.

It is important to take care of blisters because they may get infected or cause you to compensate by straining another part of your body. There are several time-proven remedies to ease the pain. A warm soak in Burows solution helps disinfect and soothe blisters and other minor skin irritations. Open blisters should be cleaned, the loose skin clipped off and an antiseptic salve applied. While they are healing, blisters should be protected by a Dr. Scholl's foam pad or a Band-Aid. A small amount of lamb's wool (paper towel will do in a pinch) should be wrapped around the tips of the toes to cushion them against the hard box of the pointe shoe. A certain amount of soreness is to be expected from pointe work, but any sharp or persistent foot pain ought to be checked by a physician.

Bunions are by no means the exclusive province of toe dancers, but they are the likeliest candidates for getting these enlarged and sometimes painful big toe joints. Technically speaking, bunions are an inflammation of the bursae (sacs of fluid which act as shock absorbers) of the first metatarsal joint of the big toe. They usually form as the result of abnormal pressure placed on the big toe due to poor foot alignment on pointe or half-toe. In moderate and severe cases the big toe is bent inward toward the other toes. Tight shoes are sometimes to blame for bunions, and some people have an inherited predisposition toward developing them. As a rule, this condition can be controlled with good technique and properly fitting shoes. Toe dancers with bunions should buy pointe shoes with a wide toe box and wear corn pads; the shoes may be slit to further reduce pressure. Bunions require medical attention only when they become incapacitating. If surgery is needed, the preferred procedure for dancers is a bumpectomy, a minor operation performed under local anesthetic.

Splits, or torn foot calluses, afflict dancers who work barefoot. Barefoot dancing produces thick calluses on the soles of the feet which, depending on the amount of moisture in your skin, can get dry. If you are dancing on a sticky floor, these overdeveloped calluses can tear open, causing painful splits. Splits should be well cleaned, applied with antiseptic, and then bandaged to promote healing. To prevent them, many dancers pare down their calluses with an emery board or pumice stone (these can be obtained at most drugstores). Afterwards a moisturizer containing lanolin is rubbed into the skin to keep it from drying.

Floor burns and bruises. Such annoyances are peculiar to modern dancers who work on their knees and practice falls to the floor. There is little you can do about floor burns and bruises except wait for them to heal. The best preventive is to learn how to fall on the fleshy parts of the body, and to support your weight correctly in the stomach, pelvis and thighs. Make sure you understand what you're doing when you work on the floor; never throw yourself around. If you bruise easily, you might try wearing athletic knee pads. They are inexpensive and they can be purchased at any sporting-goods store. Dr. Scholl's thin moleskin pads can be worn inconspicuously under tights for performances.

Cracking or clicking in the joints. Many dancers hear cracking or clicking sounds in their joints as they start to warm up. Some people even crack their joints intentionally to free their bodies of congestion. These noises are created by tendons or ligaments catching on bone and then snapping over it. As dreadful as that sounds, cracking is quite harmless so long as there is no pain. But don't get into the habit of doing it repeatedly because this may irriate your joints.

Heat stress. On hot days profuse sweating can cause dehydration, with a loss of vital minerals from your body. Drink lots of liquids and eat balanced, well-salted meals in hot weather. Watch out for excessive weight loss and indications of heat exhaustion such as muscle cramping, extreme fatigue, chills and a rapid, weak pulse. If any of these symptoms occur, stop dancing immediately; otherwise you may end up with the dangerous condition of heat stroke. Retire to a well-ventilated room and rest. Wrap yourself in a blanket if you are cold.

Skin irritations. Because increased perspiration and studio dust can irritate the skin, dancers should deep-cleanse the face often, bathe daily and wear fresh practice clothes for each class.

238

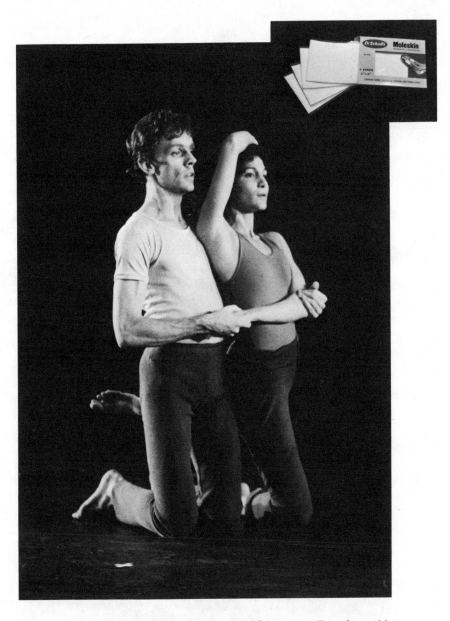

Modern dancers who spend a lot of time on the floor can easily end up with knees that look like a pair of rotten potatoes. Athletic knee guards are great skin-savers for class, but less cumbersome protection is needed for performance. Here the author, wearing Dr. Scholl's moleskin pads under her costume, rehearses with partner John Dayger. The pads, which are wafer-thin yet large enough to cover the bony parts of the knee, can also be worn invisibly under tights, provided they are not too sheer. *Philip Hiplow, John Wisdom*

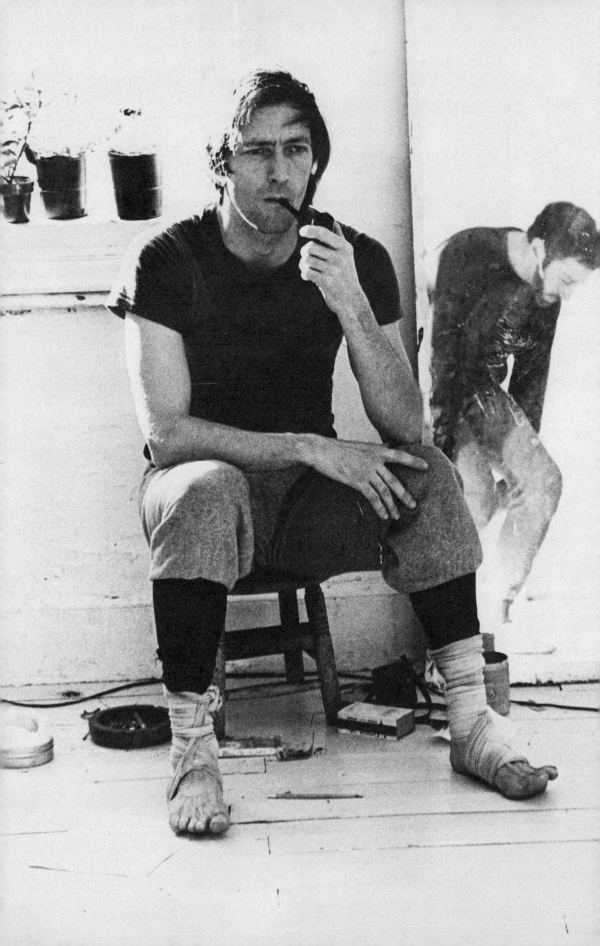

19

What to Do
About Injuries

they're not the end of the world,
but maybe a new beginning

Luck is a thing that comes in many forms. Who can recognize her?

—*ERNEST HEMINGWAY,*
The Old Man and the Sea

While onstage during a performance, the New York City Ballet's Jean-Pierre Bonnefous had a dancer's nightmare. He landed off-balance from a jump and tore all the ligaments in one ankle. Yet when he was interviewed a year later he called the period of recovery following his accident "perhaps the richest part of my life." During the time that he was unable to dance, Bonnefous taught company class and through it rekindled an old interest in choreography. He created three critically acclaimed pieces, including one for the New York City Ballet. As a result the thirty-seven-year-old Frenchman, who is back dancing with the company, has a brand new future as a choreographer waiting for him in the wings.

It is not an unusual story. Although they may be painful and discouraging, even serious injuries needn't be catastrophic. Like many setbacks in

Choreographer Cliff Keuter directs a rehearsal while an ankle injury is on the mend. *Frank Gimpaya*

241

life, they can present an opportunity to stretch ourselves and grow further. Dancers don't get injured more often than other athletes. In fact, the systematic conditioning they receive in class reduces the risk considerably. When injuries do occur, many heal nicely after a few days' rest and home care. The severest ones may require surgery, but in most cases early identification and proper treatment will prevent the damage from becoming acute or developing into a chronic condition.

Most serious injuries befall professional dancers, whose bodies are subjected to above average wear and tear over many years. They study, rehearse and perform long hours every day, often under adverse conditions. Official commitments lead them to neglect injuries by putting off needed rest or treatment, and anxiety over competition may drive them to push themselves beyond capacity. (One major ballet company disclosed that on any given day nearly a quarter of its dancers are sidelined because of injuries. The casualty list climbs even higher at the end of an extended tour or performance season.) Tap dancers sometimes boast that their way of dancing is the safest because it rarely entails unnatural or violent movement.

Strains (damage to muscle tissue) and sprains (damage to ligaments) are the most common injuries among dancers. Broken bones are rare. "This is because dancers are so loose," explains orthopedist William Hamilton, physician to the New York City Ballet. "Their muscles and ligaments are extremely stretched. People with tight ligaments break their bones; people with loose ligaments get sprains."*Injuries usually strike where there is chronic stress: Toe dancers suffer the most often from foot and ankle trouble, and men are the most likely to wrench their backs and knees from all the jumping and lifting they do. But in all dance forms, among men as well as women, nonprofessionals as well as professionals, if the body is moved with force and tension, injuries may result. Chances are that if you hurt yourself you are working in an improper or harmful way. If you approach it intelligently, recovering from an injury should help you build a stronger technique and find new, more effective ways of working with your body.

What to do if you get hurt

Stop dancing immediately. There are all sorts of heroic stories about dancers who have finished performances despite broken bones and ruptured tendons, but no Purple Hearts are awarded for valor in class. When you feel something is wrong it is wisest to retreat to a quiet spot and get your weight off the sore part as soon as possible. Trying to work through an injury is *always* a bad idea. It can only get worse and throw additional strain on other parts of the body that are forced to compensate. If, like most dancers, you think you can't afford to take a

*From David Lindner, "Dancer's Pain," in *Dance Life in New York*, Spring 1975.

few days off to properly care for an injury, think again. Can you afford the several months' recovery time you'll need if the damage becomes serious?

Tell your teacher. It is advisable to let your teacher know when you are hurt. Most dance teachers have some experience with injuries and can be helpful, if only by being a calming influence and offering a little common-sense advice.

Apply a cold compress and elevate the injury. Under normal circumstances heat is the dancer's best friend, but it is the worst thing for a fresh injury. The very property that brings blessed relief to tight, tired or spasmodic muscles—namely the ability of warmth to dilate the blood vessels and increase blood flow— merely intensifies the internal bleeding and inflammation of a new wound. Heat does promote healing, but only after the hemorrhaging and swelling have stopped. The best first aid for an injury is to elevate it and apply a cold compress or ice pack. This simple procedure shortens the total healing time by controlling inflammation. Cold reduces the swelling and internal bleeding by constricting the blood vessels at the injured site, applying outside pressure prevents the accumulation of fluids, and elevation slows down the circulation to the damaged tissue.

When you get home you can try this folk remedy: Soak a damp washcloth in apple cider vinegar and cool it in the freezer until ice crystals form (the cloth will be stiff). Hold it over the injury. You'll get a cold, then warm sensation as the compress draws the trapped blood and fluid out of the area so they can be more quickly reabsorbed into the system. When the cloth gets warm, repeat the process (you can have a replacement cooling in the fridge ready to go).

See a doctor. Mild and even some moderately severe injuries can be managed at home, but if you have any of the following symptoms, see a doctor right away:

- severe pain, swelling or discoloration
- loss of function in the affected area (i.e., inability to move or put weight on an injury); this may occur immediately or a few hours after the initial trauma
- moderate pain that doesn't subside after a few days' rest

Rather than take chances, if you have doubts about the severity of an injury get a qualified medical diagnosis. The victim is not always the best judge, since some serious injuries show no outward sign of swelling or internal bleeding; they may not even be fully incapacitating at first.

Go to a reputable orthopedic specialist, someone you trust personally and who understands the special problems incurred by dancing. The following is a partial list of orthopedic surgeons who are knowledgeable on dancers' injuries:

Dr. William G. Hamilton
343 West 58th Street
New York, New York 10019
(212) 765-2262

Dr. Barnard Kleiger
1150 Fifth Avenue
New York, New York 10028
(212) 289-1216

Dr. William Liebler
742 Park Avenue
New York, New York 10021
(212) RE4-7477

Dr. Edward H. Miller
Chairman, Department of
Orthopedics
University of Cincinnati
Medical Center
Cincinnati, Ohio 45219
(513) 872-4592

Dr. Edward Nicholas
29 Claremont Avenue
New York, New York 10027
(212) 866-6745

Dr. Alan J. Ryan
4530 West 77th Street
Minneapolis, Minnesota 55435
(612) 835-3222

Dr. Ernest L. Washington
12714 South Avalon Boulevard
Los Angeles, California 90061
(213) 756-9271, 370-8583

Dancers need to have more perfect recoveries than the average person. Your teacher or classmates should be able to refer you to a suitable physician. But if you can't get a satisfactory recommendation, as Dr. L.M. Vincent advises in his delightfully sensible *Dancer's Book of Health*, "go to the biggest jock you can find"—local college and professional athletic teams or coaches. If surgery is recommended, you should consult other doctors to confirm the opinion. Treatment alternatives are discussed at the end of this chapter.

Common dancers' injuries

Muscle pulls or strains. This injury is the most prevalent of all. It is an overstretching or tearing of the muscle fibers that is caused by a sudden abnormal stretch. Pulls occur chiefly in the muscles of the groin, foot, ankle, calf and lower back; and in the hamstrings, which run down the back of the thigh to the knee. They can be mild, moderate or severe, and they are usually attributable to poor postural alignment, insufficient body conditioning, inadequate warm-up or fatigue. The quadricep muscles in the front of the thigh, which lift the leg, are an exception. They get strained not from overstretching but from overwork.

It bears repeating: Never try to work out a muscle pull by continuing to dance with it. You risk further tearing of the muscle and more scarring when it heals. Even with a mild strain, it's best to wait until the area is pain- free before exercising. However, after healing has begun and there is a reduction in symptoms, moderate and acute strains should be kept warm and gently stretched a little each day to restore elasticity before returning to dance activities. Gentle stretching will minimize the chance of permanent muscle tightness due to excessive scarring.

Mild strains are often not noticed until the next day. They don't involve any tearing and for the most part the discomfort is due to muscle spasms. You may feel anything from a slight twinge in the muscle and soreness following activity to a local muscle spasm with associated weakness. To treat a mild strain, apply a cold compress from one-half to two hours; if spasm is present use ice massage. Then begin easy stretching of the muscle for brief intervals throughout the day. You may safely return to activity when there are no more symptoms.

Moderate strains occur when there is a tearing of portions of the muscle. You may feel it giving way, followed by spasms, weakness and a temporary loss of function. Sharp pain or a burning sensation usually come afterward, and there is swelling and discoloration. Apply a cold compress and elevate the injury on and off for the first twenty-four to forty-eight hours. Wear an elastic bandage, and avoid exercising or stretching the injured part. *If there is a loss of function for over half an hour, call in a physician.* By the second or third day, if the inflammation has subsided, soak the injury in warm water (105 degrees Farenheit) or apply a heating pad twice daily. In the days that follow, lightly massage the area above and below the damaged part during heat treatments. By the fifth day, while keeping the injured muscle warm, you can begin gently stretching it for short periods of time. The unaccustomed movement may feel strange, but shouldn't hurt. If it does, discontinue stretching until the area is sufficiently healed. Wear an elastic bandage for support.

As a general unwritten and unproven medical law, moist heat works better than dry heat. To obtain this effect when the luxury of a tub isn't available or practical, place a hot, wet washcloth on the area of misery, cover securely with Saran Wrap and a towel, and then use a regular heating pad. Since it's fairly difficult to dance while using a heat pad, Saran Wrap is rapidly becoming an indispensable first-aid item for the dancer. Wrapping a sore limb with a layer or two of Saran Wrap retains natural body warmth and perspiration: a pretty sneaky and easy way of getting fairly constant moist heat. This is particularly useful for those with chronic tendon problems.

—*L.M. VINCENT,*
The Dancer's Book of Health

Severe strains involve a rupturing, or pulling away, of muscle from muscle, or muscle from tendon, or tendon from bone. They sometimes require surgical repair. Dancers usually feel a sudden snap or tear. Pain, swelling and discoloration are intense. *Call a doctor and follow his directions.* He may prescribe a muscle relaxant or enzyme. In the meantime, apply a cold compress and elevate the injury on and off for forty-eight to seventy-two hours, and wear an elastic bandage for continuous pressure and support. Begin easy stretching of the muscle only after you are pain free.

Sprains. Sprains are a tearing of the ligaments and the surrounding tissue of a joint, usually by sudden twisting. (Remember, ligaments are the tough fibrous bands connecting our bones.) The most frequently sprained joint is the ankle, followed by the toes, knee, lower back and hip. Improper landing from jumps can cause knee ligaments to actually rupture, but fortunately this is rare. Like strains, sprains occur in varying degrees of severity, depending on how many ligaments are torn, and sprained joints should be gently exercised when healing to retain mobility. Back sprains can be eased by sleeping on a firm mattress and doing exercises to strengthen the supporting abdominal muscles.

Immediate care is even more important for sprains than muscle strains, since joints tend to swell rapidly with blood and fluid. The intensity of the injury can best be determined by the amount of pain, swelling, discoloration and loss of function. All moderate and severe sprains should be seen by a doctor because broken bones and/or tendon damage can accompany a twisted joint. It must be immobilized to prevent further harm to the ligaments and to prevent them from healing loosely, which could leave the dancer with a permanently weak or unstable joint. Heat treatments are commonly prescribed after the first few days, along with continued rest and physical therapy when the sprain is healed.

Mild sprains result from a minor twisting of the joint. This produces a slight stretching of connective tissue with little loss of function and only a twinge of pain when the joint is twisted. For the first hour or two apply a cold compress and elevate the injury. Tape or wrap the sprain for continuous pressure and avoid moving the joint for the first day. Twice daily, starting on the second day, administer superficial heat in the form of a warm soak, heating pad or lamp for ten minutes; massage above and below the injury for five minutes; and, keeping the area warm, move the joint gently to retain range of movement. If there is swelling, wrap the injury in an elastic bandage. By the third day light exercise may be resumed provided there is no pain. A mild sprain ordinarily takes one to three weeks to heal completely.

Moderate sprains often take two weeks to a month to heal. There is a more severe twisting of the joint, resulting in pain, swelling, some discoloration and a temporary loss of function. *See a doctor and follow his directions.* For the first twenty-four to forty-eight hours don't put weight on the sprain. Crutches will probably be needed until the weight can be comfortably upborne. Apply cold compresses and elevate the injury on and off for the first twenty- four to forty-eight hours. Tape or wrap it in an elastic bandage for continuous pressure and support. By the third or fourth day your physician will probably recommend some sort of superficial heat treatment, and toward the end of the first week he may have you start gently moving the joint to retain its mobility. Once the injury is adequately healed, therapeutic exercises may be prescribed to rebuild strength.

Severe sprains occur when a joint has been violently twisted, actually dislocated. There is extreme pain, a loss of function, and immediate swelling followed by discoloration. *See a doctor and follow his directions.* Severe sprains should be immobilized in a cast while they are healing, and in some cases surgery may be required to repair the torn ligaments. Cold compresses should be applied right away to control the inflammation, and the injury should be elevated. Tape or wrap the sore area in elastic for continuous pressure. If a weight-bearing joint has been sprained, no weight should be carried on it for several days. Use crutches. Once a sprain of this magnitude is sufficiently healed, physical therapy is necessary to restore range of motion and strengthen the affected ligaments and tendons. Otherwise renewed pain and swelling, or even tendinitis, may occur.

Tendinitis. Tendons attach muscle to bone, and tendinitis is an inflammation of a tendon from constant overstraining or overwork. This injury can begin as a minor discomfort but get worse with persistent activity, so it's important to nip it in the bud. Poor technique or poor leg alignment due to forcing turn-out is usually the culprit. The knee, and the Achilles tendon at the heel or surrounding tendons at the ankle, are frequent sites of tendinitis in dancers. Occasionally it flares up in the hip. Achilles tendinitis is most common in older dancers whose tendons have been weakened by wear and tear, and dancers who have a tight demi-plié. It is typically caused by failure to stretch the Achilles when coming down from jumps and relevés.

Tendinitis is characterized by swelling, irritation and pain. It starts out as a tight, burning sensation that intensifies when the tendon cools off after exercise. A dancer with Achilles tendinitis finds it difficult to relevé, and in severe cases there is often a noticeable thickening of the tendon itself directly behind the ankle joint. In all types of tendinitis consult a doctor immediately if the swelling and pain are acute; but dancers over thirty with Achilles tendinitis should be especially attentive to these warning signals, since they are likeliest to develop a complete tendon rupture. A ruptured Achilles is very painful, and a decided snap can be heard as the tendon rips apart from the bone. In rupture cases Dr. Hamilton recommends surgery to restore the normal length of the tendon, but cautions that the operation must be performed by an expert because a tendon made too long or too short will not yield satisfactory results.

If you suspect tendinitis, for the first forty-eight hours rest the injury and apply ice to it frequently. The ideal treatment is total rest until the pain goes away (normally one to three weeks), but for many dancers this is impractical. At the very least, from the third day on activity should be restricted to brief, gentle workouts with no jumps or relevés when the knee or Achilles tendon is involved, and no strenuous hip movements (i.e., extremely turned-out positions or high extensions) when the hip is affected. Prior to exercising, Dr. Hamilton advises tendinitis sufferers to soak the inflamed area in a warm bath for fifteen to twenty minutes, then massage it with a mild analgesic balm such as Ben-Gay or Heet, and cover it with Saran Wrap to hold in the heat. Heavy socks or leg warmers should be worn for extra warmth during classes. Ice or cold water should be applied for fifteen to twenty minutes immediately following each workout. The warm baths should be continued throughout the rest of the day. If the pain and swelling do not diminish after a week to ten days of curtailed activity and home treatment, see a doctor.

Dr. Vincent suggests that dancers with Achilles tendinitis use heel lifts in ballet slippers or wear jazz shoes to class to lessen the strain on the tendon. Heeled shoes or shoes with heel lifts should be worn on the street too, Vincent says.

Torn knee cartilage. Torn cartilage is usually the result of a severe sprain of the knee ligaments from repeated or violent twisting caused by incorrect landing from jumps. Once the initial symptoms have settled, it is possible to dance with minor tears so long as the dancer is well trained and scrupulously careful not to strain or twist the knee. However, most orthopedists agree that torn knee cartilage must eventually be repaired surgically, because there is always a risk that loose cartilage will get caught in the knee joint and lock the knee. It is a routine operation that takes an average of six to eight weeks to heal.

Bone spurs of the foot. Most often seen in toe dancers, bone spurs are extra bony growths that form to protect areas repeatedly subjected to stress and friction. They can also appear at the site of an old injury, such as a sprain. They are painful, restrict movement, and are commonly located in the big toe joint or the front of the ankle (in the latter case they limit the dancer's plié). Bone spurs, which may look and feel like corns, can be cushioned with corn pads and strapped to relieve the pain. Many dancers make small slits in their pointe shoes to further ease the pressure on their feet. Spurs grow slowly and sometimes disappear with rest and improved technique. If all else fails, they can be surgically removed.

Sometimes pain *behind* the ankle is attributable to an extra bone in the foot called the *os trigonium*. It limits the ability to point the foot and rise fully on the toes, and it can cause tendinitis of the Achilles or big toe. In chronic cases the surplus bone can be removed surgically, with about a three- month recovery period.

Stress fractures. While broken bones are relatively rare among dancers, stress fractures, or minor changes in a bone's structure, do occur with some frequency. As their name implies, stress fractures arise from chronic stress placed on a body part due to fatigue, poor technique, or dancing on a hard floor. They often appear in the shins, lower back, or the forefoot (in toe dancers). Stress fractures can be so mild that they go undetected; when in the shins they may be mistaken for shinsplints. If you are in good shape and experience mild to moderate soreness in the midshin area for several weeks, or if you notice a tender bump on your shinbone, you may have a stress fracture. It's best to see a doctor, for several of these tiny nicks can collect in the same area and eventually cause the bone to break. Stress fractures clear up completely after six to eight weeks of rest and curtailed activity.

Degenerated and slipped discs. Composed of spongy cartilage and gelatinous material that is mostly water, spinal discs join the bones of the spinal column (called vertebrae) together. They give the back elasticity and act as shock absorbers, protecting the nerves of the spinal cord. Any damage to the discs warrants immediate medical attention. Occasionally a suspected disc injury turns out to be a severe back sprain—which is another reason to see a doctor right away.

A *degenerated disc* is one that has become narrow or worn down by prolonged abnormal stress. Some people have an inherited predisposition toward this condition. It usually occurs in the lower spine, with radiating pain to the leg and numbness or a tingling sensation. Several days of rest, sleeping on a hard mattress, superficial heat provided by electric heating pads, heating lamps, analgesic balms or warm baths, and special exercises to strengthen the supporting stomach and back muscles are frequently successful in controlling the pain. But proceed cautiously under a doctor's care and watch the injury closely, since a degenerated disc can easily become herniated.

A *herniated* or *slipped disc* is caused by repeated or sudden trauma to the back. The disc ruptures and the cushioning fluid within spills out, subjecting the spinal nerves to extremely painful pressure. In rupture cases a disc removal or fusion operation may be recommended to relieve the pain and return flexibility to the spine, but it must be performed by a surgeon who has a good track record with dancers. Although successful surgery restores only seventy-five percent of the patient's former mobility, this amount is still functional for many dancers. Disc operations are the subject of controversy within the medical profession. Some doctors do not feel that surgery—which can be painful and dangerous—is the answer, and recommend other measures. Some spinal operations leave the patient in nearly as much pain and with less movement than ever. So before deciding on major back surgery, get a second or third medical opinion. Talk to ex-patients—preferably dancers or athletes who have undergone the same operation—and find out about alternative treatment.

Treatment alternatives

Serious injuries must be handled with tender loving care if they are to heal soundly and not adversely affect your dancing. As a rule of thumb, don't let yourself be talked into doing anything you don't feel is right. Never embark on a drastic course of treatment, such as surgery or drug therapy, without a complete explanation of the procedures and risks involved and a thorough investigation of the alternatives.

It is wise to get advice from an experienced dance teacher as well as a physician, because each knows something the other doesn't. Every now and then, it is the teacher who comes up with the best solution. A dancer I know had a severe case of tendinitis in her hip. She went to two top orthopedists. One urged her to quit dancing; the other prescribed a drug that had undesirable side effects. In desperation she saw a third doctor who gave her a steroid injection that caused the injury to flare up more. Understandably, she refused any further medication and took a two-month leave of absence from dancing. With rest, the swelling and pain in her hip receded. She then began studying with a ballet teacher who specialized in rehabilitating injuries. He traced the source of tendinitis to excessive tension in the way she was using her body. Together they corrected her faulty working habits, and she has had no trouble since.

The following are methods of treatment that don't involve the use of surgery or drugs:

Chiropractic. Chiropractors relieve pain and improve muscle functioning by releasing pinched nerves and restoring normal nerve flow throughout the body. They do this by pressing and manipulating the spinal vertebrae into correct alignment. A few chiropractors include nutrition counseling, corrective exercises and even acupressure in their treatments. There are various chiropractic methods, some of which use more force than others in making spinal adjustments. Ask about the procedures in advance, and if you are a little skittish ask the chiropractor to go slowly. Be sure to consult one who is licensed by the state and experienced in treating dancers. Some injuries, such as degenerated or slipped discs, should definitely *not* be manipulated. Do get your physician's approval before seeing a chiropractor.

Massage. Dancers go to masseurs when healthy just to relax or to relieve stiffness, soreness and fatigue. But massage is also helpful in treating injuries. It stimulates circulation, reduces muscle spasm and tension, and keeps the muscles supple while they are mending. After an injury has healed, massage therapy can aid in breaking down scar tissue. Some masseurs do minor spinal adjustments, analyze postural problems and prescribe corrective exercises. As in chiropractic, there are various massage techniques, ranging from light, general treatments to the deep, localized, close-to-the-bone kind that can be painful and leave you sore. Talk it over ahead of time. Good masseurs will work from light to deeper massage over several sessions, as your body becomes better able to tolerate it. But here too there is a need to exercise caution, since massage is not good for all types of injuries. Get your doctor's consent and try to find a masseur who has been recommended by other dancers.

Muscle relaxation and retraining techniques. Frederick Matthais Alexander (1869-1955), an Australian actor who was plagued by frequent bouts of laryngitis, invented a method of muscle relaxation based on the correct positioning of the head on the spine. This allows for the release of "holding tension" and thus the free and efficient flow of movement. The Alexander system has been particularly successful in easing back pain. Alexander taught in England and, in 1940, established a school in Massachusetts where he trained a small number of teachers. Among his grateful followers were Aldous Huxley, George Bernard Shaw and John Dewey.

In private or small semiprivate classes, the student of Alexander Technique learns to replace harmful muscular habits with healthy ones through conscious analysis and improved kinesthetic awareness. She reeducates her muscles by following her teacher's verbal directions, by visualizing the correct functioning of body parts, and by carefully practicing such basic activities as bending, sitting and standing until she is able to do them in an anatomically sound way. Qualified teachers of the Alexander Technique may be located through the American Center for the Alexander Technique, 142 West End Avenue, New York, New York 10023, (212) 799-0468. For West Coast and Mid-West teacher information, contact the following regional centers:

Marjorie Barstow	Goddard Binkley	Frank Ottiwell
1445 South 20th Street	805 Grove Street	931 Elizabeth Street
Lincoln, Nebraska 68502	Glencoe, Illinois 60022	San Francisco, California 94114

A similar muscle reeducation system was developed by Dr. Lulu E. Sweigard. Sweigard Technique employs many of the same methods as the Alexander Technique—thoughtful analysis, visualization exercises and individually supervised practice—to help students relax and move more healthfully. Sweigard's work is being carried on by her former student Irene Dowd, a faculty member at Columbia University's Teachers College and the Dance Notation Bureau in New York. André Bernard, who trained with Sweigard's colleague at Juilliard, Barbara Clark, teaches an excellent body awareness course at New York University's School of the Arts.

Alternatives to drug therapy. Doctors may prescribe drugs for severe injuries, but these should be used sparingly and only for short periods of time. Before you fill a prescription make it your business to know what the medication does, the dosage strength and the possible side effects, including addiction. Butazolidin, for instance, is an anti-inflammatory drug frequently prescribed for tendinitis. It can cause weight gain, nausea, mood swings and more serious side effects with persistent use. Valium, a sedative commonly used to relieve back pain, acts on the central nervous system and causes drowsiness, hangovers, and impaired motor functioning, among other things. Many doctors object to the use of painkillers on the grounds that they make injuries difficult to treat by desensitizing the body and masking the patient's symptoms.

The safest painkiller I know is good old aspirin, which is also an effective anti-inflammatory medication. On bad nights, a stiff drink will quiet the pain and help you fall asleep. Since dancers are in touch with their bodies and have highly developed powers of concentration, they often respond well to methods such as deep relaxation, meditation, acupuncture and self-hypnosis, which help relieve tension and discomfort and promote healing.

Rehabilitation and prevention of recurrence

Before you can rehabilitate an injury, it must heal completely. Although doctors often prescribe total body rest, depending on the type of injury and its location, they may recommend exercising healthy parts of the body or some alternate activity—such as swimming—while the injured tissue knits. Besides helping the dancer stay in shape, this Rx is good for morale.

After healing, all severe injuries leave weakened areas which must be strengthened by special remedial exercises. Doctors usually recommend a physical therapist for patients recovering from moderate to acute injuries. To be safe for dancing, the injured part has to be *stronger* than its healthy counterpart on the other side of the body.

Returning to class. After you get the go-ahead from your doctor, try these simple tests to determine whether you are ready to resume dance training:

- Compare the injured part with the healthy side of your body. It should be the same color, and there should be no swelling or uneven contours.

- Move the injured part in every way possible. There should be no pain. Have a friend apply gentle resistance while you try to move against it. There should be no pain, nor should there be pain when the injured area is gently but fully stretched.

- Run through a practice class on your own, at a comfortable pace. The injured part may feel strange or shaky as you work, but it shouldn't hurt or feel too weak to support the movement.

When you return to class after an injury, find an analytic teacher who is knowledgeable in both technique and anatomy, and who will work with you to rebuild strength and confidence and prevent recurrence (See chapter 11 on teachers). She should help you trace the cause of injury and correct whatever poor working habits, chronic physical condition or alignment problems were responsible. "An injury forces you to focus on how you work," says Paul Taylor dancer Carolyn Adams. "If the injury's source is not dealt with, you can simply continue compensating for it but never get over it, because you never get to the root of the trouble."

Start in a slow class, so you can move carefully. You and your teacher should devise a progressive regimen for getting you back into shape. You might begin by taking only the warm-up for the first week or two, and gradually add a few more exercises each week until you feel up to taking the entire class. Be sure to dress warmly for workouts and to wear supportive strapping, if needed, for strains and sprains.

Resources

Alexander, F. Matthias. *The Resurrection of the Body: The Writings of F. Matthais Alexander,* selected and introduced by Edward Maisel. New York: University Books, 1969.

Arnheim, Daniel. *Dance Injuries: Their Prevention and Care.* St. Louis: C.V. Mosby Company, 1975.

Como, William. *Raoul Gelabert's Anatomy for the Dancer (as told to William Como),* Vols. 1 and 2. New York: Danad Publishing Company, 1964.

Featherstone, Donald. *Dancing Without Danger.* South Brunswick: A.S. Barnes, 1970.

Graedon, Joe. *The People's Pharmacy: A Guide to Prescription Drugs, Home Remedies and Over-the-Counter Medications.* New York: Avon, 1976.

Hamilton, William G., M.D., "Ballet and Your Body: An Orthopedist's View," in *Dancemagazine,* February 1978 to January 1979.

Lindner, David, "Dancer's Pain," in *Dance Life in New York,* Vol. 1, No. 1 (Spring 1975).

Myers, Martha, "Body Therapies and the Modern Dancer," in *Dancemagazine,* February to July 1980.

Parish, Peter, M.D. *The Doctor's and Patient's Handbook of Medicine and Drugs.* New York: A.A. Knopf, 1978.

Sweigard, Lulu E. *Human Movement Potential: Its Ideokinetic Facilitation.* New York: Dodd Mead, 1974.

Todd, Mabel Elsworth. *The Thinking Body.* New York: Dance Horizons, 1937.

Vincent, L. M., M.D. *The Dancer's Book of Health.* Mission, Kansas: Sheed Andrews and McMeel, 1978.

Wetschler, Edward, "Chiropractic and Dancers," in *Dance Life in New York,* Vol. 1, No. 2 (Fall 1975).

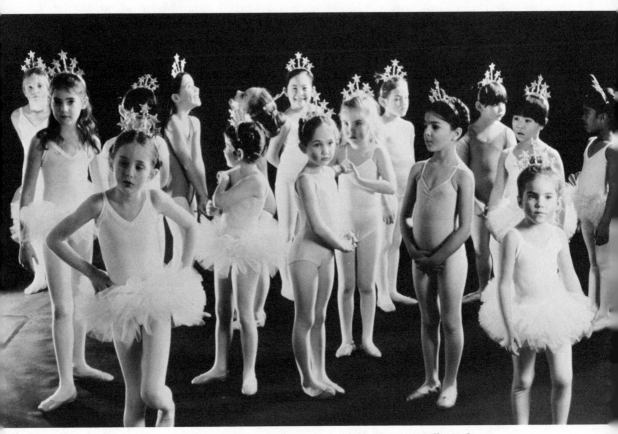

Which one is tomorrow's star? *Lois Greenfield, courtesy of Capezio Ballet Makers*

Part V

The finishing touches

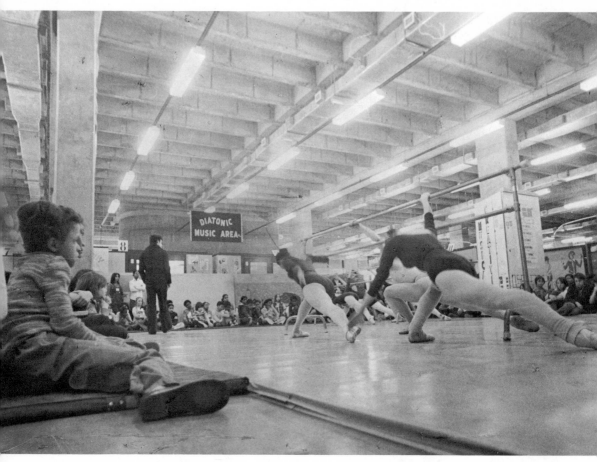

Lecture-demonstrations at public schools and other local performances give young dancers valuable stage experience while bringing dance to appreciative new audiences. *courtesy of the School of the Cleveland Ballet*

20

Launching a Performing Career

getting stage experience and making your first professional connections

The old cliché about being discovered and becoming a star overnight isn't the way it happens most of the time. As Broadway dancer Adam Grammis says, "There's no such thing as instant success. You have to make it happen step by step." The dance business depends heavily on word of mouth and personal referrals because most choreographers prefer to work with dancers they already know or who come recommended by someone they know. Careers are built on a slow accumulation of experience and a chain of personal associations made over years of performing. One thing leads to another: Someone from class is putting together a concert and asks you to be in a piece; a dancer you've performed with recommends you to a choreographer; a choreographer you've worked with uses you for another project; someone looking for dancers spots you from the audience. Luck and timing have their part to play too. However, as the father of songwriter Alan Jay Lerner once observed about his son, "The harder he works, the luckier he gets." There are probably as many different routes to the footlights as there are dancers, but most young people breaking into the profession start close to home—with school recitals and local dance companies, high school or college musicals, and home-town theater groups.

After three or four years of intensive training, a dancer should begin, however modestly, to perform and make her first connections with choreographers and other working dancers. She should begin to test herself under what

Agnes de Mille calls "the life and death conditions of the theater." This is necessary, not only because gaining experience and advancing a career take time, but from the standpoint of morale as well. In many ways performing is the culmination of all the work you have put into yourself while training. For many dancers it offers a first real glimpse of the deep personal rewards of dancing and a first true appreciation of their own performing qualities, some of which can only emerge in the transforming environment of the stage. It is very difficult to work hard in class day after day, year after year, and never know the satisfaction of dancing a finished ballet, or the exciting chemistry that sparks among performers, or the intensifying effect of an audience.

There is so much that can *only* be learned onstage. The stage, writes Doris Humphrey in *The Art of Making Dances*, "differs radically from the physical and psychological space of the studio, where [the student] has learned about her body for so many years. . . .Dance training, with its years and years of technique in a studio is very incomplete and unrealistic indeed." Not only is the performer's use of space vastly different from the student's, but her efforts have an entirely different focus. Most of the time in class, the dancer's concentration is directed inward toward herself, while onstage her concentration and energy must project outward to the audience.

Even the novice in a high school musical or a student dance company learns to maneuver cleanly in a limited space, work with other dancers and take direction. Following cues, using wings and working in lights and costumes are other aspects of learning the ropes that these early experiences provide. After many performances, the young dancer develops stage presence. Gradually she arrives at an individual performance style—her own way of communicating with an audience.

> *Technique in class and technique on the stage are two different things. Nothing can beat performing experience. The excitement of rehearsing and finally performing a variation can bring you to new heights technically and artistically. After all, dance is a performing art.*
>
> *—SARA MAULE*
> *American Ballet Theatre*

One of the nice things about dancing today is that there are more performing outlets than ever before, including student workshops and semi-professional and professional dance companies of all sizes and statures. But in order to take advantage of these, it is essential to keep an open mind and pursue all the avenues open to you. You never know which ones will pay off, and often success comes in unexpected packages. Every opportunity is a springboard that will at the very least add to your experience, broaden your exposure and introduce you to more dancers and choreographers.

It doesn't matter how or where you start performing, so long as you start somewhere. Most inexperienced dancers don't work under ideal circumstances. In your first few engagements you probably won't get paid, and you can expect some shabby performances and uneven choreography. The director may be less than inspiring—so may some of the other dancers. But it is a beginning, it is the experience you need, and what better place to get it than where you can freely make mistakes?

Of course, you should always try to work with the best available choreographers and dancers, but if this doesn't happen right away, take advantage of the openings at hand. Don't hold out for the prestigious jobs that you may not be ready for, and don't set your professional goals too soon. Frequently our ideas of how and with whom we would like to dance don't hold up under the realities of the situation.

Even if you are one of the lucky few who start out working in a celebrated company, it is usually a difficult first environment in which to grow as an artist. A young dancer can easily get lost in a big company and buckle under the strain of the competition and pressure that usually go with the territory. In the beginning, there is a lot to be said for being a big fish in a small pond. Normally it is the smaller troupes that can offer the newcomer personal nurturing and sizable roles. There are always plenty of young choreographers around, hungry for good dancers. Martha Graham, Merce Cunningham, George Balanchine, Jerome Robbins, Paul Taylor, Twyla Tharp, Alvin Ailey and Robert Joffrey started working just that way—with a small band of eager youngsters who were willing to put in long hours for little or no pay in exchange for collaborating with a promising choreographer. Indeed, some choreographers do their best work early in their careers, and to get in on the ground floor of an up-and-coming company can be the most exciting opportunity of all. There is an intoxicating sense of camaraderie in a brand new dance company. Because everyone is learning together, it is a joint venture and all are likely to care deeply about the results.

As you gain experience, you can afford to be more selective about where and with whom you perform; also you'll know better what kind of artistic environment you need. Eventually the choreographer you work with should be someone whose movement style, interests and standards of excellence enrich your own. Above all, he should be able to use your individual qualities well, while generating excitement and inspiring growth in all his dancers.

Where to start

When entering the dance profession there are no substitutes for resourcefulness and persistence, or for being in the right place at the right time. Keep your eyes and ears open and follow up all reasonable leads. Let your teachers and fellow dancers know that you are looking for work, and ask them for suggestions. The dance grapevine is fast and far-reaching. If you plug yourself into it, it will help keep you well informed.

Your dance school and teacher. An obvious place to begin establishing professional ties is your dance school. Look for a school that has a dance company affiliated with it. This will enable you to study the group's choreographic style in depth, while the school's faculty will have the chance to follow your progress in class as you develop into potential material for the company.

Dance teachers who have been performers or who are still performing have a network of professional associations. They generally know about auditions in local or even out-of-town companies, and they are often asked by colleagues to recommend students for jobs.

The biggest dance school in town. Big dance schools are a favorite site for major auditions. Professional companies on tour may give classes or hold tryouts there. Road companies of Broadway shows that need to replace cast members during stopovers also conduct auditions at big-name studios. Similarly, young choreographers looking for dancers often go where they are assured of seeing lots of talented students.

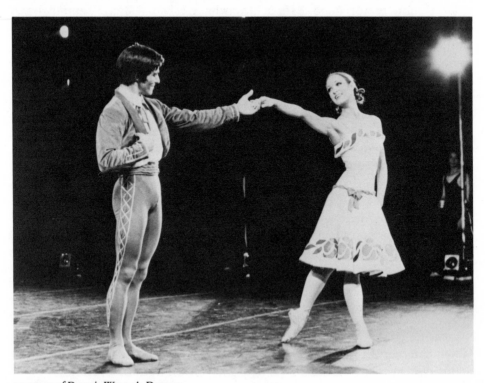

courtesy of Dennis Wayne's Dancers

If there is an active college dance or theater department nearby, it's worth your while to scan its bulletin boards now and again for audition and job notices. Colleges serve as information centers in much the same way as dance schools do.

Regional ballet companies. The ninety member companies of the National Association for Regional Ballet, all of which have affiliate schools, are rated for quality by a national board of distinguished professionals (see chapter 25). These grass-roots troupes provide first-rate performing exposure. The best of them are showcased at annual festivals, where representatives from leading ballet companies scout for new talent. A good percentage of this nation's top-ranking dancers were discovered while appearing with regional ballet companies.

Study with a choreographer you admire. Many choreographers like to teach, as a way of both developing their ideas and training dancers in their style. Some conduct classes at their own schools or rent space at local studios; others teach at colleges and summer dance festivals. An excellent way of gaining access to a choreographer is by studying with him. After you have become fluent in his movement style and he has begun to show an interest in you, tell him that you admire his work and would like to dance with him. It means a great deal to a choreographer to work with people who sincerely appreciate what he is trying to do, all the more because breaking in new company members and working them into the repertory demand a sizable investment of his time and energy. When considering dancers for his company, he is as likely to be influenced by their enthusiasm as by their technical virtuosity and prior performing credits.

After you've made your pitch, the choreographer may surprise you with an immediate invitation to audition or watch a rehearsal. On the other hand, he may not have an opening at present or feel that you are ready. He'll let you know one way or another. Don't badger him by asking repeatedly, but do give yourself a realistic time limit. If you don't get a response by then, you may want to go on studying with him but look for employment elsewhere.

Contact the company directly. If you wish to perform with a particular dance company, call or write them directly and ask whether they are teaching anywhere or holding any upcoming auditions. You may not get a reply, but it's worth a try.

Check your local newspaper and the weekly trade papers. Audition announcements are published in the theater section of local newspapers, as well as in the weekly trade papers *Backstage* and *Show Business.*

Show Business
136 West 44th Street
New York, New York 10036
(212) 586-6900

Backstage
165 West 46th Street
New York, New York 10036
(212) 581-1080

Backstage West
5670 Wilshire Boulevard
Los Angeles, California 90036
(213) 936-5200

Backstage Mid-West
1008 Bellwood Avenue
Bellwood, Illinois 60104
(312) 544-3432

Backstage South
432 Hibiscus Drive
Miami Beach, Florida 33139
(305) 532-7895

Local newspapers may list anything from dance company tryouts to notices for theater, nightclub and summer-stock auditions. The trade papers cover these, as well as casting notices for Broadway shows, bus and truck (national) tours, regional (non-commercial) theaters, dinner theaters, nightclub revues, circus shows, television productions and films. You should also thumb through *Dancemagazine*'s news section and advertisements (see chapter 26). Other places to search for jobs are the newsletters and information centers of the regional dance organizations described in chapter 25.

Look for "open call" auditions—those that are open to nonunion dancers. Until you are hired by a unionized company, you are eligible to attend open calls *only*.

Taking auditions

Auditions are regarded as a necessary evil by choreographers. They are the most expedient way of screening many dancers at once, but afford neither the choreographer nor the dancer sufficient time to get well acquainted with each other's work. Almost no one is seen at their best, and snap decisions have to be made that are bound to result in some bitter disappointments and bruised egos. Some people thrive on the pressure and excitement of auditions, but most have to learn to audition successfully.

It's best to approach auditions as learning situations and expect to take several before you land your first job. Then you can relax, enjoy yourself and benefit from them. As a matter of fact, it's wise to begin by going to tryouts you don't care about just for the experience. Arrive early enough to give yourself a good warm-up and settle down. Mixing with the other dancers helps to break the ice and may bring you some useful tips. Auditions are performances, so despite the inevitable nerves and distractions, try to concentrate on what you are doing as completely as possible. You will be given some time to practice, but if your turn is called and you are not prepared, give it your best shot anyway. Decide as best you can what the combination is and do it full out, even if you are convinced you are wrong. If you dance with clarity and conviction, your overall ability and stage presence will come through; if you try to fudge the steps or hang back in line, you won't come across at all. Be yourself.

Choreographers look for personal qualities and sense of style as much as for technical skill. Most auditors give corrections, and if you have your wits about you, you can improve in time to better your chances. If there is a choice, try to take your turn in the middle of the order so you can watch the dancers before you. When you are called to audition again, be sure to wear the same dance clothes and hairstyle each time. That way you will be easily identifiable as "the girl in the ponytail" or "the boy in the blue shirt," for example.

One valuable lesson you can learn from auditions is what to go back and work on in class. Perhaps your turns aren't as strong as they should be or your line isn't clean enough. Maybe you've got to sharpen your rhythmic attack or move more aggressively. But don't take rejection as a personal failure. Often you are being judged solely on whether you are a particular physical or personality type. Sometimes the best dancers aren't chosen because they don't fit the costumes. And sometimes choreographers are so intent on watching dancers they've invited to audition that only a real standout has any hope of distinguishing herself from the swarm of bodies in the mob. These are things you can't change no matter how many auditions you go to, so don't try and don't worry about it. Take all in stride and keep your sense of humor. In time you'll be nursing others through their first auditions.

When you register for an audition you may be asked to submit a résumé of your previous training and work experience. AGMA's Joan Greenspan advises dancers with little or no performing credits to list their dance teachers (musical-theater dancers should include their voice and acting instructors), along with any performances they might have done with school or local groups. Don't try to impress the auditors by padding your résumé with fictitious credits. It doesn't fool anyone and it can spoil your chances.

After you've chalked up enough experience, be discriminating about the auditions you attend. Think about where your qualities would be best appreciated and whose work you are genuinely interested in. Don't go to every tryout that comes along merely to bolster your morale or because you're depressed about not having a job. Auditions are the very worst places to go for ego support. Acting out of such motives puts you in a no-win predicament. If you are rejected you will probably take it as a criticism of your dancing, even if you didn't want the job in the first place; and if you get into a company you don't really care about, you won't be able to accept the work in good conscience.

A note to musical-theater dancers. Opportunities for musical-theater dancers are the most plentiful in major cities. Local theater, nightclub and summer-stock productions are the likeliest to hire inexperienced applicants. If you are not successful at open auditions, which can be out-and-out cattle calls, remember that there are other ways of getting the stage experience you need.

Several of the professionals I interviewed started performing in high school and college musicals. From there they looked for work at local clubs, coffee houses and small theater companies—door-to-door if necessary. One Broadway dancer got his first job as a singing waiter doing four shows a night at a Boston club. Gena Belkin of Actor's Equity suggests that instead of going cold to open auditions, young dancers should first get some performing experience with a dance company. Some summer-stock houses take on student apprentices, who help with the general production behind the scenes and do bit parts onstage. These apprenticeships can lead to full-time acting positions.

Resources

von Obenauer, Heidi, ed. *Dancemagazine Annual*.
A trade directory to dance artists, sponsors, services, and equipment suppliers, this annual publication lists virtually every professional and regional dance company in the country, as well as choreographers and funding sources. It costs $15.00 per copy, and can be obtained by writing to *Dancemagazine Annual*, 1180 Avenue of the Americas, New York, New York 10011; or calling (212) 921-9300.

Shurtleff, Michael. *Audition: Everything an Actor Needs to Know to Get the Part*. New York: Walker and Company, 1978.

21

New York Bound

biting into the Big Apple

What Hollywood is to the filmmaker and Wall Street is to the financier, New York is to the dancer. That city has long been the reigning capital of the burgeoning world of dance. Sooner or later every serious dancer comes to the dance mecca, or thinks about coming.

The reasons are obvious. New York City has no peer for the sheer variety and quantity of its offerings in ballet, modern, musical-theater and ethnic dance. It houses the world's largest dance library and film collection at Lincoln Center. Most of the major American dance companies either have headquarters in New York or give regular seasons there, and New York is a nonstop showcase for international dance attractions. In no other city can you study with your choice of celebrated teachers alongside principal dancers from the world's leading companies. And nowhere else on earth are there so many opportunities to perform. New York has a reputation for having not only more of everything but the best—the highest concentration of top-notch dancers, teachers, dance schools and companies.

> *I think somewhere I read that in New York City there are over two hundred dance companies—small companies, not necessarily full-time or paying. Most of them are not, but there are always people with small companies who get together for just one or two performances at a time, always. All you have to do is look around.*
>
> *—CHRISTINE WRIGHT*
> *Lar Lubovitch Dance Company*

But—and there's a big but—New York City is not the only place to make a dance career, and as many who have tried it will attest, it's not the only place to live, either. Growing numbers of talented dancers are choosing to pursue their careers elsewhere rather than cope with the professional competition and pressures of city life. Standards of dance training and performance have risen across the nation as programs such as the National Association for Regional Ballet, the National Endowment for the Arts Dance Touring Program and public television continue to expose new audiences to quality dance (see chapter 25). As dance consumers become increasingly sophisticated, they demand more and usually get it. For that matter, most of the professional dancers working in New York have received at least their initial training in other locales.

There are first-rate schools and companies in all parts of the country—witness those, for example, of the Pennsylvania Ballet in Philadelphia, the Boston Ballet, Ballet West in Salt Lake City and the San Francisco Ballet—which produce excellent dancers and attract faculties as fine as can be found anywhere. Stanley Holden, a past member of the Royal Ballet in England, has assembled a distinguished staff at his Dance Center in Los Angeles. Ian Horvath and Dennis Nahat of the Cleveland Ballet were previously associated with American Ballet Theatre in New York. Former Graham dancer Ethel Butler has been teaching for years in Washington, D.C. There is Bill Evans in Seattle, Gus Giordano in Evanston, Illinois, and other jazz pros such as Danny Daniels, Joe Tremaine, Jaime Rogers, Claude Thompson and Roland Dupree in Los Angeles. The list goes on and on.

In sum, New York is not for everyone. Some people thrive there, others find it's their Waterloo. If you don't make it in New York, it doesn't necessarily mean you aren't good. It's a tough city and you need a certain kind of temperament to survive. Ultimately you'll have to weigh the advantages over the disadvantages. You may grow and develop better in a calmer, more protective environment; or you may wish to try out the city temporarily before committing yourself to a permanent move. And you can always get a great deal from the New York dance world on a short-term basis, without having to move there lock, stock and barrel.

What to expect

> *New York is a disaster, but what a magnificent disaster . . .*
>
> *—LE CORBUSIER*

New York is a city of incongruities. *Starr and John Wisdom*

No one is ever fully prepared for New York, but it helps to know what to expect. Even for those who feel they were made for it, there has to be a period of adjustment. The city fairly teems with excitement. It is stimulating, colorful and sophisticated, and it is a cultural hotbed—the center of music, theater and art as well as dance. New York is certainly never boring, but neither is it soothing. It will keep your adrenalin flowing overtime. The screeching traffic, the relentlessly fast pace, the crowds, the pollution, the towering buildings, the lines at supermarkets, all take some getting used to. And because there is a crime problem, one has to be streetwise.

"Some of these kids are in for a big shock when they get to New York," says the New York City Ballet's Victoria Bromberg, remembering her student days at the School of American Ballet. "Picture a fifteen-year-old girl from the Midwest who goes to the School of American Ballet. She lives in one of the boardinghouses they put you up in. She calls her mom every night and dresses in pastels. All she knows is the sheltered life of classes and the residence hall. One day she goes to get an ice cream at the Carvel on Broadway. What a shock!" (Victoria is referring to the derelicts and prostitutes who habituate the area in summertime. Incidentally, the Carvel store has since closed down.)

Ellen Kogan, a modern dancer who made the move from Los Angeles, advises: "The fewer expectations you have, the better. There are no guarantees that you'll find a place to dance, paying or not. And you need time. The odds that you'll get a job right away are small. Most dancers don't have any idea of how long it is necessary to wait—it can take years. In the meantime, you need money, savings or a part-time job to support yourself. Part of the reason it takes so much time to break into the New York dance world is there is so much more competition. You have to expect some rejection and difficulty in the beginning. Then again, there are many more opportunities in New York. If it isn't happening for you at one company or school, you can try another, and another, until you find the right place for yourself."

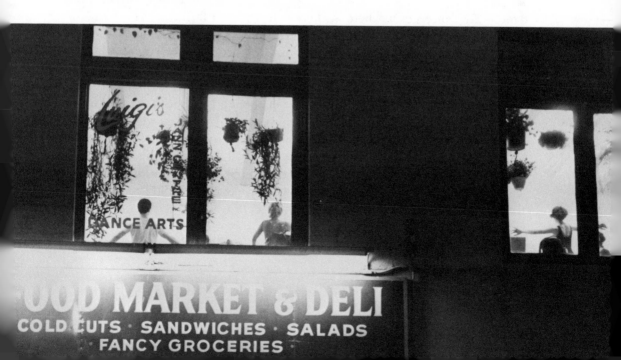

Many newcomers to the city are surprised by the range of location and ambience of New York dance schools: from the cloistered Eastside townhouses which lodge the Harkness Ballet and the Martha Graham schools, to the dingy, rundown studios in the heart of the Times Square theater district where some of the best jazz and tap classes are taught; from cooly professional institutions such as the School of American Ballet and the Merce Cunningham Studio, to the homey atmosphere of such family run "neighborhood" schools as Alfredo Corvino's Dance Circle and the New York School of Ballet; from the bewildering smorgasbord of classes at the sprawling new Alvin Ailey American Dance Center in midtown Manhattan, to the converted lofts of experimental modern dancers in Soho. Some city dance studios aren't as spacious or well maintained as those in other regions, but the cost of dance lessons in New York averages a dollar less than in the rest of the country. On the whole, New York schools take fewer vacations, too.

Like everything else, dance classes are generally crowded in the city. It is natural to need attention and recognition from your teacher, but if you don't get it right away, don't jump to the conclusion that there is something wrong with you. It just takes longer to be noticed in a crowd. Most teachers will respond to a new student after they've seen him or her for a few lessons. If this doesn't happen, look for another teacher. Some New York dance schools, especially the big ones, are impersonal. They lack the sense of support and community you might find in other cities, simply offering classes and nothing more. This is partly because they service so many dancers and partly because there is so much going on in town already. In a sense, these schools are a microcosm of city life—rich in diversity but often anonymous and potentially overwhelming. That is why it is essential to give yourself time to settle down, get to know other dancers and find your own niche.

There may also be a more serious atmosphere in New York dance classes than you're used to, and the students may seem cool or aloof to you. Often they are merely concentrating hard or trying to cover up their own shyness. But dancers are dancers everywhere in the world, and you'll find that even in New York most are friendly and helpful when you get to know them.

Once you start taking classes it may be necessary for you to adjust to different standards of quality and different values of performance, or you may discover that you have overestimated your technical level. Ballerina Patricia McBride's experience is not uncommon: "Although I had been the best in the class at Teaneck, New Jersey, I was at the bottom of the class when I came to New York. I had to work awfully hard to keep up with everybody else."* Obviously McBride was no slouch, she merely had some catching up to do. It may also be that once you get to New York and test them out, your ideas about where and with whom you should study will have to change and you along with them.

*From Cynthia Lyle, *Dancers on Dancing*.

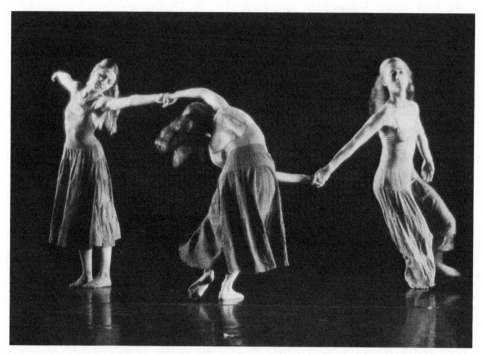

The Marcus Schulkind Dance Company is one of hundreds of small groups working in New York. *Nathaniel Tileston, courtesy of Marcus Schulkind*

Survival tips

Because a move to New York usually entails making some major adjustments, not the least of which may be leaving home for the first time, it's a good idea to sample the city for short periods first—weekends, if you're within commuting distance, or on school vacations. If you do want to relocate permanently, brief visits give you a chance to acclimate yourself in small doses.

Whether you come to New York on a temporary or a permanent basis, it will be very important to do adequate advance planning, since it is not an easy town to improvise in. It's best to take care of practical needs first, so that you are not discouraged or distracted by nondance problems. Those who are moving to the city should arrive with at least enough money to get through the first six months. If you don't have a place to stay, do some investigating ahead of time. You should be cautious about where you live in Manhattan because many of its affordable hotels and residences are unfit. Try to enlist the help of someone who has recently been to New York or who is already there. If you have any doubts about the safety of your lodgings, call the local police precinct to double check.

The St. Mary's Residence, 225 East 72nd Street, New York, New York 10021, (212) 249-6850; the Barbizon Hotel for Women, Lexington Avenue at 63rd Street, New York, New York 10021, (212) TE 8-5700; and selected branches of the YWCA and YWHA are frequently recommended for temporary housing. For further suggestions, you might inquire at the National Association for Regional Ballet office, 1860 Broadway, New York, New York 10023, (212) 757-8460; or at Dance Theatre Workshop, 219 West 19th Street, New York, New York 10011, (212)691-6500.

If you are planning to remain in temporary housing for a month or more, scour the city's newspapers (particularly the *New York Times* and the *Village Voice**) for apartments to sublet. These are especially plentiful during the summer months. Good low-cost housing for the summer is also available at some local universities, where you will be with other students in a protected environment. Columbia University, for example, offers dormitory space to students over eighteen at $6.50 per night, from May 25 to August 12. Proof of student status in the form of an I.D. card or letter from your school is required. For information, write or call the International Student Hostel, Columbia University, 125 Livingston Hall, New York, New York 10027,(212) 280-2775. From June 4 to September 3, New York University rents its vacant dormitory rooms for a fee of $8.00 per night plus the purchase of a meal plan. For an application, write to New York University Housing, 54 Washington Square, New York, New York 10012, (212) 598-2083.

Even if you are only in New York for a few days, you should allow yourself time to get acquainted with its transportation system. The numbered streets and grid design of the city make it fairly simple to find your way around, and the Metropolitan Transit Authority publishes free subway and bus maps that are distributed at many subway token booths and major railroad depots, such as Grand Central Station and Pennsylvania Station. You can send away for the maps by writing to the Public Affairs Department, New York City Transit Authority, 370 Jay Street, Brooklyn, New York 11201 (enclose a self-addressed, stamped envelop). In addition, the Transit Authority operates a telephone information service that provides directions to any street address in New York; call (212) 330-1234. Traveling by bus is more pleasant, but subways are the fastest way to go when you're in a hurry. Discount transfers are available to bus passengers.

Safety is very important in New York; you have to know how to take care of yourself. When journeying home at night from a deserted part of town, always try to walk back to your subway or bus stop with a friend. Walk in busy, well-lighted streets. Day or night, ride in subway cars that are well populated and wait for trains at the center of the station platform, near the toll booth. If you are moving into a new apartment, make sure the door and window locks are secure (the police can recommend pick-proof locks and protective window gates). To avoid petty thievery, take your dance bag and all valuables into the classroom or rehearsal studio with you. And when looking for part-time work,

---

*If you want to get a jump on other apartment hunters, at some city newsstands you can buy the *Village Voice* and the Sunday *Times* a day or two before their publication dates.

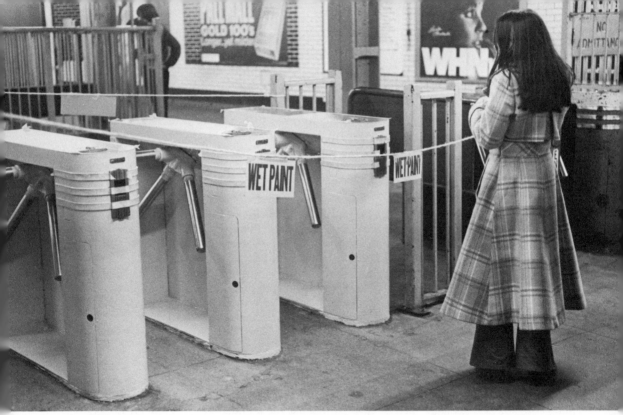

Frank Gimpaya

use common sense. Though want ads for art modeling, barmaid or go-go dancer positions may promise high pay and short hours, many of these jobs are in fact sleazy and dangerous. Be careful. There are plenty of legitimate jobs but, as the old saying goes, you don't get something for nothing.

Those making a permanent move to New York ought to take several weeks to explore dance classes thoroughly and find an encouraging teacher. New York dance schools have a reputation for being tough and cutthroat. Some of them are, and these may not be for you. But most aren't. Learn to sift through the hearsay and think for yourself. Shop around.

Men will have an automatic strength in numbers—that is, the lack of them. Women, who are likely to find themselves in the overpopulated majority, may need time to reestablish confidence—all the more reason to seek out a supportive school environment in the beginning. Remember that your special value as a dancer has everything to do with who you are and very little to do with how much you can look like someone else. Both men and women should avoid making any judgments about their dancing until they are well settled.

Temporary visitors. Try not to squeeze too much into a brief visit to New York, however tempting this may be. Even if you exhaust yourself, you won't get to see and do everything. It's better to limit your goals to those that can be enjoyably accomplished in the time you have. You can always come back for more. When you go to class, it might be helpful to introduce yourself to the teacher and explain that you are there temporarily. If possible, find a special short-term or intensive course where everyone will be starting off together in a new situation, and which you will be able to take in its entirety (intensive courses are listed in the *Dance in New York* guide noted below).

Resources

> Jacob, Ellen, and Christopher Jonas. *Dance in New York: An Indispensable Companion to the Dance Capital of the World.* New York: Quick Fox, 1980. Exactly what the title says, this comprehensive guide includes an in-depth directory of over one hundred dance schools and teachers in New York City; descriptions and locations of theaters that regularly present dance; profiles of the city's resident dance companies; plus information on New York-based dance organizations, college dance programs, dancewear suppliers, dance publications and bookstores, fitness and medical services for dancers, and temporary housing for visitors. Copies may be purchased from Danceways, 393 West End Avenue, New York, New York 10024, at $6.95 each plus $1.00 for postage and handling.

> Simkin, Margie, and Ted Striggles. *The Poor Dancer's Almanac: A Guide to Living and Dancing in New York.* New York: Association of American Dance Companies, 1976.
> A handy survival manual to what the authors call "the nonartistic side of dancing in New York," such as housing, health care, unemployment insurance, and funding and production resources for choreographers. Copies may be purchased from Dance Theatre Workshop, 219 West 19th Street, New York, New York 10011, (212) 691-6500. An updated edition is planned for 1981.

22

Is College Dance for You?

the pros and cons of college for serious dancers

When I went to college in the mid-sixties, most of the few dance programs in existence were conducted by overweight academicians in gymnasiums for the benefit of young women who got married right after graduation or became teachers themselves. A handful of programs did turn out successful performers, but they were exceptions, and by and large college was no place for serious dancers. So much so, that around the same time Agnes de Mille—an honors graduate of UCLA—was prompted to admonish readers of her book *To a Young Dancer*, ''If you wish a career as a professional dancer, you will probably have to forego college.'' A great deal has changed since then.

Experienced professionals have gradually replaced well-meaning educators in many of the more than three hundred college dance programs currently operating in America. Today, for example, you can study with former principals of the New York City Ballet and the Martha Graham Dance Company at the North Carolina School of the Arts. Tap dance virtuoso Paul Draper has been a professor at Carnegie Mellon University in Pittsburgh since 1969. Choreographer Eugene Loring is on the dance staff at the University of California at Irvine, and Katherine Dunham is associated with Southern Illinois University. Gladys Bailin, past soloist with the Alwin Nikolais Dance Theatre, is a senior faculty member of the University of Ohio at Athens, and the indomitable Harriet Ann Gray has chaired the dance department at Stephens College in Columbia, Missouri for several decades.

Many of these college programs have the autonomy, teaching staff and facilities to make them attractive training grounds for talented young performers and choreographers. Moreover, the National Endowment for the Arts

Dance Touring Program sponsors teaching and performing residencies for professional dance companies around the country, thus bringing the greater dance world to once remote campuses. In the last ten years the proliferation of dance-related careers, such as dance therapy, notation, criticism and administration, has made college more desirable for a wider range of aspiring professionals. Yet despite these and other encouraging developments, college is not for everyone. Whether or not to go to college depends very much on the individual dancer and the particular dance program under consideration.

Key issues

The strongest argument in favor of getting a college education is that it can teach you more than how to lift your leg up high or do the perfect plié. Carolyn Adams, who attended Sarah Lawrence College before joining the Paul Taylor Dance Company, explains, ''You don't go to college to study dance, you go for the other things it can offer. Early in life I knew I wanted to be a dancer, but I have always thought of myself as a person, too. And as a person I needed the rounding out that college gave me.''

College life offers a protective environment in which to grow, yet it is broadening. It brings you into contact with people of other backgrounds, interests and points of view. You'll meet scientists, psychologists and anthro-

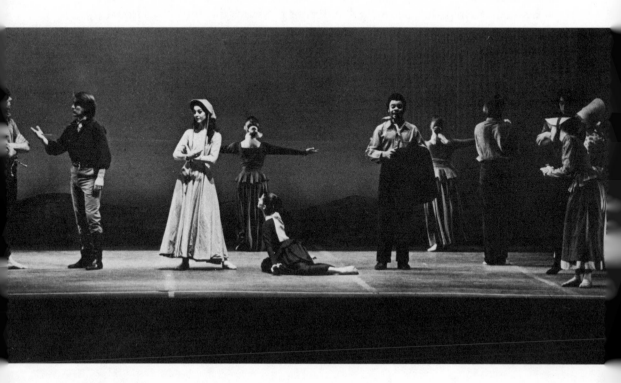

pologists there, as well as other artists. Four years of college can help give dancers the self-assurance, emotional maturity and intellectual skills to better manage their careers and handle themselves in difficult professional situations.

A good college program can broaden you immeasurably as a dancer too. Or, as one student bluntly put it, "College forces you to take subjects you might not get to on your own." Dance history, music, choreography, criticism, anatomy, and teaching methods are covered, along with various dance techniques, including ballet and modern dance and, less frequently, ethnic or musical-theater dance. Many college dance curricula also encompass courses in dance notation, acting, dance production, costume design and dance therapy.

At some colleges you can get fine performing experience, besides. Numerous dance departments hire professional choreographers to compose or re-stage pieces for student concerts; others commission reconstructions of famous historical works for students to perform. In recent years, for instance, Agnes de Mille's *Cherry Tree Legend* was mounted on dancers at the North Carolina School of the Arts; students at Brooklyn College were taught Anna Sokolow's *Moods*; and graduating seniors at Barnard College performed excerpts from José Limón's *There Is a Time*. A few college programs are affiliated with in-dependently-run professional dance companies, such as Ballet West and the Repertory Dance Theatre at the University of Utah, and the North Carolina Dance Theatre at the North Carolina School of the Arts.

In view of the general uncertainties of a performing career in dance (see chapter 9), a college degree may also prove helpful in getting needed part-time or free-lance employment, and it can lay the foundation for a second career after retirement. If you want to teach dance someday, having a bachelor's or master's degree is a great advantage and, at the college level, often a necessity.

College does not provide everything you need as a dancer, however. Although you can wait until your late teens to learn kinesiology, aesthetics or acting, in most cases it is unrealistic to begin dance training in college and expect to emerge four years later a professional. A college program, no matter how exemplary, won't make a finished performer out of a raw beginner. You'll need good training in addition to your college classes, because at this age the body needs intensive work and you cannot get a job as a dancer without a well-educated body. Those who go on to successful stage careers usually have solid outside training before, during and/or after entering college.

Furthermore, college is at best a compromise of dance and academic priorities. Dance students must divide their time between the library and the dance studio, and some find that neither their art nor their intellect is suf-ficiently satisfied by this arrangement.

Though it is a bridge to a broader world, college life can be insular in its own way. Despite the residencies by guest teachers and touring companies,

A student performance of Agnes de Mille's *Cherry Tree Legend* at the North Carolina School of the Arts.

college dance departments are often criticized for being too far removed from the realities of the professional dance world. Such isolation, says de Mille, stating the strongest case against college for dancers, "sets false standards of easy mediocrity," and "prevents the student from mixing on terms of equality with . . . ranking artists of talent and ambition." Not even the most complete college dance program can give you the experience of living and studying in a city where there are scores of good dance teachers and schools to choose from, a variety of opportunities to perform, and many top-flight professionals to watch. There is a very real danger that the college dancer can get too comfortably ensconced in a purely student environment.

One solution might be to attend a school in a city where there is a lot of dance activity, so you can see and experience dance outside the campus atmosphere. This will help keep things in the proper perspective. You'll have realistic standards against which to measure your college program and yourself. And you'll have contact with working dancers.

Is college for you?

Dancers undecided about a career. Dance may be the love of your life, but it may not be your life's work. A dance career may be easier to manage today then it was thirty years ago, but it still requires a well-considered commitment that might better be made at age twenty-one than at seventeen. A recent graduate who makes his living as a dancer told me he was glad to have his college years "to incubate." He said it gave him a chance to think about what he wanted to do with dance.

> *Let me give you an example of somebody who shouldn't go to college: A young black man from St. Louis came and auditioned here. He was wonderful, gorgeous. I asked him why he wanted to go to college. He said he wanted to be in a company. I said, if you want to be in company, why don't you go to a company school? His answer was that he didn't think he was good enough. I asked what made him think he wasn't good enough, and told him to go to the Alvin Ailey school and apply for a scholarship. He did, and he got one. Today he teaches at the school and dances with the Ailey company. His name is Milton Myers.*
>
> *—STUART HODES*
> *dance department chairman*
> *New York University School of the Arts*

276

A strong college program offers the serious dancer time to gain experience before plunging into the world of professional dance. College provides exposure to other career possibilities, and it can alert you to the opportunities that exist in dance-related fields should you decide that a performing career is not for you. Or it may let you integrate the dancing you love, as a minor concentration, into an academic degree in anthropology, physical education or psychology.

The modern dancer or aspiring choreographer. College alumni have risen to prominence in every niche of the dance profession, among them tap dancer Gene Kelly and ballet choreographers Agnes de Mille and John Neumeier; Katherine Dunham and Pearl Primus, leading exponents of Afro-Caribbean dance, both hold degrees in anthropology. But American universities have long been a stronghold of modern dance, and there are more college educated modern dancers than any other kind. José Limón, Merce Cunningham, Ethel Winter, Twyla Tharp, Don Redlich, Cliff Keuter, Carolyn Brown, Sara Rudner, Meredith Monk, Jack Moore, Lar Lubovitch, Kenneth King and Kei Takei all attended college. Erick Hawkins was a Greek scholar at Harvard. Paul Taylor was a painting major. Gus Solomons earned a bachelor of arts degree in architecture. It was early moderns such as Isadora Duncan, Ted Shawn and Hanya Holm who campaigned vigorously for dance in education, and it was a modern dancer, Margaret H'Doubler, who established the first college-level dance program at the University of Wisconsin in 1926. Early on, modern dancers found that college audiences shared many of their intellectual and social concerns, as well as their sophisticated tastes in music and stage decor.

There are some practical reasons for the preponderance of modern dance in American universities. Modern dancers generally perform longer than other dancers and thus risk less by spending four years in college. A college education may even make it easier to get work, since modern dance choreographers who teach in colleges frequently select dancers for their companies from among their students, and those who are themselves college educated often look for this in prospective company members. Choreographer Rachel Lampert says, "When I have auditions I look for dancers who can use their minds as well as their bodies. I always seem to pick people who have gone to college. It's funny, but it just turns out that way. Somehow it shows in their dancing." Over the years several graduates of the Juilliard School in New York have joined the companies of José Limón and Martha Graham as a direct result of having studied with members of these companies on the Juilliard faculty. The Pauline Koner Dance Consort was originally formed out of Koner's pupils at the North Carolina School of the Arts; Paul Taylor and Merce Cunningham have also recruited new dancers during teaching residencies at colleges.

Indeed, a large percentage of modern dancers eventually become choreographers, and here again, a good college program offers distinct advantages. The study of music, dance history, production, notation and teaching can enrich a young choreographer's background immensely. College will give her access to student dancers on whom to create new pieces, and to collaborating musicians and designers; it will give her rehearsal space, research libraries and production facilities to see her work fully realized onstage. It would be extremely difficult, if not impossible, for a fledgling to come by all this—plus qualified criticism—on her own.

The ballet dancer. The professional ballet dancer who goes to college is a rare bird. Ballet is much more youth oriented than modern dance. Due to the rigorous demands of the technique, most ballet dancers have many years of studying and performing behind them by the time they reach college age. Such a schedule leaves little room for academic pursuits. For ballet dancers, above all others, it is foolish to pretend that college can furnish the training and stage experience needed for a rising career. But if you are already strong in both areas, the right college dance program can allow you to maintain a high level of performance while finishing your education. The University of Utah, the North Carolina School of the Arts, and the State University of New York at Purchase are among the growing number of colleges that have substantial ballet departments.

The musical-theater dancer. College is also of doubtful advantage to the career of a musical-comedy dancer because the competition is so keen in that field that he needs all the practical knowledge he can get. To find work, the future Broadway performer doesn't need courses in the philosophy of dance nearly as much as he needs to learn a diversity of dance styles and gain experience auditioning and performing. More than he needs to know dance notation, he needs to study voice and acting, and to circulate among other dancers in the business. Although many schools stage college musicals, very few of them provide bona fide training in musical-theater dance. Broadway dancer Adam Grammis looks back on his college days with mixed emotions: "I did get to work with people in theater and do my own choreography in college," he says, "but I really wasn't into the academic part. It made my mother happy and I got an education, but I also wasted time there."

What to look for in a college dance program

The faculty. A college dance program can only be as good as its teachers. A department whose personnel are hired on the basis of their professional background and experience in the dance world will clearly have much more to offer an aspiring performer or choreographer than one comprised chiefly of teachers with purely academic credentials. The faculty should be large enough to afford some diversity. Be wary of understaffed dance departments. A case in point: One graduate student in the modern dance program of a large, well-known college department reported that most of the technique and choreography classes were taught by "a flabby, middle-aged woman who had never been a professional dancer herself," and whose only training outside of college was apparently limited to occasional summer workshops in Limón technique.

Fortunately, more college dance departments are enlisting the services of reputable professionals and are willing to give them the job security and salaries they require, whether or not they possess academic degrees. New York University's School of Fine Arts is a good example. Dance chairman Stuart Hodes was a leading dancer with Martha Graham and performed in a number of Broadway shows. He is also a choreographer, and he has sat on the Dance Advisory Panel of the National Endowment for the Arts. Yet Hodes has no college degree. His three "star" teachers, as he calls them, are ballet instructor Nenette Charisse, who counts among her former pupils José Limón, Jerome Robbins and Gwen Verdon; Bertram Ross, choreographer and former principal dancer with the Graham company; and Lawrence Rhodes, former principal dancer with the Joffrey Ballet, the Eliot Feld Ballet and the Netherlands Dance Theatre. None of them hold college degrees. Among Hode's younger staff, however, one instructor has her own company as well as a master's in dance, and another is a professional dancer and Bennington alumna.

Teachers who are active or past performers are not only better equipped to guide and prepare you for the professional realities you face, but as pointed out earlier, they can actually play a part in shaping your career. It is not unusual for a college teacher to arrange an audition for a promising student or, if he is a choreographer, hire the student himself.

Type of program and degree available. Dance programs occupy different places in the overall structure of universities, and this greatly influences their funding, autonomy, admission requirements and curricula. At many universities, such as North Carolina at Greensboro and Rutgers in New Jersey, the dance program is situated within the school of physical education—not surprisingly, since that is where college dance began in this country. At others, such as Northern Arizona University and George Washington University in Washington, D.C., dance is part of the school of education. At Smith College in Massachusetts and the University of California at Berkeley, it is tucked into the theater department. Sometimes, as in the case of the University of Cincinnati and Hunter College in New York, the music school houses a dance division. Many universities grant interdisciplinary degrees, whereby dance can be combined with other areas of study. If you wish to take up dance in conjunction with another interest—in theater, education, physical education, music or social science—these alternatives may work well for you.

But if it is intensive dance training and performing experience you're after, look for a program in an independent dance department, preferably one that is installed within a school of fine arts. Such programs have the most control over their own destinies, and their first priority is to turn out future performers. They select students by audition as well as by academic record, and they normally have more money for teachers, special facilities, student productions, and residencies by visiting professional companies.

You should also consider the type of degree offered, for this determines how much time you will spend on dance within the required college curriculum. Although it varies from school to school, a bachelor of fine arts degree (B.F.A.) normally permits the highest proportion of classes to be taken in dance (up to 75% of the total credit requirement); a bachelor of science degree (B.S.) calls for about 50% of the total course work to be taken in dance; and the majority of bachelor of arts (B.A.) programs allow students to devote from 25% to 40% of their undergraduate credits to dance. (Adelphi University in Garden City, New York, is an exception; B.A. candidates take 90% of their 120 credits in dance.)

Most college dance divisions confer degrees in more than one aspect of dance. For example, dance majors at the University of Wisconsin at Madison can earn a B.A. degree with an emphasis on performance and choreography, on dance therapy, or on teaching. New York University has two separate dance departments—one in the School of Fine Arts, another in the School of Education—which grant an assortment of degrees in dance performance, education and therapy.

Curriculum. Is the course work relevant to your interests? Is there enough class time devoted to technique? At this stage you should have at least two technique classes per day, which ought to include ballet (see training recommendations for career dancers in chapter 9). Are there guest teachers and residencies by professional dance companies? Are there ample performing opportunities, including chances to work with professional choreographers?

The school. Arrange to observe classes (follow the evaluation guidelines in chapter 13). Are the teachers good? Do they seem to take a personal interest in their students? Take a long, hard look at the students, too. Are they working well? Do you like what you see? Is there good musical accompaniment for classes? How are the classroom and theater facilities? Are there well-stocked research and listening libraries? Do students have access to video-and sound-lab equipment (nice but not essential)?

If possible, see a student concert at the college. It will clearly reveal the quality of the training. Ask about the program's graduates. The staff should be proud to tell you about their successful alumni. While you are there, it is also a good idea to talk to dancers already in the program you are considering. Stuart Hodes shrewdly advises prospective students to "seek out dancers who look unhappy, and talk to them alone. Find out what has gone wrong."

If you are undecided about where to apply or need advice on the

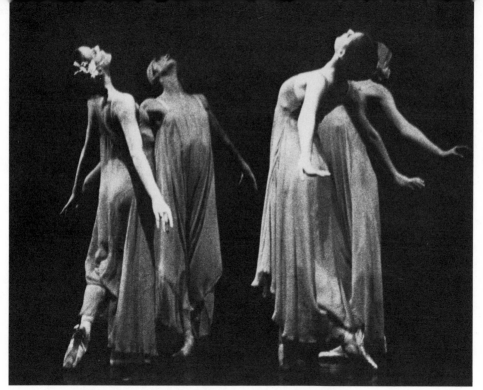

A concert by the University of Utah's Department of Ballet. *John Brandon.*

feasibility of college for you, talk to your home-town dance teacher. If the opportunity presents itself, try to get some advice from professional dancers. They are usually generous about helping others. Other places you can turn to for help are the National Association for Regional Ballet, 1860 Broadway, New York, New York 10023, (212) 757-8460; and the *Dancemagazine College Guide*, 1180 Avenue of the Americas, New York, New York 10036, (212) 921-9300.

Many college dance departments hold special summer study sessions that give nonmatriculated students a chance to try out college life on a short-term basis. There is nothing like a little active participation to help you decide if you want more.

Resources

> *Dance Directory: Programs of Professional Preparation in American Colleges and Universities*, 11th ed., compiled by Marilyn Trigg and Candy Norton. Reston, Virginia: American Alliance for Health, Physical Education, Recreation, and Dance, 1980. (At the time of our printing the price had not been fixed.)
> Not as comprehensive as the *Dancemagazine* guide below; it does, however, cover close to two hundred colleges and include faculty listings. No photographs. To obtain a copy, write to College Directory, AAHPERD Publications, 1900 Association Drive, Reston, Virginia 22070.

von Obenauer, Heidi, ed. *Dancemagazine College Guide*. New York: Danad Publishing Company, 1978. $7.50.

This biannual publication has extensive listings of undergraduate-and graduate-level dance programs. It contains information on courses, tuition, credit requirements, performing opportunities, facilities and summer study sessions, as well as helpful photographs; but does not name faculty members. To obtain a copy, write to *Dancemagazine*, 1180 Avenue of the Americas, New York, New York 10036.

23

How Others Made It: Six Paths

*career dancers
tell their
success stories*

Adam Grammis *(Broadway)*. Adam was performing onstage long before he had any formal training. Back home in Allentown, Pennsylvania, he started by doing high school shows. "We were doing simple stuff, because there were so few dancers. I just watched the choreographer. Then I saw an audition notice in my home-town newpaper for a production of *West Side Story* that a local theater group was putting on. In it I had to sing and dance. The choreographer was a neighborhood dance teacher. I got the job and did several other musicals with them. Around the same time I started taking singing lessons, and I picked up more about dancing from watching TV variety shows."

After high school Adam entered Kutztown State College near his home, where he studied eurhythmics and majored in biology. But theater proved to be his greatest love. While attending classes, he performed in college musicals, choreographing two productions himself—*Wonderful Town* and *Sweet Charity* (he choreographed the latter from notes he had taken after seeing the movie version).

During his junior and senior years, Adam used his local theater connections to get jobs with the summer-stock theater in town. At first he was hired as an apprentice doing bit parts, but he got to work with professionals. Eventually he became a full-fledged member of the company, and this enabled him to join the Actor's Equity union. "I think the fact that I could save the producers some money because I had a car and lived only a few miles away had a lot to do with my getting into the stock company," Adam adds with a grin.

After college he moved to New York. "Adjusting wasn't hard at all. I had been coming into the city on weekends before I moved. Some friends put me up in their apartment, so I could take class, eat and live on eight dollars a week. I don't know how I did it. I didn't save anything, but I managed."

At his first Equity audition in New York, Adam says he was "freaked out by the competition. It was for *Li'l Abner*, and I walked out in the middle. I suddenly realized how little experience I had and how little I knew. I decided then and there to learn how to dance and not to take another audition until I was ready. I talked to other dancers, and they showed me how to take auditions. I found out that the important thing was to be able to pick up a combination fast and give it style. They told me to wear the same dance clothes at the call-backs, so that the choreographer would remember me.

"I slowly gained confidence. I got a job in a small summer theater in New Hampshire." To support himself between engagements, Adam worked on Wall Street filing stock eight hours a day; other times he worked as a waiter. He took dance classes at night.

Things started happening. He got work with a dinner theater and another summer-stock theater. Then he landed his first Broadway musical, *Wild and Wonderful*, choreographed by Ronn Forella. The show closed after one night, but Forella, who had just opened a dance school, invited Adam to study there and to join his jazz company. "Ronn liked me and taught me a lot about dancing. I picked up more work in summer stock and, with one of the dancers from Ronn's group, put together a nightclub act. We got bookings at Caesar's Palace and other Las Vegas clubs." Next, a choreographer who had remembered Adam from a previous show gave him a leading role in a regional-theater production of *The Boy Friend*.

Adam feels that his biggest break came when he was chosen to do the prestigious Milliken industrial show, through which he met some prominent Broadway choreographers. "Once choreographers like you, they'll call you for parts. They like to work with the same dancers over and over, people who do their style well." All the while Adam kept doing nightclub stints. He appeared in a Miss America pageant, and soon afterward came featured parts in *The Shirley MacLaine Show* and *A Chorus Line*.

Sara Maule *(American Ballet Theatre).* Sara began serious ballet training at the San Francisco Ballet School, which she says "was patterned after the Balanchine School. The directors, Lew and Harold Christensen, watched your progress and asked those students they liked to join the company. I was very fortunate in that when I was thirteen, Anatole Vilzak and Ludmila Schollar from the Kirov School came to teach there. They taught us variations from *Sleeping Beauty, Coppélia* and *Don Quixote*; but most of all, they taught us about performing and artistry.

"Students from the San Francisco Ballet School performed in lecture-demonstrations, and as a child I did *The Nutcracker* every year. In that sense,

I've been treated as a professional since I was nine years old. The ballet mistress rehearsed the children like company members, bloody toes and all. At sixteen I worked in the company full time.

"I was dancing a lot, and the San Francisco Ballet had a lot to offer me. But I had grown up there. I had taken the same bus to classes and rehearsals every day since I was eight. I wanted to move to the center—to New York City—and was hoping to join Balanchine. But when I got to the School of American Ballet, I found out that I was too old for his company; he wanted sixteen-and seventeen-year-olds. So my dreams were shattered.

"Thank God I happened to take some classes with Pat Wilde at the American Ballet Theatre School. At the time she was ballet mistress for Ballet Theatre. I mentioned to her that I wanted to get into the company, and she told me to take company class. That's when Lucia* first observed me. I must have done something like fifteen auditions for Ballet Theatre before getting in. Finally, in 1973, they sent for me to audition in California, where the company was on tour. ABT was smaller then, and they needed other dancers to fill in for the ill and injured. It was a free trip home for me, so I went. I was accepted.

"It took me at least a couple of years to get used to living in New York. In some respects I'm still getting used to it. I think you either have the personality for New York or you don't. Some people seem to be born for this city; they just blossom here. For me, it took a lot of faith to get through. I spent half a year without a job, without knowing if I'd make it or if all the hard work was for nothing. I had saved some money living at home while I was dancing in San Francisco. But I was down to my last penny when I joined Ballet Theatre. Another thing that made it difficult was that it was my first year away from home. I stayed at St. Mary's Residence, a lonely place filled with other people like me.

"I found the hugeness of everything in New York overwhelming. I remember looking at all the buildings, with all their windows, and thinking: *There's a person behind each one.* San Francisco was a cosmopolitan city, but New York was still a shock. In San Francisco I had teachers who took care of me and nurtured me. What was most traumatic about New York was the anonymity. There were so many dancers, all with different reasons for being there, all going their separate ways. There were so many people in class that the teacher was more impersonal too. Joining Ballet Theatre helped. Once you're in a union company the pay is good and you have good job security. But that in itself was a shock. Ballet Theatre was such a big company—there were so many people, and everyone fighting to make it. It was a family, but after my experience in San Francisco, a big, impersonal one.

"Now, a few years later, I'm happy I did it. The struggle has paid off. I'm happy professionally and personally. I feel comfortable in the company, and I can honestly say that I'm starting to like living in New York. I've made

*Lucia Chase, the recently retired director of American Ballet Theatre.

some good friends, I've found teachers I like, and I've grown up. I know who I am and feel that others do too. I'm getting to do better parts. It's a great privilege, for example, to be working with Antony Tudor. He's a real master. His ballets are like novels, with every detail, every gesture, carefully directed and worked into the central theme. He gives us images that penetrate to the bone. He knows how to get his characters out of us.''

Carolyn Adams *(Paul Taylor Dance Company)*. Carolyn attended Sarah Lawrence College in New York, and spent her junior year abroad in Paris studying with Karin Waehner, a disciple of Mary Wigman. In 1963 Carolyn became a member of the Waehner company. "I toured Europe with them and also choreographed my own works. It was wonderful experience, and it gave me confidence in my dancing. My last year at Sarah Lawrence I auditioned for Paul Taylor. He asked me to join his company right away, but I wanted to wait until after graduation—I was so close to finishing. So Paul arranged with Bessie Schönberg, the chairman of the dance department, for me to finish school that year and at the same time work fifteen hours a week with him learning repertory. I joined Paul's company in September 1965, and have been with him ever since.

"We were one of the first companies on the National Endowment for the Arts Dance Touring Program. But the sixties were still the pioneer days of the program, and although we got grants and residencies, they were lean years. We used to work eight weeks a year, with no unemployment insurance. Somehow we managed to stay together to rehearse and create new pieces, but it was hard. I have always taught, so I could squeak by on that. Fortunately times have changed. Today we have to turn work down in order not to be over-booked.''

Richard Colton *(Twyla Tharp Dance Foundation)*. For Richard, too, the path to a career was direct and unswerving. He was a scholarship student at the American Ballet Theatre School and that led to his first stage appearance at age thirteen. "The Bolshoi Ballet put out a notice through the American Ballet Theatre School requesting young boys to perform with them at the old Metropolitan Opera House. I was one of the kids chosen." Richard also went to Indian Hill, a dance camp, for four summers. There he took classes with the late modern dance choreographer James Waring. During the school year he worked with the Waring company on weekends—the only free time he had while attending the High School of Performing Arts. This gave Richard his first steady performing experience. He describes his student days at Performing Arts as being pretty rugged: "We'd start off at 8:00 a.m. with technique classes, then break for lunch. Then we'd have our academics in the afternoon. After school I'd have another lunch and take more classes at Ballet Theatre from 4:30 to 8:00 at night. I'd come home, do my homework and fall into bed.''

When his teacher Bill Griffith left Ballet Theatre to join the faculty of the Joffrey School, Richard followed. He got a scholarship and became a member of the Joffrey II apprentice company. From there he was asked to join the Joffrey Ballet. While with the Joffrey, Richard worked with choreographer Twyla Tharp and eventually left to dance with her company.

Dru Alexandrine *(Broadway)*. Dru trained at the Royal Ballet School in England for eight years. After graduation she was invited to join the company. When they came to New York on tour, she decided to stay on and visit for three months. "Well it's been eight years now," she chuckles. "The way it happened was I started seeing Broadway musicals, which were very new and exciting to me. When I was at the Royal Ballet School all we ever saw was ballet and opera, opera and ballet. The United States has the best musical theater in the world. It made me realize that I could do something other than classical ballet that would still be rewarding and enjoyable. At any rate, I wanted to see the States, so I took a job touring here. The money was so fantastic after what I had been getting in England."

While waiting for her green card (certification as a resident alien), Dru took a year off from performing to study jazz, tap, acting and singing. She got her first job in musical theater with *Disney on Parade*. After her green card came through, Dru went to open-call auditions in New York and did three seasons at the Jones Beach Theatre, during which time she appeared in the coveted dancing role of Laurie in *Oklahoma!* As an Equity member she qualified for more auditions, which in turn brought her more work—including parts in the Broadway revivals of *My Fair Lady* and *Pajama Game*. "The competition is very stiff," Dru concedes, "but it gets easier. Once you build a reputation and choreographers work with you, they'll call you when they have a new show.

Ryland Jordan *(José Limón Dance Company)*. Ryland attributes his success to "being in the right place at the right time." He made all his important professional connections in college. While a student at Bennington College in Vermont, Ryland met choreographers Clyde Morgan and Carla Maxwell, who were looking for male dancers for a summer scholarship program at Boston University. They worked together over the summer. "Since we were all going to New York the following fall (I was planning to enter Juilliard that September), Clyde and Carla asked me to perform with them."

But in some ways Ryland's first year at Juilliard was disappointing. "I got to perform with Kazuko Hirabayashi, one of my teachers, but I was accepted only as an understudy with the student dance company. I think part of the reason that I didn't get 'discovered' my first year was that I didn't get a chance to perform, and performing was my greatest strength. The faculty saw me only in technique class, which was my weakest area. It was later, when I got to perform, that I was recognized as a good dancer."

By the end of his second year Ryland was being featured in Martha Graham's *Diversion of Angels,* which the Juilliard company presented for their annual spring concert. Twice a week he commuted to the Graham studio to learn repertory as part of an exchange program set up by the director of the dance department, Martha Hill. Ryland also worked closely with the late José Limón, who taught a repertory class at Juilliard, as well as with various members of the Graham company on staff there. After graduation he was invited to join both the Limón and Graham troupes, and he performed with both companies in subsequent years. Classmates Peter Sparling, Janet Eilber and Diana Hart found their way into the Graham company the same way.

Part VI

Talking shop

24

Conversations with Professional Dancers

fourteen professionals
give down-to-earth advice,
share experiences and
talk about their day-to-day lives as dancers

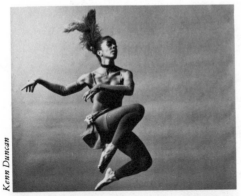

Kenn Duncan

Carolyn Adams was born in New York City and began training at the age of ten. She studied modern dance with Bessie Schönberg at Sarah Lawrence College, and she has been a featured dancer with the Paul Taylor Dance Company since 1965. With her sister Julie Adams Strandberg, Carolyn directs the Harlem Dance Studio in New York. She currently trains with ballet teacher Don Farnworth.

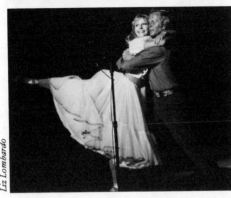

Liz Lombardo

Dru Alexandrine is from London, England, and a graduate of the Royal Ballet School. She came to America eight years ago while on tour with the Royal Ballet. Among other things, Dru has appeared on Broadway in *My Fair Lady* and *Pajama Game*; she has starred in *Oklahoma!* at the Allenberry Playhouse in Pennsylvania, and has performed in *Fiddler on the Roof*, *Carousel* and *Annie Get Your Gun* at the Jones Beach Theater in New York. She is the mother of a fifteen-month-old baby boy.

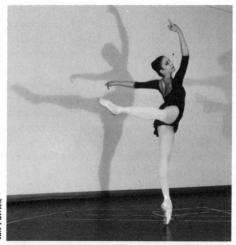

Ian Patrick

Victoria Bromberg is a native New Yorker and an alumna of the School of American Ballet, where her teachers included Alexandra Danilova, Felia Doubrovska, Muriel Stuart and Stanley Williams. She became a member of the New York City Ballet at the age of sixteen.

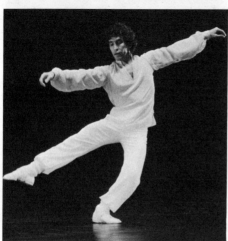

Tom Rawe

Richard Colton attended the High School of Performing Arts in New York. He was a scholarship student, first at the American Ballet Theatre School and then at the Joffrey School. Over the years his teachers have been William Griffith, Valentina Pereyeslavec, James Waring, Maggie Black and André Bernard. Richard performed with the Joffrey Ballet for four years before joining the Twyla Tharp Dance Foundation in 1977.

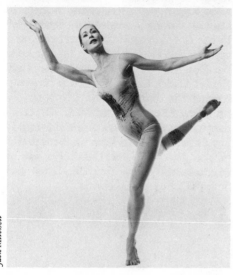

Jack Mitchell

Bettie deJong was born in Sumatra, Indonesia. She moved to Holland in 1947, where she continued her early training in ballet and mime. She went on to study at the Martha Graham School in New York and to dance with the Graham company, the Pearl Lang Dance Company and Lucas Hoving. Bettie, who became a member of the Paul Taylor Dance Company in 1962, has originated many roles in the Taylor repertory. She also acts as rehearsal mistress for the group.

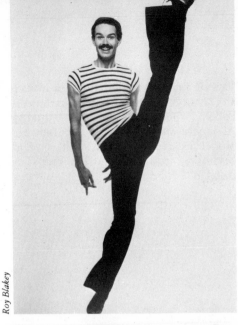

Adam Grammis is a Pennsylvania biologist who started dancing when he was twenty-two. He appeared opposite Shirley MacLaine in the Emmy-winning television special *Gipsy in My Soul*, and on Broadway in *A Chorus Line* and *Wild and Wonderful*. He has done numerous roles in summer stock and regional theater, as well as nightclub work and several Milliken industrial shows. Most recently, Adam served as choreographer Graciela Daniele's assistant for the Broadway revival of *The Most Happy Fella* and for the American Shakespeare Festival production of the *Pirates of Penzance* starring Linda Ronstadt.

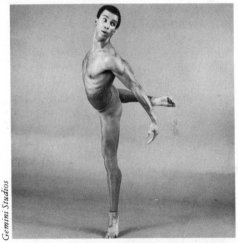

Ryland Jordan was born in Dayton, Ohio. He studied tap and jazz as a child but didn't begin serious training until his college years. He attended Williams College and Bennington College before graduating with a B.F.A. degree from Juilliard in 1972. Ryland has danced professionally with Kasuko Hirabayashi, the Martha Graham Dance Company, and he was a soloist with the José Limón Dance Company from 1971 to 1978. He has just completed a yearlong teaching stint in Puerto Rico.

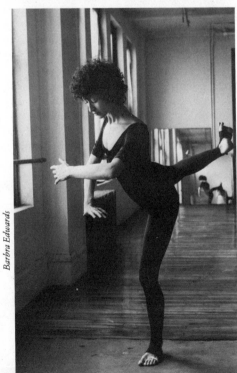

Ellen Kogan was a scholarship student at Eugene Loring's American School of Dance in Los Angeles. She has performed with the San Francisco Ballet, the Batsheva Bat-Dor Company in Israel, the Cliff Keuter Dance Company, and is currently touring the country with a solo repertory program. Ellen holds an M.A. degree in dance from the University of California at Los Angeles. She has been on the faculties of the Jacob's Pillow Dance Festival in Massachusetts, New York University and Scripps College in California.

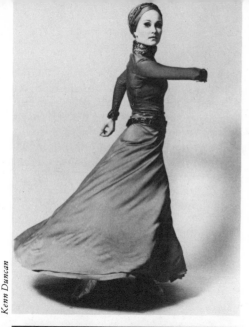

Sara Maule is originally from San Francisco. She studied modern dance with Welland Lathrop and later received her ballet training from Lew and Harold Christensen, Anatole Vilzak and Ludmila Schollar at the San Francisco Ballet School. She was a soloist with the San Francisco Ballet until 1973, when she moved to New York and became a member of American Ballet Theatre. Sara's teachers in New York have been Pat Wilde, Michael Lland, David Howard and Igor Schwezoff.

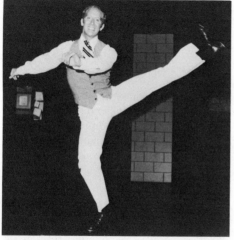

Bill Nabel entered Tufts University in Massachusetts as a premedical student and left six years later to go into show business. He began formal dance training with David Shields in Boston at age twenty-two, and he made his theatrical debut at Harvard University's Loeb Theatre playing Tony in *West Side Story* under the direction of Leonard Bernstein. Bill has worked in television commercials, summer stock, dinner and regional theater and industrial shows. He has performed on Broadway in *A Chorus Line*, *Home Sweet Homer* and *Evita*.

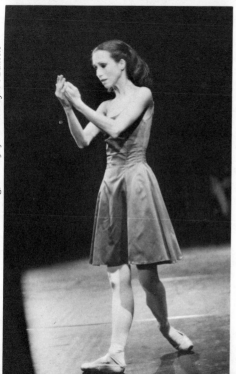

Christine O'Neal was born in St. Louis, Missouri, where she received her early ballet instruction from Carmen Thomas. After further study at the National Ballet School in Washington, D.C., she danced with the National Ballet for three years. In 1972, she won the Bronze Medal at the International Ballet Competition in Varna, Bulgaria. Following the demise of the National Ballet Company, Christine joined American Ballet Theatre. She was a soloist with Dennis Wayne's Dancers for over two years, and she is presently appearing with the National Company of *Dancin'*.

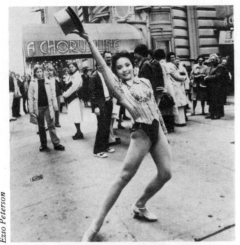

Ezio Peterson

Cynthia Onrubia, who is part Filipino, Chinese and Spanish, has been performing since she was four years old. A veteran of television commercials and specials, summer stock and several Milliken industrial shows, she made her Broadway debut at age fifteen as the youngest member of the cast of *A Chorus Line*. Cynthia is now with the national company of *Dancin'*.

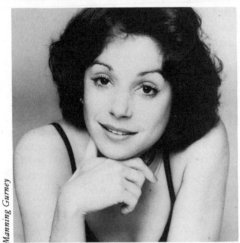

Manning Gurney

Gillian Scalici was raised in Milwaukee, Wisconsin. She trained at the Martha Graham School in London, and she has studied ballet with Alfredo Corvino and jazz with Fred Benjamin and Lynn Simonson in New York. She has been seen on Broadway in *Marvin Hamlisch in Concert*, *Very Good Eddie* and *A Chorus Line*, in summer stock, and on public and commercial television. Gillian recently portrayed Anita in a revival of *West Side Story*, choreographed by John Neumeier, at the Hamburg Opera House.

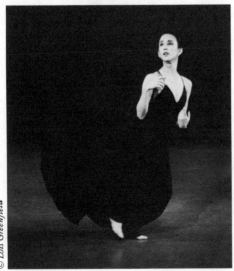

© Lois Greenfield

Christine Wright began her formal training under the direction of Mary Day at the Academy of the Washington Ballet in Washington, D.C., where she won a National Society of Arts and Letters scholarship. After studying there for four years she moved to New York to train with ballet teacher Maggie Black. Christine danced with the Eglevsky Ballet Company and with choreographers Kazuko Hirabayashi, Marcus Schulkind and Saeko Ichinohe before joining the Lar Lubovitch Dance Company in 1977.

Beginnings

Author: Do you remember when you first decided that you wanted to dance professionally?

Christine O'Neal: I was too young to really know. I was three years old when I started training, and it didn't hit me until I was thirteen or fourteen years old, when I had to take auditions. It was a question of do you want to go to that audition? And I was there. It was just a series of events, and whether or not I consciously chose to be, I was there.

Author: Vicki, you started dancing very early too, didn't you?

Vicki: I don't remember too much about my first few years at the School of American Ballet. I guess I went through it kind of unconsciously, too. But each year when it came time to pay tuition and ask myself if I wanted to sing or play the cello or do something else instead, I found myself staying. As a child at the school you get to see the company and to dance in *The Nutcracker*. You're drenched in the world of ballet and pretty soon you're hooked.

Author: Did your parents put any pressure on you to continue?

Vicki: No, it was always my decision. There were kids at the school who were trying to make their parents happy. It's so sad. I don't think it works very well because their hearts aren't really in it; they're only going through the motions. Eventually they're asked to leave, and most of the time it's probably the best thing.

Carolyn: I don't remember any specific, arbitrary moment when I started training, and I think that's because I danced so long before I ever went to class. They started us with rhythms and improvisation in elementary school here in New York, at Ethical Culture. The first time I went to a ballet class I was ten, but I had been dancing for years. I remember going to dance class to learn some very specific things about technique, but I never felt I was going to learn how to dance because that was something I already did, not necessarily well or badly, but just something I did.

Gillian: For me, dancing was the only thing I ever wanted to do. I don't remember wanting to do anything else. When I was younger it was in my dreams and it was always ballet. Now I'm not doing ballet anymore, but I am still dancing in the theater.

Author: Do you recall your first dance class?

Gillian: I come from a musical background, and my mother is a great stage mother, a frustrated actress and a very musical lady. I was always very musical, too. She took me to dance classes, which were all very poor, all very YWCA or whatever. But when I was twelve my family moved to the Midwest and I was really fortunate to find a wonderful, wonderful teacher. She was a former dancer with the Ballets Russes, Madame Zenia Custova. Here I was, a thirteen-year-old girl living in Milwaukee, and I had come upon this crazy woman in a little studio tucked away—a dark, dangerous studio. She taught with her stick and yelled and pounded the floor, and it was one way of scaring people into dancing. But she instilled a great discipline and a great love in those people who were interested in dancing. Those were the people who stayed. It was a far cry from my Miss Hoola classes on Long Island, but she was really a great influence.

Author: Did you stay with her for a while?

Gillian: All through my high school days. From the time I was thirteen until I was eighteen. She tried to teach you to have your dancing come from the heart, a dramatic way of approaching it so that your movement wouldn't be so mechanical, so technical. She worked with each student individually. She could see that I did not have it in my character or personality to be a ballet dancer. "You're too crazy to dance that way," she said. She tried to push me toward the musical world—and that's where I ended up, although much later. She always told me, "grow up, and you'll see that you're too crazy."

Christine O'Neal: In my case it was just the opposite. I wasn't a classical dancer at first, but out of everything I took, ballet was the strongest. I had good feet and legs and so my teacher allowed me to go on pointe. She had a thing about me that was really very complimentary, because she never let me go. She was always at me. It must have been that Royal Ballet or Kirov type of thing where they look at you and say, Ah ha! Those are good legs. Get her going!

Author: Did you get that kind of attention at the School of American Ballet, Vicki?

Vicki: Well, you're constantly being watched. I don't know how, but Balanchine is aware of all the students at the school. He works with the children and talks to them at rehearsals. He knows all his students, even though he doesn't teach there. He just watches you grow up. There are no auditions for the company, but he picks about five graduating students a year. Students are always being weeded out in other ways, too. Once a year the directors line you up at the barre. They decide that this one is not developing, although she works hard; that one has boyfriends and has lost interest; that one's body has changed. The school is getting bigger every year, and there may be a few students who could have developed who get passed by, but on the whole it's pretty fair.

Author: Is everyone who attends the school hoping to join the company?

Vicki: Yes. Of course, the fullest use of the technique is in the Balanchine repertory, but even if you don't get chosen—if you know yourself and know what you want to get out of the training—you can take the technique and go on from there. Marianna Tcherkassky stayed until her senior year. She's a beautiful dancer, but she knew she wouldn't get into the company because she was shorter and rounder than the typical Balanchine dancer. So now she's doing very well at Ballet Theatre.

Author: It sounds like a very competitive place. Did that bother you?

Vicki: The competition at SAB wasn't necessarily a bad thing, because it prepared you for the competition and discipline in the company. It's part of your training. You learn how to keep yourself together, as you must if you want to stay in the company. There is no probation period in the New York City Ballet as there is in the Paris Opera, where they give you a year to pull yourself together if you let yourself get out of shape or fall down on technique.

Author: Sara, whose idea was it for you to go to your first dance class?

Sara: I wanted to go, but my mother found the place. I was four years old. She was taking a modern dance class and I would tag along. Then I decided that I wanted to take class, too.

Dru: I think that most little girls have dance in their education somewhere along the line, but it's harder for boys. They have to seek it out. For girls it's always sort of there, at school or somewhere—it's available if they want it.

Ellen: My mother took me to my first class, a very typical suburban dance studio where a Miss Ballou was teaching. I don't think we did much of anything. There were a lot of little girls. I was eight. My mother kept dragging me out of these places. We would get to the point where they would have a recital and they would want you to contribute twenty dollars toward the costumes. At that point my mother would find out that I hadn't learned anything, and she would take me to a new place until the same thing happened.

Author: Do you think you would have known on your own if the training was bad?

Ellen: No, I don't think so. If you're only ten or eleven and a teacher tells you to do that, you do it. It takes a lot of experience to know what's really good for your body. But my mother finally found Eugene Loring's American School of Dance. She felt that the other places were just tiny-tot studios, but *there* was a place where you could learn something. The other places put you on pointe when you were very young and she was very upset about that. They did it, of course, because that was what brought in the students. I think that there's still too much bad training like that, particularly in small towns and suburbs.

Author: So you were fortunate that your mother had the stamina to keep trying.

Ellen: I guess so. She even gave up for a while. We lived in an area from which it was difficult to get to the American School of Dance, and so for a long time I didn't take any classes at all. I have a feeling that I was lucky not to. I could have had some very bad training if I had continued in those kinds of schools.

Author: Richard, did I hear you say that you asked your parents for dance lessons?

Richard: Yes, my parents encouraged me, but my interest in dance was something that I developed purely on my own. I had gotten a record from my uncle, who worked for UNICEF. There were recordings of folk dances and music from around the world, from Kenya and Japan, with people singing and stomping. So I ran around the living room with that music playing. Then my parents took me to a festival of Russian music where I saw the Moiseyev Company. That's when it started; I asked my parents if there was a school where I could learn more. I immediately ran back to my living room and started practicing plizzatzkies, which, as it turned out, were the first step I did as a professional dancer with the Joffrey in *Petrouchka*.

Author: Did you take to ballet right away?

Richard: The only worry I had was that if I went to dancing school I might have to wear tights. I expressed this fear to my parents and they must have spoken to the director, because I remember after the school audition he took me aside and said, "Now, Richard, I think you have talent, but if you want to study ballet we have to put you in some tights." So for the first class my father took me into the boys' dressing room and helped me into my tights, because I was the only little boy there.

Carolyn: I wonder how many of our aspirations are related to things that we saw as kids. Danny Grossman said that he was inspired by the music of Ray Charles and the circus. It's a wonderful combination. It makes perfect sense. When I was first starting my formal training there were all those marvelous circus shows on television. It wasn't any particular kind of movement or theater, but it was kind of everything. It was extreme—high-wire acts, broad musical-comedy dancing, jazz with ballet steps thrown in. In our particular generation I think there was a little of everything to be seen in an even more exciting way than now.

Gillian: I think television is definitely a strong influence. In Wisconsin there was not a lot to go and see in terms of live theater, but I remember watching Cyd Charisse and Gene Kelly dancing forever and ever and saying, I'm going to do that.

Ellen: It's an interesting thing to think about. When you're on tour, you meet people in a class and you think that they're so talented and they love to dance. But whether or not they decide to go into dancing depends on so many things. I think that for me there were a couple of turning points, moments at which I discovered that I could perform. First I found that I could reach other people, and second, that I was really able to express myself in movement. I remember once in a choreography class I took with Eugene Loring, he handed out pieces of paper and crayons and he asked us to remember a very emotional experience;

then he told us to take the crayon and put that emotional experience on paper. Then he pointed to me and said, ''Now get up and dance it.'' It was a very intense anger thing I was feeling, and I got up and let out so much emotional energy that when I finished I felt fantastic and everyone thought it was wonderful. That was expression, and I think that's what we're all trying to do. It's very hard to find training that doesn't get you so caught up with technique that you lose track of what you were trying to do in the first place. I think that's why many people turn to choreography, because someone else's movement isn't necessarily their movement and doesn't express them.

Author: Cynthia, since you're the youngest here, what was it like as a child studying with adults in an advanced class? Do you think you were treated differently?

Cynthia: Well, when I started I was in the intermediate class—you go through the levels. Then one day the head of the school saw me in class and said, ''She doesn't belong in here, she belongs in the adult class.'' So he put me there and that was when I started thinking on an adult level. Ever since then I was always treated like an adult. They never babied me in class or even outside of class. Whatever they talked about, I had to just listen to them and take it all in. So I matured very quickly; so did the other kids I was around.

Richard: Do you ever miss being a teenager?

Cynthia: I still have my average life, aside from my professional life. I like to go out with friends, to go to parties and stuff. And I'm still in school. It was difficult sometimes, but it was fun.

Author: Many men don't begin dancing until later in their lives. Is that true of anyone here?

Adam: I went to my first dance class when I was twenty-two. It was at Herbert Berghoff's acting studio, of all places. I was in college in Pennsylvania studying biology, so I took the bus into New York City on weekends for about six months. Once I moved to New York I found out who were the right teachers to go to. Before that I can always remember moving or dancing. I had done some shows in high school and choreographed some college musicals, but I didn't study dance until I came to New York.

Bill: My first class was a ballet class, in 1972. Boy, was I brave! I took an advanced class. Not only was I brave, I was embarrassed.

Author: How did you end up there?

Bill: I had started messing around with tap dancing, and having learned that the only way to get into it is to get into it, I said well, let's walk into a class. Ballet was the only thing around at the time (I was in college in Boston). Well, I took that class and I took another class and soon I was up to two or three classes a day. I realized that floundering around was kind of an integral process in learning. It's nice if you can get into an elementary class and progress gradually, but I started very late and I couldn't do that. I had done sports and was coordinated. I had reasonable extensions and all that.

Author: Is that when you decided to make dancing your career?

Bill: Yes. Once I had a taste of it I realized that it was for me. All of a sudden I didn't want to be a doctor anymore, I wanted to be in the theater. It was a very conscious decision. As I look back and remember how much dancing has always been a part of me, it wasn't so surprising. Even in high school I loved to social dance. I went to every dance in sight.

Author: Was it a tough choice to make?

Bill: When I was in college—in the late sixties and early seventies—there was quite a bit of thought at that time about where our country was going. If I were growing up now I'm not so sure I would have gone out and done what I really wanted to do. I think there's a lot of pressure on kids today to do something that will ensure their future, their security—which is something I never felt I had to deal with. I just don't think my decision would have been as easy to make now as then.

Author: Did your parents support your decision?

Bill: My parents came to this country from Poland. They were very proud of the fact that their son was going to be a doctor, and I'm sure this played a very big part in my growing up. When I decided to go into theater it was not at all a popular decision.

Gillian: I had a little bit of trouble with that also. Not from my mother, she was rather unusual, but from the other members of my family. I was always very good at subjects in school like math and business, and the response from my family was, "Dance? Theater?" My grandmother would say, "Do you make any money in that field? So she wants to be a movie star, huh?"

Chris Wright: I almost had to split with my family to get to New York. My father had a very puritanical viewpoint; he didn't want me to be a dancer. I was very good in school, so he wanted me to go to college so that I could get a good job so that I could give my kids an education so that they could get a good job and so on, with nobody getting the chance to do what they wanted to do. So when I said I wanted to be a dancer he didn't take me seriously. Actually I never came right out and said I wanted to be a dancer, I just said I wanted to go to New York. I was sixteen then, and I didn't feel I was getting what I wanted in Washington. I went to New York for some summer courses and found a great teacher. I really had to stay, but my parents didn't approve of my moving because I was so young.

Author: How do they feel now that you've made it?

300

Chris Wright: Even though I am vaguely successful in his eyes now, it's still difficult for my father to understand what I'm doing. He grew up during the Depression. He wasn't raised in a cultural atmosphere. To him the arts are unnecessary. So he can't understand what I'm doing, and that I'm making a living at it at the same time is totally unfathomable to him. If I told him I was on unemployment he'd die! To him that would be like coming full circle. He'd think, Oh my God, my daughter is on the dole!

Adam: I didn't have the same problem because dancing has always been a commercial art form to me. When I went to class I knew I was going to make a career out of it and that I had to get a job. I thought, I'm going to have to make some money, because I was already twenty-two. Like Bill, I couldn't fool around ten years learning how to dance. It was strange listening to everyone talk about their classical training because I haven't had any at all. In the eight years I've been in New York I have only taken about three years of dance training, and I have studied with maybe four teachers, all of them jazz teachers. It was enjoyable, and I was lucky—I never had any problem with stretch. I could do splits and get my legs up high. My ballet training was nothing. I hated it. For what I'm doing now I don't need it. When I do something balletic I will watch the choreographer do the movement. I don't know any of the terms. But he'll do it and I'll mimic it and it will look like his. It won't have the placement; it won't have correct positions, but.it will look exactly like the person who showed it to me. And then on top of that I'll say, Now what can I do to put it across? Right from the beginning, I tried to produce a product that would be marketable.

Image of yourself

Author: How has your image of yourself as a dancer evolved over the years? Has your notion of the kind of dancer you are, or would like to be, changed?

Carolyn: I never really had a very clear notion of what kind of dancer I wanted to be or what company I wanted to be in. And because of that I was open to the various opportunities that came along. I think it's an advantage sometimes not to try to make decisions in advance about what you can do or should do. You never know how much stuff you've got in you.

Christine O'Neal: When I started off I didn't have any image of myself. I was just a dancer. As different dance styles came my way, I found they were either easy to do or hard to do. Only much later was I able to understand my capacity to take on a great variety of movement. Some people find it more comfortable to stay in one form of dance, but I think the ideal is to get yourself to the point where you can take on any form. I think that if I had to train young dancers I would tell them that they shouldn't close themselves off. It's too boring that way.

Bill: I try to do a lot of different types of movement. And the more I do that, the more I find that it's all movement: It's all mass in space; it's line; it's energy. As we get into different techniques and different inputs it all simply becomes just movement.

Author: Bettie, your early training was in ballet. How did you get into modern dance?

Bettie: In Europe at the time I studied, only ballet was taught, and so of course I had a good ballet background. I was very tall, almost as tall as I am now, and the boys came up to my shoulder. But I had a good body for ballet: I had the stretch for it and a perfect turn-out. I sleep in a turn-out. But I didn't want to perform ballet because it wasn't for me personally; it didn't fit my mind. I felt that there had to be another way for me to move. It was maybe because I had known Javanese dancing and mime that I knew there had to be somewhere else I could fit. I also knew that I had to come to America. I did, and I studied at the Graham school in New York. But the Graham style was not for me either. I had to have somewhere in between ballet and Graham that let me breathe. I think it's a very personal thing, which style of dancing is right for each individual.

Chris Wright: In a way that's what happened to me also. When I first came to New York I wanted to be a ballet dancer. I had been so classically oriented that I thought it was the only thing I could be. I'd never really seen modern dance before—I thought it had to be crawling on the floor. And it wasn't until a couple of years later that I discovered it purely by accident. A friend of mine asked me to do a concert with him. He was a modern dancer. So I said, "Well, I'm not performing, I'd like the experience. Sure!" And a whole new world opened up for me. After that I saw all sorts of modern dance performances in New York and I could finally understand where I belonged.

Gillian: At eighteen, for me too, it was ballet classes all the time. Twice a day, that's all I ever did. I left high school early every day and all I did was dance. Then I left and traveled around the world for two years and discovered that there were a lot of other things to do. I got away from ballet more and more, and from the technical discipline of it. Once I started working in muscials I found out that that was the kind of dancing I wanted to do.

Author: What about you, Cynthia? Are you still in the process of changing?

Cynthia: Until I was about twelve or thirteen I was always studying ballet with this one teacher. That's where I really got my basic technique. I learned a lot from him. My mother wanted me to take from other teachers, to get other ideas. I took one class somewhere else and he found out. He said, "What's this, you're taking from all over the city?" and he got all flustered. From the time I was about four I started doing commercials, so I had two different worlds. I had the classical ballet world and the show-business world. I was trying to do both at the same time and my ballet teacher would say, "Oh, you're doing all this commercial garbage.'' By the time I was twelve I was still in that school studying his technique all the time. My mother made me go to other teachers, and I also wanted to take from other people. That's when I started into jazz and tap, singing and acting. Now I take my jazz—because in the show we do mostly jazz—and I have my singing lessons. I still would like to do ballet, that's my main interest. But I'm open about it.

Bill: The more you study, the easier it becomes to do different styles because you have all that input, all that experience. You have that clearer idea of your instrument moving in space, and that's what dancing is.

Carolyn: The mind is really the essential element in our growth as dancers. It makes the trip, too. That's how you're able to go on year in and year out and to perform at the various stages of development. I think we're talking about various doors and openings. But in order to free, to liberate, ourselves— whatever the movement styles are—the mind has to make the trip.

Bill: It's interesting. We're a product of anyone who has ever trained us, of anyone we've ever seen and of anything we've observed. It all becomes part of your dancing. You, as a dancer, become everything that's fed into you.

Carolyn: Yes, if you can find a teacher who helps you function more effectively through the technique they teach you, so that the technique is a vehicle for you, then that's fine. But I've always felt it was important to avoid becoming a particular kind of dancer. There are a lot of dancers who have a Graham look or a Limón look, which is absolutely stunning, but personally I've always wanted to hold on to who I am as an individual.

Ellen: I'm now trying to change in a bigger way, aside from the question of what kind of dancer I'm going to be, ballet or modern or show business. I think there is a way that you see your body, and in order for you to grow you have to be able to let go of that, to soften it, and to move on to another way of looking at yourself, to move on to another plateau. That's what I'm trying to do now.

Author: What you're all saying, I think, is that you have to be flexible about how you see yourself in order to continue to develop as a dancer.

Teachers

Author: What makes a good teacher, in your opinion?

Bill: I remember when I first started dancing the teachers I had may not have been that good technically, but they loved dancing and they instilled that in their students. That was the biggest thing I got out of it.

Chris Wright: I was fortunate in that when I began studying in a professional sort of way my teacher had a great sense of dance and movement, even though she did not have the greatest technique. When she demonstrated, it was very much with the emphasis on quality, quality, quality. Beautiful, beautiful, beautiful. It was almost like a performance in class.

Bettie: I think that's the best teaching to begin with.

Richard: When I was studying, about the age of seven, we all just loved our ballet teacher Madame Youskevitch.* The game at the end of class was who could run up to her and kiss her first. Everyone waited until she said "Plié," and we did our changes,† and then everyone dashed off. She was also one of those teachers who emanated a love of dancing. That's the most important thing, I think. That's how quality expresses itself and where discipline begins.

Chris Wright: Yes, and a lot of it is also seeing the teacher dance. I remember when I first came to New York I happened by accident to take a class from Madame Swoboda.†† She had this little voice, and if you were new you spent the whole lesson—

Richard: —trying to figure out who the demonstrator was.

Chris Wright: Right. But at the end of the class she got up and did a révérence, or she might do a little Spanish thing, but I remember just sort of standing there, not knowing what I was doing and just watching her. The joy she had in dancing and the extreme artistry and beauty in what she was doing gave me so much.

Bettie: One thing that kept us going in class—even without a piano—was my teacher's wonderful sense of completion. He was an excellent choreographer, and he'd always figure out some kind of variation for us toward the end of the day in which to *dance*. It's terribly important that dancing comes first and then technique.

Author: What else goes into making a good teacher?

Bettie: It's very individual. I may be a good teacher for tall people, but I don't understand a short body too well—because they're so coiled. I had the hardest time getting this Bambi body together to one straight line, so I can see the problems of a tall person. But I cannot see the problems of a tight-hipped, coiled, short body. That's my shortcoming because I put all my heart into the former. When I get older maybe I can learn, but I haven't yet put my mind to it, to really look at a short body and what the problems are for a short body. I think that's why people choose, and should choose, different teachers, not to get hung up on one.

Chris Wright: Well I certainly don't have the same body structure as my present teacher, but if it weren't for her I probably wouldn't be dancing today. She has, if you look at her, far from a perfect body. But she had to find a way to make it

---

*Wife of the former Russian premier danseur Igor Youskevitch.
†Changements, small jumps in which the dancer changes his feet in fifth position in the air.
††Former Ballets Russes dancer Maria Swoboda.

304

work because she wanted to dance so badly. And so she worked very hard. Now she has an extraordinary knowledge of a body that did not work. She probably tried many different ways, and now she can look at a body—almost by instinct—and understand it and know how to work with it, because she has gone through it herself. Whereas another teacher of mine had a beautiful body—she is in her sixties now and she still has beautiful turn-out and extensions—but she couldn't help me with problems of technique.

Dru: I agree. When you get a beautiful dancer with a perfectly formed body in front of a class they often don't know how to explain what they do, because they've always just done it.

Bettie: The teacher I've taken the most ballet with in this city was someone who had polio, a short man. He rehabilitated himself, and now he has become a very good teacher for any type of body. It's very valuable to study with him because the main emphasis is on how to stand up on your own two legs and move yourself—not correctly, but efficiently.

Author: What do you mean by "not correctly but efficiently?"

Carolyn: Someone who gets you to understand how to do it, not what it should look like.

Ellen: Somebody who deals with function, not what is beautiful. That kind of teacher usually has a class that's mentally healthy. I think that there are a lot of classes that may be technically all right, but they don't create a good learning atmosphere. A good teacher is someone who doesn't lay a lot of trips on you about "the foot going like this is beautiful, do it like this," when in fact it doesn't have anything to do with being able to do the movement. I think what's important is *how* to do it. And also someone who is going to understand that your body is your body, it's not their body. We can't all do it the same way. An image or approach that works for one person doesn't always work for someone else.

Bill: A good teacher is a very rare thing—a real *teacher* as opposed to a dancer who no longer dances. You know you have a good teacher because everything's right. It's very obvious.

Bettie: There are so few born teachers who really look at every individual clearly and know what that body requires as an image to be able to get all the potential out. You're all put into a mold.

Chris Wright: Exactly. A lot of teachers don't teach the student to understand her own body, and that's what you have to look for. It was only when I came to that kind of teacher that I finally began to understand my body, and she began to teach me how to teach myself.

Adam: But once you know your own body it's important to find other teachers so you can pick up other styles, do what they do and learn how they do it. The first teacher is the most important because he's the one who teaches you about your own instrument. Then when you have the knowledge and self-confidence, you can take your instrument and make what someone else has done look good on you.

Author: Are there any other qualities you can think of?

Vicki: I would say a good eye is important, the ability to pick up mistakes that the student is making. And fairness, a teacher who doesn't play favorites. A good teacher should also be able to keep the energy of the class high and keep up interest. If kids are dizzed out in the back of the class, it isn't doing them much good. And an individual who is open, who keeps growing and changing—maybe he watches other teachers or sees other performances. Good music and good movement, giving students a chance to move and to do nice movement is important, too.

Chris Wright: I'd just like to add that I think there should be some sort of certification for dance teachers. Despite some of the good things I got from my early training, it took me five or six years to get rid of the effects of poor training in technique—and I was lucky. There are so many dance teachers who do real physical damage to a dancer's body because they don't have a basic knowledge of technique and anatomy. One of my first teachers, in Paris—we were there because my father is in the foreign service—had us jumping on a cement floor. Can you believe that? But even though dance teachers can do so much harm to naive students, particularly children whose bodies are still forming—I mean like changing their bone structure—they don't have to be licensed in any way.

Limitations

Author: How much do you think training can change your body?

Bill: My body has changed dramatically since I started dancing. I played quite a bit of basketball and I also swam. I used to be much bigger in the chest and shoulders. I didn't have a dancer's body when I began. The definition of the muscles in my legs and upper body has changed tremendously in the past six years.

Gillian: Since I left behind my ballet training I've had a great deal of Graham, and that has changed my whole movement style a lot. It changed me physically too—my body line, my muscular shape.

Christine O'Neal: It's interesting. Depending on which kind of class you go to you can see the way the students pick up different things from their teacher. You can see the muscles change. If you go to a heavy Russian class, the women are going to develop stronger thigh muscles; if you do a lot of jumps, it's going to be something else. If you dance with a teacher who is not relaxed, you're going to have tension and sheer gut force. If you learn from someone who has a naturalness about their dancing, you'll get that kind of flowing quality—like what Balanchine has created. You can see it a mile away in any of his dancers.

Author: Are there certain physical limitations you've had to accept?

Chris Wright: I think there are limitations, but there's usually a way to work with them. For instance, when I was in Washington, D.C., I wasn't getting the best training. I have a tendency to have a large muscular structure, and not knowing about turn-out and a lot of other things, I had the idea of just grinding it out even harder. I was just a mass of tension and terribly, terribly frustrated. Everywhere I went they would say, "Well, you have to do something about those thighs." I tried everything, but of course nothing worked until I found the proper way to work with my body. A friend of mine told me to go to my present teacher in New York, and she taught me how to use my body in an efficient way. I think that we all might have certain limitations—I mean, I'll never be able to kick my leg up to my ear—but I was amazed at the ability of my body once I was calm.

Richard: I think it has a lot to do with the teacher making you feel that it is possible. In your case, until you found the right teacher your mind had been telling you, Maybe I won't be able to do it.

Chris Wright: Maybe. I'd go to classes and the teachers wouldn't really give me any useful corrections. At the end they'd say something like, "When you come back, maybe you should do something with your legs." I didn't know what to do. I wished I knew. I was working the only way I knew how. But since then I've seen many people who have a lot of limitations, but in the right atmosphere it's unbelievable what they can do with themselves once they know how.

Author: A good teacher does that for you. She stops the franticness. She gives you the confidence that she will help you overcome the problem, that there is a solution.

Bill: Usually the nervous anxiety and muscular tension that go with a physical limitation are worse than the limitation itself. It's like insomnia: The more you fixate on the problem, the more you tense up and the worse it gets. What you need are some solutions. And the mental state of panic or futility you're in makes it impossible to see solutions.

Carolyn: It's also important for us to be as generous with ourselves as we are with other people. We don't think anybody else has to be perfect, and so we can appreciate the things they do well. It's very important to be able to build on our strengths.

Ellen: I know when I started out I tried to do everything, and I never thought about whether or not I should. I think that as you grow older you still try to do everything, but you become kinder to yourself. I think that one of the things you're trying to do as a dancer is know yourself. That means knowing when to leave yourself alone, when not to kill yourself and when to kill yourself. It's a very important part of staying in the field.

Sara: And you have to believe in those good things about yourself.

Richard: Yes. It's not only a matter of believing in the good things, but of finding what makes dancing vital and interesting to you. Focusing on your limitations isn't what made you interested in dancing in the first place.

Chris Wright: But when I was in the ballet world it was very easy to find yourself focusing on your limitations, because they were always being brought to your attention. You looked around the class and there were all those perfect bodies, perfect feet and whatever. And there you were. In a school situation that focus is almost always there. It's not the adult situation, the professional atmosphere which I feel a good teacher is able to bring about. Usually there's so much pressure that you're always aware of your limitations and you're not able to get over that. It wasn't until I went into modern that I realized that it didn't matter so much that I didn't have great feet and beautiful legs and beautiful line.

Richard: Or maybe you discovered that the beauty of your line was something else. You find that there are lots of different kinds of beautiful line, and different ways of approaching it. I took a class with Twyla Tharp yesterday which was quite an experience. I've been doing tendus*for years and years, but she made me see something new in them. She said, "Okay, think of tendus dégagés as your first exercise in seeing how gravity pulls the leg down and how you release the breath." So I was stimulated to think of tendu in a different way. There's a great excitement when you can feel a movement internally— where it comes from. This has nothing to do with beautiful line, but more to do with focus, concentration, momentum and weight and, perhaps, phrasing. A good teacher, I think, can see small internal movements *toward* the correct line and not only the line itself. That is an invaluable help in getting there.

Author: Do you think that physical limitations become more or less important depending on the type of dancing you do?

Sara: As far as ballet goes, I think that there are limitations that can prevent you from pursuing it. The Kirov Ballet, for example, chooses their dancers from the beginning, so they're not later fighting bad feet or no turn-out. Today in ballet the competition brings us to such a high level that the people who are hiring are only interested in absolute perfection. I know in my case, I have very long toes and I don't have enough flexibility there. People told me that I'd never be able to dance on pointe. Well I was determined, and so I fought the problem. But I still have problems sometimes, and it's a limitation that has hindered me.

Bettie: In ballet you just have to have a certain line, and when you start at an early age your bones are still pliable enough to do that. Did you ever have any foot X rays, Sara? Do you have bone spurs?

---

*A ballet exercise designed to stretch and strengthen the feet and ankles.

Sara: I have. I have calcium deposits in my left foot, which is where I have the problem. But I've learned to work with my feet, such as they are, though they're my cross to bear. Some things are just more difficult for me to do, they take a little more effort and concentration. But I've accepted it. I still can—and want—to dance.

Author: Vicki, did you have problems fitting into the Balanchine mold?

Vicki: Well to get into the company you need nice arched feet, long legs, good turn-out, a small head and high extensions. It's very sad to see some students always rubbing their feet with Tiger's Balm, wrapping them in towels and trying to stretch their arches. That doesn't help very much. I don't have a perfect turn-out and my legs don't fly up to my ears, either. At the school everyone could do splits—I couldn't. But I have a good jump, and I've worked to have nice arms and a free and open upper body. To a certain extent you can compensate for some limitations as a performer. For example, you can turn your standing leg in slightly so that you get more rotation in the working leg, to give the illusion of more turn-out.

Ryland: I think I agree about accepting your limitations. My feet aren't great, my line isn't great, and so I have to do something else with my dancing. In your first year at Juilliard there are juries that you have to perform for who decide whether or not you will go on to the next level or leave. I did a duet with Clyde Morgan and we finished and I sat down and watched everyone else do their things. Then Martha Hill—the director of the dance department—spoke to us out loud with absolutely no privacy about it at all. She said, "Ryland, your technique is terrible! But put you and Clyde on a stage with some lights and you're wonderful." I was terrible in class, but I could make the magic happen for her onstage. And I was still terrible when I left Juilliard—I learned more about technique after I left—but I got to dance when I was there.

Sara: Just look at the films of Ulanova. So many things are wrong with her technique, as we would judge it today, but she's a great artist.

Carolyn: I guess I have a different approach to limitations. I think that at least mentally one works for absolute perfection in class. I think that if we ever get to the point that we can assume there are certain things we'll never be able to do, then that's the end of the road. Of course, there are days when one thinks, Well anyway, I'm a nice person, I have a great family. But essentially I'm always working as if the ultimate is going to happen and I'm always surprised if it doesn't. That's the mentality you have to keep alive and that's the hard part about it. Somebody recently said to me, "You know, I'm going to retire from the stage. The mind gives out long before the body."

Author: You've touched on a major point, Carolyn. A well-known hypnotherapist in New York—his name is Herbert Spiegel—has had enormous success in helping people overcome all sorts of psychosomatic disorders. Basically his philosophy is this: The way to get over a problem is not to focus on the negative aspects but to keep thinking of the positive goal—for instance, that you want to kick your leg up as light as a feather, instead of fixating on how hard it is to lift—because, even if you don't achieve your goal entirely, it will prevent you from getting bogged down in panic and preoccupation.

Carolyn: It's really true. This unbelievable optimism and determination and concentration is what I find the most wearing. But that's what makes it all possible, and everything you do in the right direction is a source of improvement. If you try for absolute perfection, you can go a long way on whatever results from that effort. The important thing is to be going in the right direction. And the trick is to maintain some kind of equilibrium while you're in a constant state of flux.

Richard: I think one of the things about learning how to dance in class is just learning how to dance when you feel a hundred different ways—if you're sick or if you're tired or if you're feeling wonderful. You learn how to perform when you do that. It's that daily consistency.

Bill: But you also have to be realistic in terms of your body.

Author: Did you discover that early because you started dancing at a late age?

Bill: No, because I got a few injuries. You learn very quickly if you're not working correctly because you get hurt. It's really a kind of paradox, I think. You have to be realistic about your limitations and at the same time—as Carolyn says—keep trying to do better.

Working in class

Author: Do you think you've developed a way of working in class over the years?

Ellen: There's an attitude I've learned to strive for that's very important in order for me to be able to work well. I always attempt to learn something about myself instead of becoming dead. In a way, when you keep forcing yourself harder and harder, it leads to a kind of deadness because you're not really thinking about how to make it work best for yourself. I try to learn about myself when I'm taking class, to work with knowledge rather than just driving myself. Otherwise, I'm just grinding away with a lot of tension and I don't get much accomplished.

Carolyn: I think what Ellen is saying is that one doesn't go into class with a pure dead instrument. A totally pure instrument is an instrument without a soul in it, without a mind in it. There's a lot of baggage that you take with you to class. If somebody shoves you in the subway on the way to class, you're going to be tenser than if they don't. That's a very superficial example. But as you get older you have more and more baggage, so there are more and more obstacles. And it's a constant battle to get back to the basic thing: Lift your leg and do it. The more stresses and strains you have placed on your life—they don't have to be monumental but they add up—the more you have to fight to rid yourself of the extraneous things, to be able to simply respond as directly as possible. That's a very important thing to be able to do, particularly if you're working with a choreographer or if you're auditioning.

Bill: You know, I find it nice sometimes, because in spite of my troubles I go to class at one or two o'clock every day, and the one constant thing in my life is the plié. No matter what else is bothering me, I go back to pliés and everything is back to normal. It's almost therapeutic.

Carolyn: Yes, but what I'm talking about is the buildup, the loss of innocence that happens as you mature. We all know that children are glorious. I teach children a lot, and they all have perfect turn-out and most of them have beautiful feet. They don't know that they're not *supposed* to get their legs up, so they do. They're not afraid of turning because no one ever told them that they'll fall down, and no one told them that falling down is a disgrace. It's more that kind of thing one is constantly fighting. For a professional, it could be that the stakes get higher, or that we have a reputation to maintain, or that we have to think about the next role. Those things can all potentially get in the way of our thinking of ourselves as children walking into a class simply to execute what we are asked to do without expectations.

Bill: Recreational dancers may be lucky. They don't have to go to class to become professional dancers. And they may possibly be getting more out of it because they're not so hard on themselves.

Gillian: I know what you mean by expectations. When I'm working I can't get to class as often as I would like. I feel the expectations that I impose on myself. I think, Oh my God, I haven't been to class in three weeks. I go into class with a slight depression ahead of time because I know I have these expectations of myself that I'm not going to live up to. There's the pressure of people around me knowing I'm dancing in *Chorus Line* and I'm falling off my turns or whatever, and I'm not that child. I'm embarrassed. I'm a little nervous sometimes before going to class. I'd like to take a class where nobody knows me.

Ellen: I think the problem of being totally there, of having body and mind come together so that you are totally involved in the movement, is what we're all talking about. How to do that, how not to let the unpaid telephone bill, or the subway or whatever interfere. Because that's not what you're doing when you're dancing. You're doing the movement. The greatest times in dancing come when you are just doing the movement, and that's that. I don't have that all the time in class, either, but that's what makes it all meaningful to me. Those are the times when dancing is wonderful.

Author: Ellen, I'd like to get back to something you said earlier. You said that you've learned to dance with knowledge only recently. But you've been performing quite a long time.

Ellen: When I was younger I worked hard, terribly hard, but I didn't learn very much about mechanics. By sheer force and will and a lot of dance classes I learned how to dance. I don't think I learned how to dance with knowledge for years afterward. Even after I joined a company, I got by with sheer brute force. I feel that just now, in the past few years—and after a couple of injuries—I'm learning to dance with knowledge.

Author: Do you think you got away with it for so many years because dancing was physically easy for you?

Ellen: I may have been lucky, because I have a very good body for dance and I could get away with a lot. I am thin and I have length to me and very good feet. But I have often thought that in another way this may not have been so fortunate. I didn't realize that I had to learn to use my feet properly, for instance, since they always seemed to look good no matter what I did. I really didn't have to point; now I know that you have to point in order to feel your leg the right way.

Bettie: It's important to begin your dance training in a situation where dancing comes before technique, but you eventually find that you've learned everything the wrong way first and then you have to unlearn it all. You may be forty years old by the time you can say, Now I know what I'm talking about, technique and dancing.

Ryland: Yeah, and by then you're too old.

Ellen: When I was eighteen and first started dancing seriously, there was a kind of abandonment and naiveté and pure sweat that I would have in class. I mean I was just throwing myself around. I had a very flexible body that was strong and healthy. But as you get older you do things with more knowledge—perhaps there's a kind of sadness to that. You don't run around and skip in the street anymore. With knowledge and with age and with discipline you lose a kind of energy of abandonment that you had when you were naive.

Author: It sounds as though dancing isn't as much fun, now that you're a trained dancer.

Ellen: No, I wouldn't say that. There's a feeling of totality that comes over you as a dancer when you're doing well. It's that feeling of being totally involved—whether it's at the barre or on the stage—that I consider to be dancing. I suppose that's why I say this initial feeling I had as a young person dancing is what I remember with such love. I didn't know enough to tear things down. In fact, maybe I've come full circle because that's what I'm enjoying now, that totality. And that's the same feeling I enjoyed when I was eighteen. Maybe in between you tear everything down.

Author: Sara, you're nodding your head. Did you have a similar experience?

Sara: Very similar. I had Harold and Lew Christensen as my teachers in San Francisco, and they were very technical, "hip down" sort of teachers. That was what was important. Then Anatole Vilzak and Ludmila Schollar came along. They were from the Russian tradition and they gave beautiful, dancy combinations. For the first time I realized that there was more to dancing than technique. I figured out by myself how to do these things. I was never told how to do a pirouette correctly or anything like that, but because I had to do it and I wanted to do it, I figured out the most efficient way. That was the beginning of my joy of dance. It wasn't until after I got into a company that I went back and learned the mechanics of it in the right way. At the time I was really having trouble with my ankles. I looked good from the outside, but then I had to go through a remaking of the thing.

Author: Like so many dancers, you started to learn about technique when you started hurting.

Sara: I didn't think I needed to learn technique before, I just thought I could figure it out myself, and it worked. Many of the things I was doing were right. In fact, I started to dissect too much when I first got to New York. New York is so much more technically oriented than I was ever brought up to be in San Francisco. Don't talk about dancing, just do it—that's how I was brought up. When I came to New York my first impression was that everyone was so technical they didn't dance. There was a lot of tension and I got very critical, very analytical. My natural sense of movement and my natural way of figuring out how to do things were destroyed. It's very difficult to recapture that once you start to analyze. It wasn't until I went to David Howard that he was able to talk to me. He was able to communicate to me with his system of counterweights and pulleys and things, and somehow or other it clicked in my mind. I could do the same things I was doing before, only know that I was consciously doing them. You can do a double pirouette, but to *know* how to do it, that's a different story, to work on that level.

Ellen: I think that you have to lose some of your natural spontaneity—at least temporarily—in order to go forward and get something else. A lot of the things that come with that early feeling of totality are not necessarily good in the long run. They're not sustaining. There's a lot of tension, excess tension, that you can't use for the next ten or twenty years, or you won't have anything left. You'll just beat your body to a pulp if you try to dance that way for twenty years. I have wonderful times dancing now—surely as wonderful as then—but as a performer you can't just walk onstage and look into the lights and go, Ah, lights! You don't do that, you don't blind yourself by looking into the lights. You think about what you're doing and you do the movement, and then you feel that you're dancing. All these things are going on together.

Author: Here's one from left field: How do you learn new movement?

Carolyn: I always go for two things: the movements that are most familiar and the rhythm. I think that in any learning process the initial impression is the total foundation. For example, when we revived a ten-year-old repertory piece recently I found that I remembered the first things that I had learned—the original version. And this is very typical. So I try to trust the indelible impression of the things that strike me first, and then solidify the spaces between the familiar shapes and times. It makes for very quick learning, but that's just because it works for me. I do feel that whatever you see first makes the most lasting impression and you don't have to worry about it.

Bill: Being in musical comedy I find that I'm confronted with an incredible variety of dance styles. I find that the more I do, the easier it is for me to pick up things. The more movement you've done, the more styles you've seen—again it becomes a process of association.

Author: You mean the more memory pegs you have to hang the new movement on?

Bill: Yes, the first thing you go to is something that's familiar, but that can come from your background, what you've seen and done. Styles are such a hard thing because they so frequently have nothing to do with technique but so much to do with the choreographer's body. That's where you have to rely totally on your impression.

Ellen: Someone once told me that the best thing is to learn the beginning and the end of the combination first, and then fill in the middle. For me what works is an incredible amount of sticking to it—never letting my mind go anyplace else. As the choreographer is working and trying things, I'm trying things. I move with him as he's doing it. Then I find that I pick it up very quickly. If my mind wanders even for a second and then comes back, I have too much to deal with. So again, it's constant concentration. But in class I think it helps a lot to remember the first and last steps. And then you can just follow everyone else in the middle [laughs].

Staying in shape

Author: How good are you about going to class and keeping up your technique?

Gillian: Once you start working steadily, it's hard to keep up the same technique. Working on Broadway and doing musicals, you're constantly going away, working here for six weeks and there for eight weeks. It's been seven or eight years since I went to class every day. I'm definitely not the dancer I was then in terms of technique. If I could go back to the kind of dancer I would like to be, I would go back to when I was eighteen years old and a ballet dancer. Now it's a matter of trying to get back to the dance classes, to try to get that technique back again. I'm not disappointed with where I am now, it's just that I've changed my priorities.

Author: That's one of the little ironies of success. When you work a lot and can't go to class, your technique suffers, at least in some ways. Performing and rehearsing aren't enough to keep you in top shape.

Dru: It's very unfortunate that we have to go to class, that we have to have a technique, that we have to do a plié every day. After so many years you don't really get a thrill out of doing your first plié of the day. When I first started to dance back home I loved it, and slowly I began to hate it. It was such a bore. But you have to have that technique. It's very sad that we can't just get up and dance and go home.

Author: What do you do to stay in condition?

Dru: Before a show I can do a fifteen-minute to a half-hour warm-up, which is enough for the show but not enough for my body. I have to do a ballet class to be in shape. I mean I could get through the show every night just warming up, but in a few weeks if I went to an audition I would just flunk. My body would fall apart.

Adam: Now because I work a lot and for long periods of time, the only time I go to class is when I feel like I'm in trouble, when I feel like I can't hold my turns and I'm really in bad shape. Only when I'm not working. Then I'll go back to class to get it together for another job or something. And only because I know I just have four or five weeks—a limited time—and then I'll be finished and ready to work again.

Author: Well, there you have a completely different point of view!

Dru: I think it's easier for men to stay in shape than women. I think we lose our muscle tone much more quickly than you guys

Author: But most men aren't as flexible.

Dru: I don't mean flexibility but muscle tone, don't you think?

Bettie: You probably think that because men have a taut muscle structure, which is easier to maintain. The longer your muscles are, the harder they are to rebuild. I had that experience after a knee injury. It took me so much longer to get the muscle tone back than any of the male dancers I knew with the same injury, because they have shorter, bulkier muscles.

Dru: My husband is ten years older than I and he has a great pair of legs. He doesn't do anything for it. If I don't go to class for a week I start getting all sloppy.

Richard: I think there are lots of things that dancers can do to maintain themselves. It's a very individual thing. I'm still experimenting myself. Besides going to class, I think it's important to take some time and work on your own, at your own pace; to take one part of what you've worked on in class and concentrate on that, for instance, or to take a phrase from a piece you're learning and try doing it different ways. Especially in New York, with the fast

315

pace of the life here, it's easy to spend your whole day just running—to the bank, to class, to rehearsal or whatever, without really taking time to absorb what you've learned. You don't always have to be moving, either. Lying down at the end of the day and just thinking about movement can be helpful too. I've found that it's good for the muscles to have a slight change of schedule every so often. Some days I want to get the blood circulating, so I start out running— especially when it's cold outside. Other days I begin by just lying on my back quietly and feeling the length of my spine. I've also discovered that it's good to stretch out my muscles at the end of the day, so I do that religiously every night.

Closing thoughts

Author: Would anyone like to offer a final piece of advice?

Bettie: I would not like to give people advice on where to take class, but to tell them to go to as many places as they wish. The people who are going to be dancers will do it anyway, and the people who only *think* they want to dance are not going to.

Richard: Don't lose yourself in eight classes a day. There are things to learn about movement in the street, on the train. It's not only in the classroom that you learn about dancing.

Bettie: I think you have to keep on shifting. Whatever's best for you at the time. If it fits you, it's right for that time. And then you sometimes have to leave and go to another plateau. When I know my feet are losing strength, I go to ballet. When I know my torso isn't functioning so well, I go to modern. When I know nothing is working anymore, I work on my own because I have gotten bored with all those pliés. When that happens I think it is important to go to a totally different thing, like swimming or pushing springs, where you can use your muscles efficiently and correctly and get yourself out of this rut.

Ryland: I got an incredible lift from taking balalaika lessons. All of a sudden a port de bras meant something because I could hear this instrument playing, and somehow it fit. My legs felt better and my head felt better.

Richard: What Ryland said is really fine. Even if you have your main focus on ballet or a modern technique I don't think taking three or four classes a day in that technique is necessarily good. Speaking of balalaikas, when I visited the Soviet Union with the Joffrey Ballet we saw that in all the ballet schools the students had classes in music, gymnastics, mime, character dancing, art history and anatomical exercise (like blowing through tubes into water to help breathing). In New York and other big cities there is an abundance of classes. Finding the right combination of classes (which usually means running around a little because it's not all at one school) will reflect itself in your dancing.

Carolyn: I would advise everybody to explore and to go see a lot of dancing, to develop personal opinions and to develop taste—not channel themselves in one direction prematurely.

Bettie: I studied at the Martha Graham School for quite some time. The technique was very beautiful, but I didn't know what it was for—besides getting into the Graham company—until I went outside. I didn't know that you can use a contraction to propel yourself into space, or to get speedily down to the floor and up again. It's a difficult style for some body types. In Graham class you start your warm-up sitting on the floor. But after these floor exercises I was so stretched out that I could not use my legs and move in space. I'd stand up and feel like Bambi on ice.

Ryland: That fourth position on the floor always destroyed me because I don't have much turn-out. Once I got up off the floor, though, I was fine.

Bettie: Graham floor work is difficult for many men. After all, the technique was built on a female body. But I think that happens in ballet class too. I was brought up in a very strict sense in ballet, from ten to one o'clock, and from two to five o'clock every day—without a piano. There were eight students in a class. When you didn't do your jumps in first position correctly, you did them over and over again until you were blue in the face. You start to think that's all there is to dancing. Every day, six days a week. That's why you have to get out and see, to try different things.

Bill: Yes, because then not only do you have the wherewithal to judge other people's work, but you also develop the honesty within yourself to know what you as a dancer need to do. You can't avoid making mistakes. In the learning process I think you have to make mistakes.

Carolyn: Don't close the door on possibilities. I think that's the big no-no— going from your neighborhood dancing school to one teacher and not seeing anything else. There are whole studios where they simply don't go to see certain kinds of dance. You should avoid that kind of attitude.

Ellen: Dance studios tend to be very cultish, and particularly when you're young and impressionable it's very easy to fall into that way of thinking because it's comfortable.

Author: How do you know when a school or teacher isn't right for you?

Carolyn: The same way you decide that you like or don't like anything— strawberries—through experiencing. That's why you have to get out and around and see what's going on and see what ways there are to move, the same way that Richard got turned on by the Moiseyev or Gillian got inspired by watching Moira Shearer.

Bill: Trust your instincts. If it doesn't feel good try something else, but don't be afraid to try something else. It may be hard after being ensconced for a long time. You feel secure, and that's usually so hard in this business, to feel secure. So once you finally find something you become very avid, but you have to be careful just then. There's the problem of getting too comfortable in someone's class, which can be really dangerous.

Adam: Then you're afraid to go somewhere else. But when you do go to another teacher and he does the same exercise a little differently, all of a sudden you discover that you're feeling new things and using muscles you haven't used for years. It's important to go to teachers who are different shapes and sizes so you can learn to pick up different styles of moving, because you're not going to work with that one person or a body like yours the rest of your life.

Ryland: The one thing that I've always had and I wish I could communicate and I never can, but I feel we all have, is that love for doing what I do. As long as I keep that there I know that I'll find the right teacher, that I'll be doing the right thing. You have to trust that little lightbulb or whatever it is inside of you that says you're right. And don't worry that your parents are going to be upset or that you've changed your school again.

Part VII

The
dancer's
yellow
pages

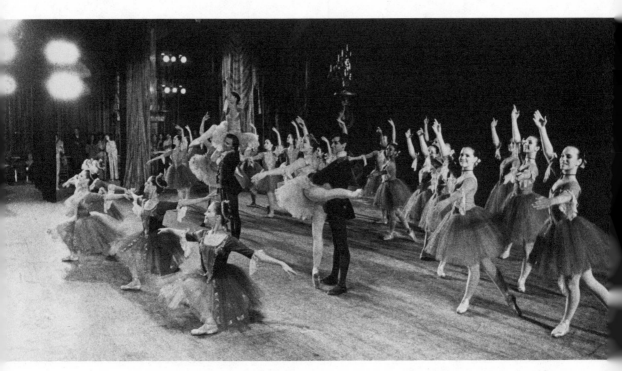

Few people know that the Atlanta Ballet, a regional company founded in 1929, is the oldest ballet troupe in the United States. *King Douglas*

25

A Dance Map
of the Country:
Where to Find Quality
Dance in Your Area

some simple strategies;
organizations that can help

The surest way to find a good dance class is the simplest: Ask around. Whenever possible, get recommendations from other dancers because they speak from experience. Once you start to inquire, you'll be surprised how many people study dance or know someone who does. Keep your eyes and ears open. Dance schools and teachers advertise in nationally sold periodicals such as *Dancemagazine* and *Dance News* (see chapter 26 for a complete listing), in local newspapers and the yellow pages of the phone book, on dance school bulletin boards, and even in shop windows. These sources will help keep you abreast of upcoming concerts, auditions and other dance events too. Dance school dressing rooms are great places to pick up information, and most dance teachers will be glad to refer you to someone else they respect if their own classes aren't suitable. Follow up suggestions that sound promising, but don't feel compelled to stay with an unsatisfactory teacher just because she or he has a big reputation.

As John Dayger of the Lar Lubovitch Dance Company advises, "Look for dancers you like and find out where they study. You've got to like the end product the class produces." If a performer catches your eye, check your theater program. It is likely to contain biographies of the cast that tell about their training. If you have the chance, in class or at a lecture-demonstration, do not hesitate to ask dancers where they have studied. They are usually very obliging about sharing this kind of information.

Dance organizations that can help

The following service organizations can save you precious time by steering you to the best available dance teachers, companies and resources in your area.

The National Association for Regional Ballet (NARB). It used to be that a dancer with any serious aspirations toward a career was forced to leave home at a tender age and head for a big, bad city like New York where the training, professional opportunities and pay were supposed to be superior. If she was successful, sooner or later she would probably have to choose between dancing and marriage because the demands of performing wouldn't allow both. In most parts of the United States those who wanted to see reputable dance companies, or even to take up dancing recreationally, had to be content with occasional visits from the New York troupes and exercise classes at the neighborhood YWCA.

But in the past two decades the National Association for Regional Ballet has made the dream of decentralized dance in America a reality. It has made it possible for serious dancers to get good training and stage experience at home, for professionals to continue working without having to sacrifice a family life, and for increasingly sophisticated dance audiences to enjoy first-rate performances at nearby theaters.

The NARB was founded by people who wanted to stay in their own communities to dance, and who believed that dance of high technical and artistic merit could and should exist everywhere. It got started in much the same way as civic orchestras and regional theaters did. In the 1940s and 50s a few stalwart malcontents and married couples from the big professional companies sought work outside of New York. These dancers and teachers became the first dance settlers in the regions. They opened schools—some of them in their living rooms—in Tucson, Fort Worth, Tulsa, Miami and Dallas. Later they formed companies to give talented students a chance to perform.

For a long time these little dance outposts fended for themselves as best they could. Then in 1956, Dorothy Alexander, director of the Atlanta Ballet, organized a gathering of eight local dance companies to perform for each other and share information. This grew into the Southeastern Regional Ballet Association. The practice of attending annual ballet festivals took hold as more and more companies banded together for mutual support and assistance. Four other regional associations were founded: the Northeastern, Southwestern, Pacific and Mid-States. Finally, in 1963, the National Association for Regional

Ballet was officially incorporated as a nonprofit organization governed by a board of directors with representatives from each of the five regions. Today there are ninety regional ballet companies and schools throughout the fifty states.

NARB schools and companies are good starting places for dancers, because the organization is above all a qualitative one which sets standards and guides the development of its members. It provides expert assistance to teachers and company directors on everything from technique and choreography to management and funding. Since they are linked together both regionally and nationally, NARB schools are well informed of dance classes and performing opportunities in their locales *and* around the country.

Although the Association defines "ballet" as including all forms of theatrical dance, the majority of NARB companies are ballet oriented; but most of the schools offer classes in modern dance, jazz or tap as well. In keeping with the main objective of the regional ballet movement, NARB companies perform mostly in and around their own communities, often in cooperation with civic orchestras and opera companies. About one-third of the groups tour on a limited basis, and several of them have works by the likes of George Balanchine, John Taras and Leonide Massine in their repertories.

Regional ballet companies vary widely in performance level, from fledgling amateurism to solid professionalism. Each one is periodically evaluated on the excellence of its training, repertory and service to the community, and these ratings are made available to the public. There are four NARB ranks. The highest is Major Company, of which there can never be more than ten; next is Regional Honor Company, then Performing Company and lastly, Intern. A Professional Wing was recently established for companies that pay their dancers the federal minimum wage for at least 30 weeks a year and maintain an annual budget of $250,000. There are currently five: the Atlanta Ballet, the Dayton Ballet, the Indianapolis Ballet Theatre, the Louisville Ballet and the Santa Barbara Ballet Theatre. In order to qualify for professional status, NARB companies must give at least ten full-length performances at home.

Sponsoring annual spring festivals where companies congregate for three and a half days of master classes, workshops and panel discussions continues to be a central function of the NARB. The festivals, which culminate in public performances, are held in each of the five regions, with different companies acting as hosts each year. Among the guest faculty at these gatherings are such celebrated teachers as Robert Joffrey, Arthur Mitchell, Mary Hinkson, Gus Giordano, James Truitte, Maria Tallchief and Ethel Winter. Specialists lecture on topics ranging from make-up to injury prevention and dance notation. But for many young dancers, the most valuable and exciting part of the regional ballet festivals is the performances. One participant told me, "Being able to see yourself in relation to other dancers of the same age puts things in perspective. It lets you see your own strong and weak points more clearly." This is especially important for males, who may be isolated in their home towns.

Regional festivals give dancers as much chance to be seen as to see. It is a tribute to the overall caliber of the dancing that scouts from major companies such as the American Ballet Theatre and the New York City Ballet regularly attend NARB galas to recruit new talent.

For information on the NARB school and company nearest you (including their official rank), contact the national office:

Doris Hering, Executive Director
National Association for Regional Ballet
1860 Broadway, Room 410
New York, New York 10023

For information about dance classes, performances and related activities in your area, contact your region directly:

Mid-States
Julia Bennett, Director
Dance Theatre of the Hemispheres
117 Third Avenue Southeast
Cedar Rapids, Iowa 52401
(319) 362-0529, 365-5133

Northeast
Jozia Mieszkowski, Director
Wilkes-Barre Ballet Theatre
102-104 South Main Street
Wilkes-Barre, Pennsylvania 18701
(717) 824-8602

Pacific
Paul Curtis, Director
San Jose Dance Theatre
115 Cherry Wood Court
Los Gatos, California 95030
(408) 354-3930, 379-8901

Southeast
Norman Shelburne, Director
Lexington Ballet
140 Indiana Avenue
Lexington, Kentucky 40508
(606) 233-3925, 272-3002

Southwest
Mascelyne Larkin, Director
Tulsa Ballet Theatre
5414 South Gillette Street
Tulsa, Oklahoma 74105
(918) 742-5425, 747-0370

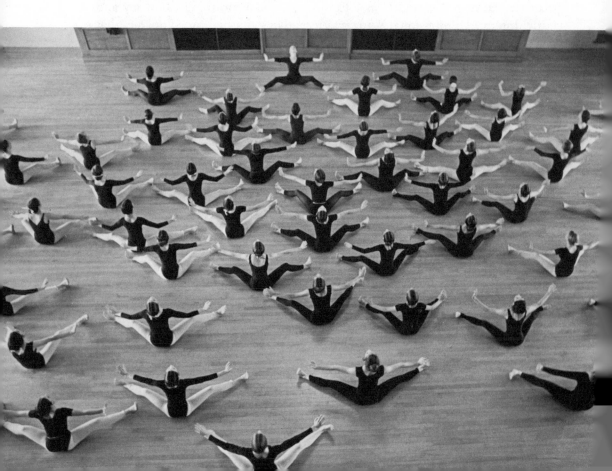

Community and state arts councils. Community arts councils are local organizations that sponsor and promote the arts. There are about 1800 of them in the United States and they range considerably in size and scope of services, particularly with regard to dance. Some arts councils are shoestring operations run by one or two dedicated volunteers; others have annual budgets of over $100,000 and paid employees.

Many of these groups got started in parts of the country where fine arts performances and training were scarce. They were created to fill the gap between what was needed and what was already provided by the community. Thus, in culturally active cities, arts councils simply act as clearing houses by publicizing dance events, dispensing information and advising sponsors, performing groups and other existing arts organizations. In cities where there is very little arts programming, community arts councils frequently set up community arts centers that hire performers and in some instances offer dance classes themselves. Some local arts councils even raise scholarship funds for promising young dancers.

Like community arts councils, state arts councils differ in budget size and range of services. All states receive a yearly start-up allowance of about $230,000 from the National Endowment for the Arts, which they must match with their own revenues. The largest agencies — the New York State Council on the Arts, for example — maintain budgets in the millions. State Arts councils distribute government money to community arts councils, individual artists and arts organizations. They also publicize arts activities and in various ways increase performing opportunities. Some state councils publish calendars of events and listings of arts organizations and resources in their states. The agencies listed below (with their directors) will be able to refer you to the community arts council best suited to your needs.

State Arts Councils

**Alabama State Council
on the Arts and Humanities**
M.J. Zakrzewski
114 North Hull Street
Montgomery 36130
(205) 832-6758

Alaska State Council on the Arts
Ronald L. Evans
619 Warehouse Avenue, #220
Anchorage 99501
(907) 279-1558

American Samoa Arts Council
Enosa Pili
P.O. Box 1540
Office of Governor
Pago Pago 96799
(684) 633-4347

**Arizona Commission
on the Arts and Humanities**
Louise Tester
6330 North 7th Street
Phoenix 85014
(602) 255-5882

Arkansas Arts Council
Carolyn Staley
Continental Building, #500
Main and Markham streets
Little Rock 72201
(501) 371-2539

California Arts Council
Bill Cook
2022 J Street
Sacramento 95814
(916) 445-1530

**Colorado Council
on the Arts and Humanities**
Ed Harrison, Acting Director
Grant-Humphreys Mansion
770 Pennsylvania Street
Denver 80203
(303) 839-2617

**Connecticut Commission
on the Arts**
Anthony S. Keller
340 Capitol Avenue
Hartford 06106
(203) 566-4770

A master class in modern dance at a Southwestern Regional Ballet Festival. The teacher is Dallas-based Jerry Bywaters Cochran. *King Douglas*

Delaware State Arts Council
Joseph Brumskill
State Office Building
820 North French
Wilmington 19801
(302) 571-3540

**D.C. Commission
on the Arts and Humanities**
Mildred Bautista
1012 14th Street, #1200
Washington 20005
(202) 724-5613

Fine Arts Council of Florida
Rebecca Kushner
Division of Cultural Affairs
Department of State
The Capitol
Tallahassee 32304
(904) 487-2980

**Georgia Council
for the Arts and Humanities**
Frank Ratka
1627 Peachtree Street Northeast
#210
Atlanta 30309
(404) 656-3967

Insular Arts Council of Guam
S.M.Callista Camacho
P.O. Box 2950
Agana 96910
(671) 447-7413, 447-9845

**Hawaii State Foundation on
Culture and the Arts**
Alfred Preis
250 South King Street, #310
Honolulu 96813
(808) 548-4145

Idaho Commission on the Arts
Carl J. Petrick
c/o State House Mall
Boise 83720
(208) 334-2119

Illinois Arts Council
Clark Mitze
111 North Wabash Avenue
#700
Chicago 60602
(312) 793-6750

Indiana Arts Commission
Janet Harris
Union Title Building, #614
155 East Market Street
Indianapolis 46204
(317) 232-1268

Iowa State Arts Council
Sam Grabarski
State Capitol Building
Des Moines 50319
(515) 281-4451

Kansas Arts Commission
John Reed
112 West 6th Street
Topeka 66603
(913) 296-3335

Kentucky Arts Commission
Ms. Nash Cox
302 Wilkinson Street
Frankfort 40601
(502) 564-3757

Louisiana State Arts Council
Al Head
Division of the Arts, Box 44247
Baton Rouge 70801
(504) 342-6467

**Maine State Commission
on the Arts and Humanities**
Alden C. Wilson
State House
Augusta 04330
(207) 289-2724

Maryland Arts Council
Kenneth Kahn
15 West Mulberry
Baltimore 21201
(301) 685-6740

**Massachusetts Council
on the Arts and Humanities**
Anne Hawley
1 Ashburton Place
Boston 02108
(617) 727-3668

Michigan Council for the Arts
E. Ray Scott
1200 6th Avenue
Executive Plaza
Detroit 48226
(313) 256-3735

Minnesota State Arts Board
John Ondov
2500 Park Avenue
Minneapolis 55404
(612) 341-7170
1-800-652-9747

Mississippi Arts Commission
Lida Rogers
301 North Lamar Street
Box 1341
Jackson 39205
(601) 354-7336

**Missouri State Council
on the Arts**
Mary DeHahn
706 Chestnut, Suite 925
St. Louis 63101
(314) 241-7900

Montana Arts Council
David E. Nelson
1280 South Third Street West
Missoula 59801
(406) 543-8286

Nebraska Arts Council
Robin Tryloff
8448 West Center Road
Omaha 68124
(402) 554-2122

**Nevada State Council
on the Arts**
Jacqueline Belmont
329 Flint Street
Reno 89501
(702) 784-6231

**New Hampshire Commission
on the Arts**
John G. Coe
Phenix Hall
40 North Main Street
Concord 03301
(603) 271-2789

**New Jersey State Council
on the Arts**
Eileen Lawton
109 West State Street
Trenton 08608
(609) 292-6130

New Mexico Arts Division
Bernard Lopez
113 Lincoln
Santa Fe 87503
(505) 827-2061

**New York State Council
on the Arts**
Beverly D'Anne
80 Centre Street
New York 10013
(212) 488-5222

North Carolina Arts Council
Mary Regan
Department of Cultural Resources
Raleigh 27611
(919) 733-2821

**North Dakota Council
on the Arts**
Glenn Scott
Box 5548, University Station
Fargo 58105
(701) 237-7674

Ohio Arts Council
Wayne Lawson
50 West Broad Street, #3600
Columbus 43215
(614) 466-2613

State Arts Council
of Oklahoma
Ben DiSalvo
Jim Thorpe Building
2101 North Lincoln Boulevard
Oklahoma City 73105
(405) 521-2931

Oregon Arts Commission
Peter Hero
835 Summer Street Northeast
Salem 97301
(503) 378-3625

Commonwealth of Pennsylvania
Council on the Arts
Peter Carnahan
3 Shore Drive Office Center
2001 North Front Street
Harrisburg 17102
(717) 787-6883

Institute of Puerto Rican Culture
Luis M. Morales
Apartado Postal 4184
San Juan 00905
(809) 723-2115

Rhode Island State Council
on the Arts
Robin Berry
334 Westminster Mall
Providence 02903
(401) 277-3880

South Carolina Arts Commission
1800 Gervais Street
Columbia 29201
(803) 758-3442

South Dakota State
Fine Arts Council
Charlotte Carver
108 West 11th Street
Sioux Falls 57102
(605) 339-6646

Tennessee Arts Commission
Arthur L. Keeble
222 Capitol Hill Building
Nashville 37219
(615) 741-1701

Texas Commission on the Arts
Allan Longacre
P.O. Box 13406
Capitol Station
Austin 78711
(512) 475-6593

Utah Arts Council
Ruth Draper
617 East South Temple Street
Salt Lake City 84102
(801) 533-5895

Vermont Council on the Arts
Ellen McCulloch-Lovell
136 State Street
Montpelier 05602
(802) 828-3291

Virginia Commission
for the Arts
Jerry Haynie
400 East Grace Street
Richmond 23219
(804) 786-4492

Virgin Islands Council
on the Arts
Stephen J. Bostic
Caravelle Arcade
Christiansted, St. Croix 00820
(809) 773-3075, Ext. 3

Washington State Arts
Commission
James L. Haseltine
9th and Columbia Building
Mail Stop FU-12
Olympia 98504
(206) 753-3860

West Virginia Department
of Culture and History
Arts and Humanities Division
James B. Andrews
Capitol Complex
Charleston 25305

Wisconsin Arts Board
Jerrold Rouby
123 West Washington Avenue
Madison 53702
(608) 266-0190

Wyoming Council on the Arts
John Buhler
122 West 25th Street
Cheyenne 82002
(307) 777-7742

Local dance organizations. The latest outgrowth of the dance explosion, these grass-roots groups are comprised of dance sponsors, teachers, choreographers and dancers who have joined forces to promote dance events, showcase local dance companies, and pool information and resources. Most of them publish calendar/newsletters that cover area dance activities, upcoming concerts, residencies by visiting artists, auditions and other newsworthy goings-on (*Contemporary Dance News*, put out by the Massachusetts Contemporary Dance Association, is a handsome example). Local dance organizations often sponsor master classes and educational workshops, and all function officially or unofficially as referral services for dancers seeking good training and job opportunities. Several have begun to compile videotape and research libraries. Dance Theatre Workshop in New York, the San Francisco Bay Area Dance Coalition, the Massachusetts Contemporary Dance Association in Boston, the Los Angeles Area Dance Alliance and the Philadelphia Dance Alliance are among the oldest and most active of the groups noted below. Keep an eye out. New ones emerge every year.

Association of Ohio Dance Companies
Phyllis Levine, Director
3570 Warrensville Center Road
Suite 202
Cleveland, Ohio 44122
(216) 491-9169

Dallas Dance Council
Mrs. Mary Bywaters, President
P.O. Box 17034
Dallas, Texas 75207
(214) 361-0663
For Dallas, Fort Worth, Houston and San Antonio, Texas.

Dance Concert Society
Jerry Kvasnicka
8338 Big Bend Boulevard
St. Louis, Missouri 63119
(314) 968-4341

Dance in Canada Association
100 Richmond Street East
Suite 325
Toronto, Ontario
Canada M5C 2P9

Dance Theatre Workshop
David White, Director
219 West 19th Street
New York, New York 10011
(212) 691-6500

Dance Umbrella
Eve Larson, President
P.O. Box 1352
Austin, Texas 78703
(512) 478-0047

Los Angeles Area Dance Alliance
Betty Empy, Director
5820 Wilshire Boulevard,
Suite 300
Los Angeles, California 90036
(213) 937-9586

Massachusetts Contemporary Dance Association
Gail Glick, President
Box B
Babson Park Branch
Boston, Massachusetts 02157
(617) 868-1676

Michigan Dance Association
Jeanette Abeles, Director
953 Rosewood
East Lansing, Michigan 48823
(517) 351-0454

Mid-America Arts Alliance
Jerry Kvasnicka, President
20 West 9th Street, #550
Kansas City, Missouri 64105
(816) 421-1388
For Missouri, Kansas, Nebraska, Oklahoma and Arkansas.

Minnesota Independent Choreographer's Alliance
Judith Mirus, President
400 First Avenue North
Minneapolis, Minnesota 55401
(612) 340-1900

Philadelphia Dance Alliance
Lois Fischer
260 South Broad Street
20th Floor
Philadelphia, Pennsylvania 19102
(215) 546-7240

San Francisco Bay Area Dance Coalition
Sukey Lilienthal
Building C, Fort Mason
San Francisco, California 94123
(415) 673-8172

Southern Arts Federation
Wayne Birt
225 Peachtree Street, Suite 712
Atlanta, Georgia 30303
(404) 577-7244
For Alabama, Florida, Georgia, Kentucky, Louisiana, Mississippi, North Carolina, Tennessee and Virginia.

The National Endowment for the Arts Dance Touring Program. Over the last fifteen years the National Endowment for the Arts Dance Touring Program has probably done more for dancers and dance audiences than any other government endeavor. It has made it possible for concertgoers all over America to see a great variety of top-quality professional dance, and it has ensured the survival of many worthy companies by enabling them to work steadily and cultivate new audiences. It is largely due to the support of the Dance Touring Program that, for the first time in our nation's history, concert dancers are able to make a reasonable living.

In the past the Touring Program shared the cost of engaging dance companies with sponsors. (Sponsors are organizations that hire companies for performances, classes and lecture-demonstrations; they are usually colleges, community arts councils, local dance schools, public schools, theaters, or parks and recreation departments.) For their part, sponsors had to hire at least two dance companies a year for residencies of two and a half days each. Under this system, dancers could avoid dreaded one-night stands, while audiences got more in-depth exposure to visiting companies, and local sponsors could afford to book more dance events.

But since 1978 the Dance Touring Program has been undergoing extensive bureaucratic restructuring. Budgets have been drastically cut; so, unfortunately, has the number of dance companies funded. The reordering is expected to continue until 1982, when there is a distinct possibility that the Dance Touring Program will be merged with another National Endowment program.

Despite the uncertainties of the future, the majority of companies that have toured under the Dance Touring Program in the past are continuing to tour with or without government assistance. Many of them hold classes and auditions at home, and their travel itineraries are published monthly in *Dancemagazine*. For a partial listing of professional touring companies, see the *American Dance Directory*, obtainable from:

The Association of American
Dance Companies
162 West 56th Street
New York, New York 10019
(212) 265-7824, (800) 223-6573

For information on companies currently performing under the National Endowment for the Arts Dance Touring Program, contact:

Nello McDaniel, Tour Coordinator
Dance Program
National Endowment for the Arts
2401 E Street Northwest
Washington, D.C. 20506
(202) 634-6383

Dance teacher organizations. Dance teacher organizations have existed since the mid-nineteenth century. They were established to educate teachers and upgrade dance instruction. There are dozens of teacher organizations with hundreds of chapters throughout the United States. The trouble is that requirements for membership and standards of quality vary widely among them. Some teacher organizations, for example, spend a good deal of their time running beauty contests and talent shows; others raise scholarship funds and sponsor legitimate teacher-training courses for which college credit is given.

These groups probably do the most good for teachers isolated in remote areas, by putting them in touch with other teachers and providing guidelines for instruction. Many local branches offer technique classes and special workshops to members. They give advice on business ethics and studio management, and supply teachers with choreographic material for school recitals. Every summer dance teacher organizations hold conventions in major cities, where teachers and their students attend master classes conducted by prominent guest faculty, performances, and awards ceremonies.

Listed below are the national headquarters of some of the more serious dance teacher groups. They can put you in touch with the chapters nearest you. Be aware, however, that the competence of these teachers does vary and apply the same criteria you would in evaluating any other dance instructors.

Cecchetti Council of America
Marjorie Hassard, President
17725 Manderson Road
Detroit, Michigan, 48203
(313) 864-2197
The Cecchetti Council of America was formed in 1939 to perpetuate the training method of the Italian ballet master Enrico Cecchetti. The emphasis is on learning set classroom syllabi. Certified members must pass through eight grades of study, successfully complete an examination and take refresher courses.

Dance Masters of America
William A. Royal, National Secretary
923 West Smith Street
Orlando, Florida 32804
(305) 425-3049
The oldest and largest dance teacher organization in America. Its teacher-training course can be taken for college credit.

Dance Educators of America
Skip Randall, Secretary
Box 470
Caldwell, New Jersey 07006
(201) 228-5547
The Dance Educators of America operates a summer training school at Western Kentucky University. Among the master teachers at its conventions have been New York-based Don Farnworth and Charles Kelley, Gus Giordano from Chicago, and Joe Tremaine from Los Angeles.

National Association of Dance and Affiliated Artists
Patti Lewis, President
163 DuBois Avenue
Sea Cliff, New York 11579
(516) 671-7681
This group has no teacher-training course per se, but publishes a quarterly "Extension Course" booklet containing teaching tips, business advice and general dance news. They also have a teaching exchange program through which instructors from various chapters guest teach at each other's schools.

The Royal Academy of Dancing U.S. Branch
Elaine H. Keller, Secretary
8 College Avenue
Upper Montclair, New Jersey 07043
(201) 746-0184
The Royal Academy of Dancing was founded in London in 1920 to establish standard class syllabi, train teachers, regulate dance school curricula and award scholarships to talented students and potential choreographers. Since 1954, the president of the Academy has been Dame Margot Fonteyn. Once a year examiners from England come to test and evaluate teachers in the American branch.

Other organizations of interest

American Dance Therapy Association (ADTA)
2000 Century Plaza, Suite 230
Columbia, Maryland 21044
(301) 997-4040

The American Dance Therapy Association was founded in 1966 to establish and maintain high standards of professional education and competence in the field. It defines dance therapy as "the psychotherapeutic use of movement as a process which furthers the emotional and physical integration of the individual." The ADTA holds an annual conference and publishes *The American Journal of Dance Therapy*, several monographs and pamphlets, a code of professional ethics and a newsletter. Its helpful brochure "Educational Opportunities in Dance Therapy" includes a current listing of approved college programs as well as institutions that offer internships and ongoing courses and workshops in dance therapy. One of the Association's most important services is the upkeep of a registry of dance therapists who have met its professional standards of education and clinical practice. Registered dance therapists are identified by the initials "D.T.R." after their name.

Dance Notation Bureau
505 Eighth Avenue
New York, New York 10018
(212) 736-4350

The Dance Notation Bureau documents choreography, does research in movement analysis and trains professionals in dance notation and reconstruction. It reconstructs major works by choreographers such as George Balanchine, Antony Tudor, Doris Humphrey, Paul Taylor and Jerome Robbins for dance companies and college dance departments at a modest fee. Courses in Labanotation (an extremely precise system of scoring movement devised by Rudolf Laban), Effort/Shape (the qualitative analysis of movement), music, anatomy and kinesiology for dancers, injury prevention, choreography, and historic dance forms are regularly offered by the Bureau's seasoned faculty.

National Dance Association
American Alliance for Health,
Physical Education, Recreation
and Dance
1900 Association Drive
Reston, Virginia 22070
(703) 476-3400

An organization dedicated to raising the level of dance in education and promoting dance in the American educational system. It grants interest-free loans to students preparing for dance-teaching careers, holds conventions, and issues publications on dance education, dance therapy, children's dance and college dance programs, among other subjects. The National Dance Association also maintains a library of oral tapes of outstanding dance educators.

26

Finding Out More About Dance

tips on dance viewing,
where to find dance films
and publications;
suggested reading

Seeing more dance for your money

Next to dancing yourself, the best way to learn about dance is to see it performed — all kinds — in a variety of settings. And the best way to watch a dance performance is to sit back, relax and enjoy. Let yourself respond instinctively, the way you would automatically reach out to shake a hand extended in friendship. We see dance with our bodies as much as with our eyes. "If the dancer's body is erect, do we see merely an upright figure or do we recognize — because we have felt it ourselves — pride or assurance or authority?" writes Walter Terry in *The Dance in America*. "And if the dancer's muscles are contracted, bending his body low, do we see simply a bent pattern or do we remember the spasm which afflicted us, the broken arch of the spine when we ourselves experienced loss or pain or defeat?" Dance can be enjoyed on many levels, but it is primarily a physical communication.

In many ways looking at dance for the first time is like watching a sport whose rules you don't understand. To the unaccustomed eye the stage seems a chaos of scrambling bodies. But in time the eye takes in more of the action. The viewer begins to perceive the intent of the choreography and to appreciate the subtleties of the dancers' interpretations. For this reason it is good to see dances more than once. If a piece is well crafted, the more you see it, the more you see in it.

New-to-dance audiences are commonly under the impression that all dances are supposed to mean something. Actually, there are several kinds of ances. Some present movement for its own sake, for the sheer invention of motion and music; others evoke a strong atmosphere of mood; others tell a story, and still others combine elements of all three. No matter how sophisticated the choreography, all a dance demands of the viewer is that he trust his senses and, as choreographer Erick Hawkins recommends, "try to enter into it fully and innocently as a child and simply see what is in front" of him.

It needn't cost a small fortune to be an avid concertgoer. There are many ways to cut expenses. Theaters often give special discounts to students and senior citizens. In a few cities you can buy subsidized ticket vouchers that enable you to see many dance companies for as little as $2.00. At present, there are voucher programs in Boston, Minneapolis, New York and San Francisco, with others planned for Los Angeles, Toronto and Chicago:

Arts/Boston
73 Tremont Street
Boston, Massachusetts 02108
(617) 742-6600

Theatre Development Fund
1501 Broadway
New York, New York 10036
(212) 221-0013

Twin Cities Metropolitan Arts Alliance
310 Fourth Avenue South
Minneapolis, Minnesota 55415
(612) 332-0471

Performing Arts Services
1182 Market Street, Suite #311
San Francisco, California 94102
(415) 552-3505

If you're game, you can also try buying twofers or inexpensive standing-room tickets on the chance of finding some empty seats in better locations later; or that ancient ploy, second-acting — sneaking into a theater by mingling with the crowd in the lobby during intermission.

Dance films

Unlike painting, music or literature, dance is an ephemeral art. Prior to the use of film and videotape, the dance usually died with the dancer — unless it was recorded by expensive and cumbersome notation methods, which were imperfect at best because they were always subject to interpretation. Film allows us the luxury of viewing and reviewing great works from the past as well as the present. Thanks to modern technology, dances can be preserved and reconstructed with their original flavor and performance quality intact. Besides films that are straightforward records of performances, there are films on dance instruction and appreciation, and dances made expressly for the film medium.

Dance films can be viewed, borrowed or rented at low rates from many public and university libraries and some state arts councils. Foreign consulates and local ethnic societies sometimes lend out films of ethnic dances, and a number of regional dance organizations have their own videotape archives (see chapter 25)—the Minnesota Independent Choreographer's Alliance in Minneapolis and the San Francisco Bay Area Dance Coalition, for example. Professional film distributors are another source, and dance film series are presented in several cities.

The most comprehensive catalog of dance films to date is John Mueller's *Dance Film Directory*. It can be found in many libraries or purchased directly from the publisher.

> Mueller, John. *Dance Film Directory: An Annotated and Evaluative Guide to Films on Ballet and Modern Dance*. Princeton, New Jersey: Princeton Book Company, 1978. $9.95.
>
> The *Dance Film Directory* catalogs three hundred films and videotapes of ballet, modern dance and, despite its title, Hollywood musicals, mime and ethnic dance. In addition to basic information on rental fees and distributors, Mueller provides helpful descriptions and critiques of each film listed. The book is also a user's guide to finding inexpensive film sources, ordering films, getting a projector and planning a film series. Available from the Princeton Book Company, 20 Nassau Street, Princeton, New Jersey 08540, (609) 924-2244.

Ernie Smith has assembled an extraordinary assortment of rare film and still photographs (some of which are reproduced in chapter 10 of this book) of jazz and tap dance from 1903 to the late 1960s. Included are snippets of Bill Robinson's famous step dance, Snake Hips Tucker at the Cotton Club and Whitey's Lindy Hoppers dancing up a storm at the Savoy Ballroom in Harlem. Although his archive is not open to the public, Smith, who has meticulously researched his material and who has an endless reserve of colorful anecdotes about the performers, is available on a limited basis for film showings and lectures.

The Ernie Smith Jazz Dance Collection
601 West End Avenue
New York, New York 10024
(212) 724-9196

The Dance Collection at Lincoln Center

A permanent film library for our nation's theatrical and folk dances is a dream come true for generations of American choreographers. Ted Shawn foresaw the possibility in 1938 in a book called *Dance We Must*:

> *I visualize it thus: One enters the museum, fills out a card saying: "I wish to see Ruth St. Denis in* Liebestraum*" and is taken to a special room where that sound film can be projected for the applicant.*

The Lincoln Center Library and Museum for the Performing Arts in New York

City, which houses the world's largest dance film archive, has realized Shawn's vision in full. Anyone can arrange for a private screening of most of the thousands of films and videotapes in store at the Dance Collection. Visitors are encouraged to make a preliminary trip to look through the library's catalog listings beforehand, however, because some films have union restrictions or can be seen only with permission from the choreographer. Viewing appointments should be made at least two or three weeks in advance.

Among the treasures preserved on reels at the Dance Collection is footage shot by Douglas Fairbanks of Anna Pavlova while she was on tour in California, and a 1908 short subject called *Animated Picture Studio* which is believed to feature Isadora Duncan. José Limón can be seen with Pauline Koner and Lucas Hoving in *The Moor's Pavane*, Agnes de Mille is shown in her own ballet *Three Virgins and a Devil*, and there is a videotape of Twyla Tharp in an early choreographic effort, *Tank Dive*.

That's not all. There are hundreds of recorded interviews with dance celebrities in the library's oral history archive. The Dance Collection is also the world's largest library of dance literature and iconography. Every aspect of dance is covered: ballet, modern, theater dance, ethnic, ritual and social dance. Over 28,000 books and pamphlets crowd its shelves, including biographies, critical writings, notebooks and memoirs, dictionaries, anatomy studies, and works on dance history, technique, education and notation. There are rare manuscripts, photographs and prints, scrapbooks and other memorabilia from the private collections of Isadora Duncan and Gordon Craig, Ruth St. Denis and Ted Shawn, Agnes de Mille, Lincoln Kirstein, and Jerome Robbins, among others. Current and back issues of all the dance periodicals are on hand, too. Special photographic exhibits are frequently on display in the informal surrounds of the Dance Collection reading room. It is not unusual to see a college student hunched over a term paper seated next to a well-known critic researching his latest book or a ballet superstar boning up on a new role.

The Dance Collection
Library and Museum of the Performing Arts
New York Public Library at Lincoln Center
111 Amsterdam Avenue at 65th Street
New York, New York 10023
(212) 799-2200
Open Monday to Saturday, noon to 6:00 p.m.

Right next door to the dance research library are the equally impressive Theater and Music collections. The Rodgers and Hammerstein Archives of Sound is the largest listening library in the world, containing over 200,000 recordings.

Dance books and periodicals

It seems that every month new books on dance appear, and there is a host of dance periodicals that carry reviews and articles on just about every facet of the art. Numerous public and university libraries today have a healthy selection of dance books. If you would like to start a dance library of your own, many bookstores, including large chains such as B. Dalton, stock dance books both in hardcover and inexpensive paperbound editions. Certain dancewear suppliers — Leo's Advance Theatrical Company and Taffy's, for instance — sell dance books and records too. If you are unable to find a local bookseller that stocks dance publications, you may want to write the following dance ''specialists'' for a catalog and mail-order form:

Alfred A. Knopf
201 East 50th Street
New York, New York 10022
(212) 751-2600
Mostly biographies, photograph books and esoterica.

The Ballet Shop
1887 Broadway
New York, New York 10023
(212) 581-7990
New and out-of-print titles from all over the world; largest selection of dance books, periodicals and records in the country.

Children's Book and Music Center
5373 West Pico Boulevard
Los Angeles, California 90019
(213) 937-1825

Da Capo Press
227 West 17th Street
New York, New York 10011
(212) 255-0713
Reprints of old titles.

Dance Horizons
1801 East 26th Street
Brooklyn, New York 11229
(212) 627-0477
Historical books and reprints of old titles.

The Dance Mart
Box 48, Homecrest Station
Brooklyn, New York 11229
(212) NI5-9607
Mail order house selling current and out-of-print books on all aspects of dance.

Dance Notation Bureau
505 Eighth Avenue
New York, New York 10018
(212) 736-4350
Books on dance notation and movement analysis.

Danceways Books
393 West End Avenue
New York, New York 10024
(212) 799-2860
Practical guides to dance and dancing.

The Drama Bookshop
150 West 52nd Street
New York, New York 10019
(212) JU2-1037
Books on dance and theater arts.

George Sand Bookstore
9011 Melrose Avenue
Los Angeles, California 90069
(213) 858-1648

Mayfield Publishing Company
285 Hamilton Avenue
Palo Alto, California 94301
(415) 324-8673
Books on dance training and children's dance.

Paperback Traffic
1501 Polk Street
San Francisco, California 94109
(415) 771-8848

Wesleyan University Press
Distributed by Columbia University Press
136 South Broadway
Irvington, New York 10533
(914) 591-9111
Historical dance books.

Westwood Bookstore
1021 Broxton Avenue
Los Angeles, California 90024
(213) 473-4644

Other sources of dance publications

American Dance Guild Book Club
20 Nassau Street
Princeton, New Jersey 08540
(609) 924-2244, 924-2251
The only book club exclusively for dance. Members receive advance descriptions of the monthly selections and can buy books at a substantial savings.

Dancing Times Book Center
18 Hand Court
High Holborn
London WC1V 6JF, England

For dance books published abroad. Write to the above address for their catalog and price list.

Dancemagazine
1180 Avenue of the Americas
New York, New York 10036
(212) 921-9300
Dancemagazine is the publisher of the *Dancemagazine College Guide*; *Raoul Gelabert's Anatomy for the Dancer*; the *Dancemagazine Annual*, a directory of resources and services for dancers, dance companies and dance sponsors; and *Pas de Deux*, a textbook on ballet partnering.

National Dance Association
AAHPERD Publications
1900 Association Drive
Reston, Virginia 22070
(703) 476-3400
The National Dance Association of the American Alliance for Health, Physical Education, Recreation and Dance (AAHPERD) publishes studies on dance therapy, aesthetics, dance education and children's dance, and a directory of college dance programs. Their free brochure lists titles, descriptions and prices.

Footnotes Buyer's Guide
F. Randolph Associates, Inc.
1300 Arch Street
Philadelphia, Pennsylvania 19107
(215) 567-6662
A performing arts shopper through which hundreds of dance books, records, novelty items and supplies may be ordered by mail.

Suggested reading

Periodicals

Ballet Review
Marcel Dekker, Inc.
270 Madison Avenue
New York, New York 10016
(212) 889-9595
subscriptions:
Marcel Dekker Journals
Box 11305
Church Street Station
New York, New York 10249
Francis Mason, Editor
quarterly; $5.00/issue, $21.00/year
Ballet Review was founded by Arlene Croce to encourage dance criticism and scholarship and open up a "lively discussion of the state of the art." Intelligent and well written, it contains an interesting mix of essays, critical reviews and interviews.

Contact Quarterly
Box 603
Northampton, Maine 01060
Nancy Stark Smith and Lisa Nelson, Editors
quarterly; $3.00/issue, $9.00/year
A beautifully designed and produced journal, *Contact Quarterly* addresses itself to the body therapies, applied kinesiology and contact improvisation, both as an educational tool and a performance technique. Contents range from biographical sketches of outstanding contributors to the field, such as Ida Rolf and Moshe Feldenkrais, to practical advice on rehabilitating injuries, photo essays, drawings and fiction.

Dance Chronicle
Marcel Dekker, Inc.
270 Madison Avenue
New York, New York 10016
(212) 889-9595
subscriptions:
same as for *Ballet Review*, above
Jack Anderson and George Dorris, Editors
quarterly; $5.00/issue, $21.00/year
Dance Chronicle has a strong historical emphasis. It covers ballet, modern dance, folk dance, stage decor, dance books and music.

Dance in Canada
100 Richmond Street East
Suite 325
Toronto, Ontario
Canada M5C 2P9
(416) 368-4793
Michael Crabb, Editor
quarterly; $2.00/issue, $7.50/year
Naturally, much of *Dance in Canada* is concerned with developments on the home front (interesting in their own right, for dance in Canada is growing by leaps and bounds), critiques of local dance concerts, and stories on Canadian dancers, companies and dance schools. But the magazine's substantial book reviews and feature articles—Rhonda Ryman's twelve-part series on "Training the Dancer" is a fine example—are relevant to dancers everywhere. An attractive, well produced publication.

Dance in New York
Danceways Foundation, Inc.
393 West End Avenue
New York, New York 10024
(212) 799-2860
Ellen Jacob and Christopher Jonas, Editors
biannual; $6.95/issue
An in-depth guide to the dance capital of the world, with evocative photos. *Dance in New York* contains comprehensive profiles of New York's dance theaters, schools, teachers and professional dance companies — fully indexed for convenient use. It also includes vital information on city-based dance organizations, college dance programs, dancewear suppliers, dance publications and bookstores, medical and therapeutic services, and even temporary housing for visitors.

Dancemagazine
1180 Avenue of the Americas
New York, New York 10036
(212) 921-9300
William Como, Editor-in-Chief
Richard Philp, Managing Editor
monthly; $2.00/issue, $20.00/year
Dancemagazine is the world's largest dance publication, and it has, without a doubt, the most complete coverage of nationwide dance news. Included are performance calendars, dozens of concert reviews, a coast-to-coast dance school directory and a plethora of ads for upcoming dance events, auditions, and dance supplies of all kinds. The magazine reports on regional ballet and college dance, and carries articles on dance history, education, injury rehabilitation, dance technique, and dance films and books, as well as interviews with eminent dance personalities. Lots of photos.

Dance News
119 West 57th Street
New York, New York 10019
(212)PL7-6761
Helen V. Atlas, Editor
monthly except July and August;
$1.00/issue, $10.00/year
A sixteen-page newspaper containing news briefs on dancers, dance companies and schools around the world. Its performance calendar and school directory are less extensive than *Dancemagazine*'s, and the reviews tend to be cursorily written.

Dance Scope
American Dance Guild
1133 Broadway, Room 1427
New York, New York 10010
(212) 691-4564
H.B. Kronen, Editor
quarterly; $2.50/issue,
$10.00/year, $18.00/2years
A serious journal, but quite accessible. *Dance Scope* treats a diversity of dance-related subjects, from critical writings and historical pieces to book reviews and interviews with prominent dance figures. It is one of the few periodicals that seems to give equal space to ballet, modern and musical-theater dance. Recent issues have featured a survey of black dance in America, an interview with ice dancer John Curry and "Ballet Student Confidential," an inside look at the School of American Ballet. Sparsely but nicely illustrated.

Dance Teacher Now
SMW Communications, Inc.
1333 Notre Dame Drive
Davis, California 95616
(916) 756-6222
Susan Wershing, Editor
bimonthly;$10.00/year, $17.00/2 years
This new publication focuses on the practical aspects of teaching dance and running a dance studio. Whether you're thinking of becoming a teacher or simply curious, *Dance Teacher Now* offers a glimpse of the work-a-day world of

the rank-and-file teaching profession. The magazine touches on such subjects as nutrition, injury prevention, college dance, buying stereo equipment, tax management, teacher certification, scholarships, preparing students for auditions, and school recitals. There are interviews with successful teachers and an advice column on typical teaching problems, such as how to remember students' names.

Dance West Magazine
479¾ Washington Street
Marina del Rey, California 90291
(213) 821-1124
Martin A. David, Editor
monthly; $1.00/issue, $10.00/year
Energetic reportage of dance in California, the western United States and Canada. *Dance West* is packed with reviews and photos of local and visiting dance companies, extensive news sections, and articles on such topical issues as theater techniques for dancers and how to evaluate dance schools. Conferences, workshops, auditions and college dance events are covered, along with current dance books, films and records. *Dance West* also publishes interviews of local dancers and national dance personalities, and it runs a monthly performance calendar.

Performing Arts Journal
928 St. Marks Place
New York, New York 10009
(212) 260-7586
Bonnie Marranca and Gautam Dasgupta, Editors
triannual; $4.00/issue, $11.00/year
Since 1976, the *Performing Arts Journal* has been covering theater, dance, music, opera, video and film the world over. There have been articles on dance celebrities such as Edwin Denby, Kenneth King, Bob Fosse, Jerome Robbins, Merce Cunningham, and Meredith Monk; concert and book reviews; a survey of current dance photography; and reports on dance festivals and conferences. Illustrated.

Washington Dance View
1909 Baton Drive
Vienna, Virginia 22180
Alexandra Tomalonis, Editor
bimonthly; $1.00/issue, $4.50/year
The *Washington Dance View* primarily features lengthy concert reviews and one or two news items. A calendar of upcoming events and a directory of dance schools complete its format.

Books

General interest

Anderson, Jack. *Dance*. New York: Newsweek Books, 1974.

Chujoy, Anatole, and P.W. Manchester. *The Dance Encyclopedia*, revised and enlarged ed. New York: Simon and Schuster, 1978.

Clarke, Mary, and David Vaughan. *The Encyclopedia of Dance and Ballet*. East Rutherford, New Jersey: G.P. Putnam's Sons, 1977.

Cohen, Selma Jeanne. *Dance as a Theater Art*. New York: Dodd Mead and Company, 1974.

de Mille, Agnes. *The Book of Dance*. London: Paul Hamlyn, Ltd., 1963.

_____. *Dance to the Piper*. Boston: Little Brown and Company, 1952.

_____. *To a Young Dancer*. Boston: Little Brown and Company, 1962.

Emery, Lynne. *Black Dance in the United States from 1619 to 1970*. Palo Alto: National Press Books, 1972.

Guest, Ivor. *The Dancer's Heritage*. London: Dancing Times, 1960.

Herrigel, Eugene. *Zen in the Art of Archery*. New York: Vintage Books, 1971.

Kirstein, Lincoln. *Dance*. New York: Dance Horizons, 1969.

_____. *Movement and Metaphor*. New York: Praeger, 1971.

Lazarus, Arnold. *In the Mind's Eye*. New York: Rawson Associates Publishers, 1977. Using mental imagery to grow and change.

Lyle, Cynthia. *Dancers on Dancing*. New York: Drake Publishers, 1977.

Martin, John. *Introduction to the Dance*. New York: Dance Horizons, 1965.

Sachs, Curt. *World History of the Dance*, trans. Bessie Schönberg. New York: W.W. Norton, 1965.

Terry, Walter. *The Dance in America*. New York: Harper and Row, 1956.

Walker, Katherine Sorley. *Dance and its Creators*. New York: John Day Company, 1972.

Photograph books

Baryshnikov, Mikhail. *Baryshnikov at Work*, ed. Charles Engell France. New York: Alfred A. Knopf, 1977.

Hughes, Langston, and Milton Meltzer. *Black Magic: A Pictorial History of the Negro in American Entertainment*. Englewood Cliffs, New Jersey: Prentice-Hall, 1967.

Kahn, Albert E. *Days with Ulanova*. New York: Fireside Books, 1979.

Kirstein, Lincoln. *Nijinsky Dancing*. New York: Alfted A. Knopf, 1975.

Klosty, James. *Merce Cunningham*. New York: E.P. Dutton and Company, 1975.

Mitchell, Jack. *American Dance Portfolio*. New York: Dodd Mead and Company, 1964.

_____. *Dance Scene U.S.A.* Cleveland: The World Publishing Company, 1967.

Morgan, Barbara. *Martha Graham*. New York: Duell, Sloan and Pearce, 1941.

Philp, Richard, and Mary Whitney. *Danseur: The Male in Ballet*. New York: McGraw-Hill, 1977.

Reynolds, Nancy. *Repertory in Review: Forty Years of the New York City Ballet*. New York: Dial Press, 1977.

Spencer, Charles. *Leon Bakst*. New York: St. Martin's Press, 1974.

Ballet

Balanchine, George. *101 Stories of the Great Ballets*, ed. Francis Mason. Garden City, New York: Doubleday, 1968.

Beaumont, C.W. *Fanny Elssler.* London: C.W. Beaumont, 1931.

_____.*Michael Fokine and His Ballets.* London: C.W. Beaumont, 1935.

Benois, Alexandre. *Reminiscenses of the Russian Ballet,* trans. Mary Britnieva. New York: Da Capo Press, 1977.

Blasis, Carlo. *The Code of Terpsichore.* London: James Bulcock, 1823.

Fokine, Michel. *Memoirs of a Ballet Master,* ed. Anatole Chujoy and trans. Vitale Fokine. Boston: Little, Brown and Company, 1961.

Grant, Gail. *The Technical Manual and Dictionary of Classical Ballet.* New York: Dover Press, 1967.

Gruen, John. *The Private World of Ballet.* New York: Viking Press, 1975.

Guest, Ivor. *The Dancer's Heritage.* London: The Dancing Times, 1977.

Karsavina, Tamara. *Theatre Street.* New York: E.P. Dutton and Company, 1931.

Kerensky, Oleg. *Anna Pavlova.* New York: E.P. Dutton and Company, 1973.

Krementz, Jill. *A Very Young Dancer.* New York: Alfred A. Knopf, 1977.

Lifar, Serge. *Serge Diaghilev: His Life, His Work, His Legend.* New York: Da Capo Press, 1977.

Magriel, Paul, ed. *Nijinsky, Pavlova, Duncan: Three Lives in Dance.* New York: Da Capo Press, 1977.

Migel, Parmenia. *The Ballerinas: From the Court of Louis XIV to Pavlova.* New York: Macmillan Company, 1972.

Moore, Lillian. *Russian Ballet Master: The Memoirs of Marius Petipa.* London: A. and C. Black, 1960.

Nijinsky, Romola. *Nijinsky.* New York: A.M.S. Press, 1934.

Noverre, Jean Georges. *Letters on Dancing and Ballets*, trans. C.W. Beaumont. London: C.W. Beaumont, 1930.

Stevens, Franklin. *Dance as Life.* New York: Avon, 1976.

Taper, Bernard. *Balanchine.* New York: Harper and Row, 1963.

Terry, Walter. *The Ballet Companion.* New York: Dodd, Mead and Company, 1968.

Ballet Technique

Beaumont, Cyril, and Stanislas Idzikowski. *A Manual of the Theory and Practice of Classical Theatrical Dancing.* New York: Dover Press, 1975. Cecchetti technique.

Bruhn, Erick, and Lillian Moore. *Bournonville and Ballet Technique.* London: A. and C. Black, 1961. The Danish school.

Stuart, Muriel, and Lincoln Kirstein. *Classic Ballet.* New York: Alfred A. Knopf, 1952. The Balanchine School.

Vaganova, Agrippina. *Basic Principles of Russian Ballet Technique.* New York: Dover Press, 1969.

Modern Dance

Armitage, Merle, ed. *Martha Graham*. New York: Dance Horizons. 1966.

Banes, Sally. *Terpsichore in Sneakers: Post-Modern Dance*. New York: Houghton Mifflin Company, 1980.

Cohen, Selma Jeanne. *The Modern Dance: Seven Statements of Belief.* Middletown, Connecticut: Wesleyan University Press, 1966.

Cunningham, Merce. *Changes: Notes on Choreography*, ed. Frances Starr. New York: Something Else Press, 1968.

Duncan, Isadora. *The Art of the Dance*. New York: Theater Arts, 1977.

_____.*My Life*. New York: Universal Publishing and Distributing, 1968.

Forti, Simone. *Handbook in Motion*. Halifax, Nova Scotia and New York: Nova Scotia College of Art and Design and New York University Press, 1976.

Fuller, Loie. *Fifteen Years of a Dancer's Life*. Boston: Small, Maynard and Company, 1913.

Graham, Martha. *The Notebooks of Martha Graham*. New York: Harcourt Brace Jovanovich, 1973.

Halprin, Anna. *Movement Ritual I*. San Francisco: San Francisco Dancers Workshop, 1975.

Hawkins, Erick. *The Dance of Choreographer Erick Hawkins*. New York: Guinn and Company, 1964.

Horst, Louis. *Pre-Classic Dance Forms*. New York: Orthwine, 1937.

_____,and Carroll Russell. *Modern Dance Forms*. San Francisco: Impulse Publications, 1961.

Humphrey, Doris. *The Art of Making Dances*, ed. Barbara Pollack. New York: Grove Press, 1959.

Johnston, Jill. *Marmalade Me*. New York: E.P. Dutton and Company, 1971.

Laban, Rudolf. *The Mastery of Movement*, 2nd ed. London: Macdonald and Evans, 1960.

Lloyd, Margaret. *The Borzoi Book of Modern Dance*. New York: Dance Horizons, 1974.

Martin, John. *The Modern Dance*. New York: Dance Horizons, 1965.

Mazo, Joseph H. *Dance as a Contact Sport*. New York: Saturday Review Press, 1974.

_____.*Prime Movers: The Makers of Modern Dance in America*. New York: William Morrow and Company, 1977.

McDonagh, Don. *Don McDonagh's Complete Guide to Modern Dance*. New York: Popular Library, 1977.

_____.*The Rise and Fall and Rise of Modern Dance*. New York: New American Library, 1970.

Rainer, Yvonne. *Work 1961-73*. Halifax, Nova Scotia and New York: Nova Scotia College of Art and Design and New York University Press, 1974.

St. Denis, Ruth. *An Unfinished Life*. New York: Harper and Brothers, 1939.

Shawn, Ted. *Dance We Must*. Pittsfield, Massachusetts: The Eagle Printing and Binding Company, 1940.

_____.*One Thousand and One Night Stands*. New York: Da Capo Press, 1960.

Sherman, Jane. *Soaring*. Middletown, Connecticut: Wesleyan University Press, 1976. The diary of a Denishawn dancer.

Sorell, Walter. *Hanya Holm: The Biography of an Artist*. Middletown, Connecticut: Wesleyan University Press, 1969.

Terry, Walter. *Miss Ruth*. New York: Dodd Mead and Company, 1969.

Warren, Larry. *Lester Horton: Modern Dance Pioneer*. New York: Marcel Dekker, 1977.

Wigman, Mary. *The Language of the Dance*, trans. Walter Sorell. Middletown, Connecticut: Wesleyan University Press, 1966.

Tap and jazz

Ames, Jerry, and Jim Siegelman. *The Book of Tap*. New York: David McKay, 1977.

Audy, Robert. *Jazz Dance*. New York: Vintage Books, 1978.

_____.*Teach Yourself How to Tap Dance: Bob Audy Method*. New York: Vintage Books, 1976.

Croce, Arlene. *The Fred Astaire and Ginger Rogers Book*. New York: Random House, 1977.

Draper, Paul. *On Tap Dancing*. New York: Marcel Dekker, 1978.

Giordano, Gus. *Anthology of American Jazz Dance*. Evanston, Illinois: Orion Publishing House, 1978.

Stearns, Marshall, and Jean Stearns. *Jazz Dance*. New York: Shirmer Books, 1979.

Traguth, Fred. *Modern Jazz Dance*. New York: Dance Motion Press, 1978.

Criticism

Croce, Arlene. *After-Images*. New York: Alfred A. Knopf, 1977.

Denby, Edwin. *Looking at the Dance*. New York: Horizon Press, 1968.

Jowitt, Deborah. *Dance Beat: Selected Views and Reviews*. New York: Marcel Dekker, 1977.

Siegel, Marcia. *At the Vanishing Point*. New York: Saturday Review Press, 1972.

_____.*Watching the Dance Go By*. New York: Houghton Mifflin Company, 1978.

Index